Queer Psychology

Kevin L. Nadal • María R. Scharrón-del Río
Editors

Queer Psychology

Intersectional Perspectives

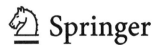 Springer

Editors
Kevin L. Nadal
John Jay College of Criminal Justice
City University of New York
New York, NY, USA

María R. Scharrón-del Río
Brooklyn College
City University of New York
New York, NY, USA

ISBN 978-3-030-74145-7   ISBN 978-3-030-74146-4   (eBook)
https://doi.org/10.1007/978-3-030-74146-4

This Springer imprint is published by the registered company Springer Nature Switzerland AG
The registered company address is: Gewerbestrasse 11, 6330 Cham, Switzerland

To our children and to the next generation of trans and queer youth. May they always know their worth and may they always be surrounded by people who remind them.

Foreword

Reflecting on my own graduate training in the late 1970s and 1980s, the closest we ever came to any discussions on LGBTQ training and scholarship was the result of discussions organized around clients presented at case conferences. Invariably, if someone presented a case about a client who was a sexual minority group member, the comments which were made by some of the students and the faculty clinical supervisor—which I think were actually intended to be helpful and presumed to be expressions of liberal tolerance—were actually very destructive. I distinctly recall a professor, who was a significant leader in the field of psychology at the time, proudly demonstrating what I am sure he thought was his tolerance when he pointed out that he saw sexual minority clients and that he "would never force or press them to undertake conversion therapy." Instead, he said that he would tell them that he felt sorry for them if they did not wish to change their orientation. Yet another response was a supervisor's perplexity when describing his work with a gay man who was struggling with his need to come out to his family, that his gay patients always seemed to have the need to "expose their families to their homosexuality." Why, he reasoned, couldn't they just keep it to themselves? At the time, there really was no space to safely challenge such homophobic or transphobic commentary, as it was simply part of the dominant cultural narrative that was normalized and supported by organized psychology at that time. There was no acknowledgement of the subjective cultural positioning of the discipline.

Simultaneously, discussing racism as a systemic inequity that might be affecting clients' lives (or therapist's perceptions) was also unwelcome. Students who were members of racial and ethnic minority groups had to be very strategic about how we raised questions about race, as well as in sharing some of the therapeutic work we were doing with people of color, if it openly examined the matter of race and racism. Demonstrating that racism often played a role in the presenting problems of our clients would often be interpreted as overidentification or something undesirable in a clinician. It was clear that the very paradigms we were using at the time were infused with racist, sexist, heterosexist, ableist, and ageist thinking, frequently supported by empirical research that was riddled with methodological errors and presumptions based on social bigotry wrapped in psychological accoutrements. At that time, many of our professors and supervisors were completely oblivious to these realities. There was no awareness of legitimate nondominant cultural voices.

In the earlier stages of my own work, one of the things that concerned me—as someone who had no inclination toward the academy at all, as someone who felt like a stealth intruder, and as someone who identified primarily as a clinician—was how to treat people in therapy in ways that were helpful and were not damaging. It was important for me that therapists did not reinforce the very traumatic and harmful experiences that brought clients into therapy in the first place. And while I had some ideas about how to do that in my own practice, I believed that in order to really create substantive change, psychologists and other mental health practitioners needed to be trained in how to work effectively with sexual minorities, people of color, and people of color who also identified as members of sexual minority groups. That became the impetus for some of my early work.

For the most part, my scholarly work is anchored through the lens of a clinician, rather than through a research scientist. Because there was little work in the literature at the outset of my career that one would want to use as guidance about practice in working with historically marginalized groups, a cohort of us took on the task of developing that literature. We knew that this literature needed to be out there, that these discussions needed to take place, and the only way for the field to change was if we wrote this scholarship ourselves. While there was burgeoning work on specific ethnic groups, Vickie Mays and Susan Cochran at UCLA were among the very few who were first addressing these issues with clients who were members of both ethnic and sexual minority groups in their empirical studies of Black lesbians. Finding their research was like finding gold in the wilderness.

In the earlier attempts at this multicultural scholarship—within LGBTQ psychology, within ethnoracial psychology, and within feminist psychology—there was a tendency for each group to want to operate on its own little island—as if these identities were isolated and consolidated into a master identity that could be separated from the others. It suggested that you could compartmentalize identity and come away with a realistic sense of what a person's experience was. At the time, I certainly understood that this was one way to enter into the discussion; however, I tried to embed a lot of my work with at least some notion that these things are intersectional. If you are working with clients, you simply cannot look at identities, as if they are in silos. While it is not a good idea in research either, it certainly was not beneficial within clinical work. It would be too reductionistic to capture the complexity of human beings by not considering how individuals navigate their multiple identities, alongside their unique lived experiences.

The types of struggles that came up for the LGBTQ people of color who came to me for therapy were never really articulated in either ethnoracial research or sexual identity research. And while this condition has improved somewhat over the years, it is still problematic. There are still many research studies in which there is a really insignificant number of LGBTQ people of color, but yet the research is presented as if it generalizes to them and in the same way as it may apply to their white counterparts. In erasing or minimizing these experiences, researchers do not get a sense of how people's identities, experiences, and struggles complicate their sexual orientations and gender identities. Theoretical paradigms fail to capture the complexity and the uniqueness of LGBTQ people of color and their experiences. Quantitative empirical research models were also very reductionistic, in that they studied human identities and struggles as separate compartments, instead of interrelated parts of complex and authentic selves.

At some point, I was introduced to Feminist Psychotherapy Practice and Theory, which despite its own limitations in its need to initially prioritize gender as the primary location of marginalization for all women, was the first theory that I experienced as a clinician that created a space to overtly examine social context and a wide range of social marginalizations as contributing factors to mental health problems as a required part of the analysis of any kind of clients dilemma. Because Feminist Therapy and Theory has a tendency to understand that women's mental health problems were often connected to the disparaged status of women—not something intrinsic about women or something individually pathological about a given woman—it opened the door to understanding how similar forms of social marginalization contributed to mental health problems. The theory posited that social marginalization based on systemic inequity creates problems for people from which they cannot escape by their own efforts alone. That social marginalization creates stressors that we now understand as minority stress that contributes to mental health problems for people. Such an idea was novel at that time because other psychological paradigms used to establish psychotherapy practice did not do that. In fact, there was not much of a space for examining the influences of systems and oppressions—unless you chose to depart from the dominant cultural narrative (which many of us did). As a trainee, it was difficult to depart from the dominant assumptions about the world and not get penalized for it, but when I was no longer in training, I learned that I could make my own decisions about such matters and that in fact I had a responsibility to do that.

At some point, there was also an emergence of Black, lesbian, feminist narrative writings, including Kimberlé Crenshaw's work on intersectionality. Such scholarship created this kind of wedge effect in the scholarship—allowing the creation and opportunity for a lot more of these complex and nuanced understandings of people to become part of the clinical and scholarly conversation. I greeted these readings with welcome eyes, as they gave me the affirmation that our multiplicities were valid and that our stories were important.

Decades later, a new generation of LGBTQ scholars of color have emerged—many psychologists—still challenging the many paradigms and teachings of psychology that we were fighting against too. While I am moved that Drs. Kevin Nadal and María Scharrón-del Río have invited me to write the foreword for *Queer Psychology: Intersectional Perspectives,* I am also moved that there has been so much literature and research for the authors and contributors to write about and pull from. It is wonderful that a comprehensive text like this has been able to emerge and that it has captured the many ways that we can queer or challenge the field of psychology. I am humbled that our early ideas as early career psychologists have expanded into a subfield that covers topics like clinical work, identity development, research methods, career counseling, mental health and health disparities, and more.

I commend the many contributors for their diligence in reviewing these various topic areas, while providing recommendations for clinicians to improve their approaches—particularly for LGBTQ people (and LGBTQ people with multiple marginalized identities). I also commend Drs. Nadal and Scharrón-del Río for their assemblance of premiere scholars, psychologists, and activists, and for being the leaders of the next generation.

Finally, I must recognize that while we have made important strides, we still have a lot of work to do. There is the unfinished business of the past, as well as the current backlash that seeks to erode the hard won, previously acquired civil rights for marginalized group members. As I write, we live in the aftermath of a polarizing and divisive presidential administration that overtly supported increased attacks on the civil rights of sexual and ethnic minority group members as well as other vulnerable populations. Transgender youth have been particular targets of state legislation that removes protections from their involuntary subjection to conversion therapies. Voter suppression and police brutality against Black citizens is disturbingly all too frequent. All of this takes place in the midst of a major public health crisis that disproportionately negatively affects the groups that are this book's focus.

Dr. Martin Luther King, Jr once said "Progress does not roll in on the heels of inevitability. We can ill afford to relinquish our vigilance." This text is just the tip of the iceberg. Psychologists and mental health practitioners must continue to challenge the ways that heterosexism, transphobia, racism, sexism, ableism, ageism, and other forms of oppression harm our fellow citizens and infiltrate our field. But, for now, I am grateful to see the continued evolution in thinking. We remain challenged in this work, but nevertheless this book is evidence that we persist.

Beverly Greene
Department of Psychology
St. John's University
Queens, NY, USA
greeneb@stjohns.edu

Acknowledgments

This book would not be possible without all of the people who have supported us throughout our lives and our careers. We want to especially thank our families (both families of origin and chosen families) for always believing in us and pushing us to reach our fullest potentials. We thank Dr. Beverly Greene not just for writing an amazing foreword but for blazing the trails for all of us to follow. Queer Psychology would not exist without you. Black, Indigenous, Latinx, Asian, and Pacific Islander queer and trans people would not have what we have without your work and advocacy.

We thank all of the authors who contributed to this book. *Salamat* and *gracias* to Angela Ferguson, Angelica Puzio, Alexis Forbes, Hector Adames, Nayeli Y. Chavez-Dueñas, Ethan Mereish, M. Son Taylor, Brandon Velez, David Zelaya, Jillian Scheer, Anneliese Singh, Rebekah Estevez, Natalia Truszczynski, Alison Cerezo, Roberto Renteria, Darren Freeman-Coppadge, Khashayar Farhadi Langroudi, Nic Rider, Jieyi Cai, Leonardo Candelario-Pérez, Jan Estrellado, Lou Felipe, Nadine Nakamura, Amanda Breen, maria torre, Shéár Avory, Christian Chan & Nicole Silverio, Sarah Baqet, Vincent Marasco, Jehan Hill, David Ford, Kendra Doychak, and Chitra Raghavan. You are a true "dream team" of queer psychology. Thank you for giving voice to our communities and for ensuring that our field does a better job of serving them and future generations.

We would like to thank our spouses (Kaleohano and Yvonne) for being our biggest cheerleaders—even when we find ourselves being overcommitted and overwhelmed. We sincerely appreciate all that you do for us and we know we can never fully repay you for all that you do for us. And finally, we thank our children (J, T, and E). Thank you for reminding us why we do this work. Thank you for giving us joy. Thank you for inspiring us to keep fighting.

Contents

The original version of this book was revised. The correction is available at
https://doi.org/10.1007/978-3-030-74146-4_18

Introduction to Queer Psychology

Kevin L. Nadal and María R. Scharrón-del Río

1   Introduction

According to Queer Theorists, to "queer" something means to disrupt it. It means to challenge the status quo, particularly as it relates to gender, sexual orientation, and other social identities (Mayo, 2007). Queering means to question, and to be critical of, all of the things that people of a given society have been socialized to learn and believe, while also centering and uplifting the experiences of the most marginalized people. For instance, it is a call for people to critically examine what they have learned about topics and belief systems involving sexuality, romance, monogamy, family structures, success, and happiness—recognizing that common experiences of lesbian, gay, bisexual, transgender, and queer (LGBTQ) people have been typically pathologized, criminalized, or victimized, while experience of cisgender and heterosexual people have been celebrated, honored, or deemed as the standard. Relatedly, queering methods means to acknowledge the limitations of rigid categories and to consider or implement new approaches to normalized thoughts, behaviors, or understandings (Brim & Ghaziani, 2016). For instance, Butler (2011) describes the ways in which gender is a mere social performance—one that people have been taught to believe and accept as the norm; because gender it is a social construct and not based on any biological or innate determinants, it is one that we should constantly question and critique. (Fig. 1).

K. L. Nadal (*)
Department of Psychology, John Jay College of Criminal Justice—City University of New York, New York, NY, USA
e-mail: knadal@jjay.cuny.edu

M. R. Scharrón-del Río
Brooklyn College—City University of New York, School of Education, Brooklyn, NY, USA
e-mail: mariaRS@brooklyn.cuny.edu

K. L. Nadal and M. R. Scharron-del Río (ed.), *Queer Psychology*,
https://doi.org/10.1007/978-3-030-74146-4_1

1

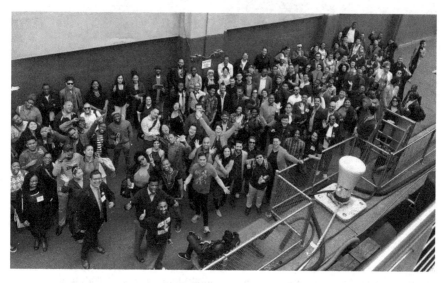

Fig. 1 Participants of the Lesbian, Gay, Bisexual, Transgender and Queer Scholars of Color National Network, taken at their 2017 Conference in New York City. Photo Courtesy of Kevin Nadal

To "queer" psychology would be no different. It would mean that it is important for psychologists to reflect upon all that has been taught in our education, training, and supervision and to challenge the status quo in the field. It would mean to question the theories and concepts that we have learned and studied—from our introductory psychology undergraduate classes to our advanced doctoral-level courses. It would mean to recognize that the earliest musings of Western Psychology have centered (and continue to center) the perspectives and experiences of White, cisgender, heterosexual, male, European and European American people. It means to make ample and overt efforts to decolonize and resist Western and hegemonic standards—despite the decades of complacency or the fact that we were professionally trained in these standards ourselves. In doing so, we must question if psychology teachings were (or are) relevant for people who identify as Black, Indigenous, or other people of color (BIPOC), transgender or nonbinary people, queer people, women, non-White immigrants, non-Americans, or any other historically marginalized group in the US or across the world.

2 A Brief History of LGBTQ People in Society

Before we even begin to delve into the field of Queer Psychology, it is crucial to understand the experiences of LGBTQ people throughout history and how this history had shaped the ways that LGBTQ people are treated today. In doing so, it is important to acknowledge that the actual history of LGBTQ people is incomplete or unknown—mainly because LGBTQ people of previous generations were not able to live in their truths—out of fears of being ostracized or being targeted by violence. While it is presumed that LGBTQ people have been present in every culture and society throughout history (with some documentation in many parts of the world), most LGBTQ people in previous centuries may have never disclosed their identities publicly. And those who did were criminalized, hospitalized, or even killed. So, while many historians begin "LGBTQ History" with the narratives of the uprisings in San Francisco and New York in the late 1960s, LGBTQ people have actually been part of both world history and American history, even if there are limited records of their existence.

With that being said, there are some hints of LGBTQ people who existed (either proudly or in secret) throughout the world. Nadal (2013) describes how LGBTQ people have been depicted throughout history—beginning in the hieroglyphs in Ancient Egyptian pyramids to biblical stories of same-sex romances in the Torah or the Old Testament (e.g., David and Jonathan, Ruth and Naomi). Further, in Ancient Rome, people like Mark Antony and Julius Cesar are depicted as being bisexual, in that they had both male and female lovers and romantic partners. In places like Thailand, precolonized India, and precolonized Philippines, transgender people were integrated members of society, and in some cases, were even revered and celebrated as spiritual leaders or prophets. In the land that is now known as North America, transgender and queer people were accepted and celebrated across various tribes. Known as "two-spirited" people, these individuals were and are seen as a third gender of people who may demonstrate both male and female traits.

Nadal (2020) provides a history of the criminalization and persecution of LGBTQ people in the United States and across the world—based primarily on their sexual orientations and gender identities. When English colonizers came to escape religious persecution and formed what is now known as the US on indigenous North American lands, they brought with them the Christian values that persecuted sodomy (which was legally defined as anal sex, oral sex, or sex between a man and an animal). The earliest American writings on the group of people who would later be considered LGBTQ involved men in the 1800s who were charged for sodomy and later sentenced to death. As state sodomy laws were enacted, death penalties were no longer used as punishment; however, for decades, people who were arrested or charged with sodomy were either bribed, jailed, or forced into psychiatric institutions for their sexual orientations and gender identities (which were legally considered crimes or mental illnesses). Because homosexuality and transgenderism were considered "moral turpitudes", being convicted of—or even presumed to be participating in—such acts were justifiable reasons for termination of employment, denial of immigration into the country, and even deportation.

Besides being criminalized for sodomy and other "lewd" behaviors, state and local jurisdictions enacted "crimes against humanity" laws—or general governmental legislations that were used to target LGBTQ people. For instance, if LGBTQ people gathered in public spaces, they could be arrested or imprisoned—even if they were not engaging in sodomy or any sexual activity. Further, if businesses were known to overtly support LGBTQ patrons in any way, they would be raided or shut down by law enforcement. Further, different jurisdictions passed "masquerade laws" in which police officers arrested and jailed people who dressed in clothing that did not match their sex assigned at birth. As an example, in New York City, transgender and queer people describe an unofficial "three-article" rule, in which people were expected to always wear three gendered items or fear being arrested; as a result, people who dressed in drag or whose gender presentation did not align with their birth sex were arrested (Nadal, 2020).

In addition to law, societal stigma had also contributed to an array of psychological stressors for people who did not conform to heterosexuality or cisgenderism (Herek, 2007; Nadal, 2013). Within families and communities, messages about LGBTQ people being immoral, evil, or pathological were influenced by religious dogma that had been passed down across generations. When children were outed or suspected of being LGBTQ, parents or families would send them to places where they would be treated with conversion therapy—or efforts to attempt to change one's sexual orientation or gender identity. For centuries, LGBTQ people endured some of the most tortious forms of treatments—ranging from electroshock therapy, lobotomies, and castrations. With the knowledge of this stigma and violence, most LGBTQ people knew to conceal their identities—out of fears of violence, death, or being rejected or disowned by their families and loved ones (Herek, 2007).

What is often identified as the impetus of Queer Psychology is Evelyn Hooker's foundational research from the mid-1950s that challenged the societal notion that gay men were mentally ill. Despite the presumed psychopathology of gay men, Hooker (a developmental psychologist) compared the mental health symptoms of gay and bisexual men with heterosexual men—finding no significant differences in mental health adjustment between the two groups (Hooker, 1993; Nadal, 2017). Hooker's work was used as an empirical foundation for successfully advocating for the removal of homosexuality in the American Psychiatric Association's *Diagnostic and Statistical Manual of Mental Disorders (DSM)* in 1973. Despite this advocacy, the U.S. government still viewed sexual orientation as a mental deficiency for almost two decades—barring all LGBTQ people from immigrating into the US until 1990 (Nadal, 2020).

It was also around the time of Dr. Hooker's work that the LGBTQ Civil Rights began to take form. In the 1950s and 1960s, protests against police brutality and police harassment emerged in metropolitan cities across the country. For instance, in May 1959, at Cooper's Doughnuts (a diner in Los Angeles) a group of trans women and gay men began an impromptu uprising against a group of harassing police officers by throwing doughnuts and other objects at them. In August 1966, a group of trans women resisted violent police officers at Compton's Cafeteria (a diner in San Francisco) by first throwing a cup of coffee at them. While both events were documented via oral histories, they were never covered by the media (nor recorded in police records) and were generally erased from history (Nadal, 2020; Stryker, 2008).

However, in June 1969, in New York City, a routine police raid at the Stonewall Inn (a bar that served LGBTQ patrons) yielded an uprising that would change American (and world history; Stein, 2019). While such raids would typically result in arrests and fines, queer and trans patrons resisted arrest. Hundreds of protesters (many who were queer and trans people of color) gathered outside of the bar and fought back against police too—throwing bricks, Molotov cocktails, garbage cans, and whatever else they could find. More law enforcement was called (as were other protesters), and the resistance lasted for several days. Unlike the previous two events (and other potential resistances that occurred), the Stonewall Uprising was documented by both mainstream media (e.g., *The New York Times*) and alternative media (e.g., *The Village Voice*). It also resulted in mass community organizing and the Gay Liberation March the following year. That march would become the impetus for LGBTQ Pride Parades in the US and around the world. Thus, Stonewall is typically viewed as the event that jumpstarted LGBTQ activism across the US (Nadal, 2020; Stein, 2019).

Shortly after Stonewall, LGBTQ people across the country—particularly in major metropolitan hubs like New York, Washington DC, San Francisco, Los Angeles, and Chicago—began to organize and advocate for civil rights in masse. Within the field of psychology, specifically, activists in the early 1970s began to form coalitions as a way of addressing homophobia within professional psychology organizations. For example, within the California Psychological Association, a group called the Association of Gay Psychologists (later referred to as the Association of Lesbian and Gay Psychologists) was formed and met regularly to tackle the notion that homosexuality was still considered a mental disorder. Through lobbying and public protest, the group was instrumental in pushing the American Psychological Association (APA) to take public stands against homophobia. After the American Medical Association declassifying of homosexuality as a disorder in 1973, the group further pushed for the APA to publicly reject homosexuality as a psychological disorder too. The group's advocacy also resulted in APA's inclusion of sexual orientation as a protected class in the organization's nondiscrimination policy (Kimmel and Browning, 1999).

Activism within the American Psychological Association continued in the 1980s and 1990s—mainly via the creation of organizations and long-standing committees dedicated to issues around sexuality and gender identity (Kimmel & Browning. 1999). For instance, in 1985, the APA first created the Committee on Lesbian and Gay Concerns as a way to standardize its commitment to issues involving sexual orientation. Over the decades, the committee was renamed several times to be more inclusive of bisexual people and transgender people; it is currently called the Committee on Sexual Orientation and Gender Diversity (CSOGD).

Concurrently to the formation of what is now known as CSOGD, a group of lesbian and gay psychologists advocated for the creation of the 44th division of the APA, or the Division on the Psychological Study of Lesbian and Gay Issues (Kimmel & Browning, 1999). Divisions were a way for formalized groups with the organization to coordinate efforts based on specific missions of psychology—from identity-based issues (e.g. race and ethnic minorities, women, etc.) to subfields (e.g., counseling psychology, psychology and law). Over time, Division 44 had also been renamed several times to be more inclusive; it is currently known as the Society for the Psychology of Sexual Orientation and Gender Diversity.

With both CSOGD and Division 44, advocacy for LGBTQ people grew significantly within APA (and the field as a whole) in the 1980s and 1990s. Further, psychological research involving LGBTQ people began to flourish too. While feminist psychology researchers like Carol Gilligan and Sandra Bem published on issues like girls' development and the influence of sex roles, some researchers began to study sexuality (Nadal, 2017). In 1979, Vivienne Cass first published her identity development model, which highlighted hypothesized stages of sexual orientation identity formation and acceptance. In 1991, Anthony D'Augelli, a clinical/community psychologist, published a sexual orientation identity development model for lesbian, gay, and bisexual people, which was supported by empirical data. One critique of both of these models was that they were not inclusive of transgender identities, nor did they focus on other intersectional influences (e.g., race, disability, social class, immigration status, religion, etc.).

Beyond identity development, psychology research in the 1990s and early 2000s began to focus on the detrimental effects of discrimination on LGBTQ people. Gregory Herek contributed a prolific body of research on lesbian, gay, and bisexual people's experiences of heterosexist violence and discrimination—coining terms like sexual stigma and sexual prejudice. He also is credited as first writing extensively about anti-gay hate crimes—a topic that had been largely missing in academia. Not long after, Ilan Meyer (a social psychologist and an epidemiologist) published his minority stress theory, which described the multiple ways in which discrimination negative affects the psychological health of LGBTQ people and people of other historically marginalized groups. The work of Herek and Meyer were instrumental in advocating for numerous LGBTQ issues at the time—from the bans on gays in the military to the fight for marriage equality (Nadal, 2017).

Beginning in the 1990s, some psychology scholars began to describe the influence of intersectional identities, as they related to LGBTQ people. Beverly Greene, a Black lesbian clinical psychology professor first published an article entitled "Ethnic minority lesbians and gay men: Mental health and treatment issues" in the Journal of Consulting and Clinical Psychology (Greene, 1994) and a book titled *Ethnic and cultural diversity among lesbians and gay men* (Greene, 1997). Dr. Greene also wrote specifically about clinical issues related to Black lesbians and lesbians of color. Similarly, Eduardo Morales, a gay Puerto Rican clinical psychology professor published on ethnic minority families and LGBTQ people, as well as experiences of LGBTQ Latino Americans in the early 1990s (see Morales, 2013). Lester Brown, a two-spirit Native American professor of social work edited *Two Spirit People: American Indian Lesbian Women and Gay Men* (Brown, 1997). Barry Chung (a gay Asian American counseling psychology professor) published on the experiences of lesbian and gay Asian American (see Chung & Singh, 2009 for a review). These pioneering scholars- along with others like Connie Chan, Oliva Espin, and Mark Pope opened doors for many others to write about psychology-related issues amongst queer and trans people of color (QTPOC).

Finally, it is important to note how the integration of LGBTQ issues had been infused into the field of psychology today. In 2000, APA published the *APA Guidelines for Psychological Practice with Lesbian, Gay, and Bisexual*

Clients—describing the ethical obligations for psychologists who work with non-heterosexual clients or constituents. The document was later updated in 2011 (APA, 2012). In 2006, the APA established the Office of LGBT Concerns, which later became the Office on Sexual Orientation and Gender Diversity. In 2013, APA (spearheaded by Division 44) launched *Psychology of Sexual Orientation and Gender Diversity*—the first journal to focus explicitly on issues related to LGBTQ issues in psychology. Finally, the APA published the *Guidelines for Psychological Practice With Transgender and Gender Nonconforming People* in 2015—providing ethical codes for working most effectively with TGNC people (APA, 2015) (Fig. 2).

3   Queer Psychology Today

Today, LGBTQ psychology or Queer Psychology is a thriving force with in the field. While LGBTQ scholarship was once rare (and even frowned upon), LGBTQ scholarship persists among many subfields of psychology, including counseling psychology, clinical psychology, and social psychology. Multiple psychology books have been written about LGBTQ people and issues, and LGBTQ-related psychology courses have emerged across the United States. As an example, "Queer Psychology" is a doctoral-level course that has been taught at the Graduate Center at the City University of New York since 2016.

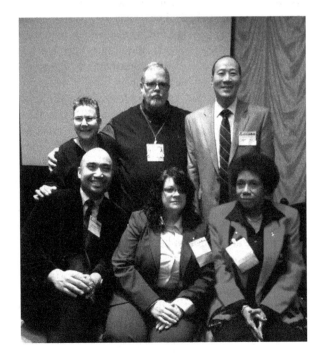

Fig. 2 LGBTQ psychologists of color panel taken at the National Multicultural Conference and Summit. Clockwise from top left: Dr. Vic Munoz, Dr Mark Pope, Dr. Barry Chung, Dr. Beverly Green, Dr. Arlene Noriega, Dr. Kevin Nadal. Photo Courtesy of Kevin Nadal

Despite this growth, Queer Psychology is still continuing to expand as a field. While academic scholarship on Queer Theory has been flourishing in the humanities for decades, it is still minimally integrated into psychology. While LGBTQ community organizations have been at the forefront of training others on topics like inclusive terminology and the proper use of gendered pronouns, these concepts have only recently been introduced to the field of psychology. Finally, while psychology has begun to delve into work reversing racial justice and intersectionality, topics related to sex positivity (e.g., polygamy, sex work, BDSM, etc.) are still relatively taboo across psychology training programs (Burnes et al., 2017). The lack of integration of sex psychology is embedded in systemic heterosexism; because American society in general is derived from white, Western puritan thought, the act of embracing or celebrating one's sexuality and engaging in consensual and pleasurable sexual behaviors is stigmatized. Thus, if heterosexual or cisgender sexuality is stigmatized, queer or trans sexuality would even more stigmatized. Thus, queering psychology must include integrating of sex positivity and the normalization of conversations on sexual desires and behaviors.

Further, LGBTQ people with multiple marginalized identities (e.g. LGBTQ people of color, LGBTQ people with disabilities, LGBTQ immigrants) are still typically overlooked in psychology and mental health literature (Cyrus, 2017; Nadal, 2013). Because LGBTQ people of color may experience multiple forms or marginalization—including racism with LGBTQ communities, heterosexism and transphobia within their racial and ethnic communities, and double marginalization in general society, they are at risk for developing negative mental health stigmas, while also receiving substandard mental health treatment—if they are able to access treatment at all (Cyrus, 2017). Thus, when psychologists do not discuss issues related to race and ethnicity among LGBTQ people, nor do train their students and trainees on how to do so, they may inadvertently perpetuate false narratives of a universal LGBTQ experiences and even contribute to the negative mental health experiences of queer and trans people of color.

Similarly, queer and trans people with disabilities still remain fairly invisible in psychology—despite the pushes for disability to be integrated into multicultural psychology curricula (Williams, 2019) and the emergence of Queer Crip Theory in other disciplines (Kafer, 2013). So, although, queer and trans people with disabilities may encounter an array of difficulties, ranging in disclosing their identities to navigating multiple forms of systemic and interpersonal oppression (see Miller et al., 2019), there is a dearth of psychological literature that highlights their experiences. Accordingly, psychologists and others may not be providing the most effective or accessible care for LGBTQ people with disabilities—resulting in their further marginalization in both psychology and general society.

Given all of these factors, it is evident that psychologists (especially psychology leaders) have a reached a critical point. They (or we) have to decide whether we want to maintain the status quo, or if we are truly ready to "queer" everything we have ever learned about, and from, this field. They (or we) have to decide whether we are comfortable in accepting our complicity in promoting a universal LGBTQ community, or whether we are committed in acknowledging and advocating for diverse LGBTQ communities. They (or we) have to decide whether we are willing to teach future generations the same materials—some which have and may continue to harm certain communities—or if we want to revamp our curricula in order promote the most inclusivity and the most equity for people of all historically marginalized groups.

4 Why We Wrote This Book

There were many reasons why we decided to write this book. First, we recognized the need for a comprehensive text that covered psychology-related issues involving LGBTQ people. Throughout our careers, we have witnessed the ways that historically marginalized groups have been underrepresented in general psychological research, or the ways that minoritized people have treated as mere afterthoughts. For instance, when multicultural considerations are included in textbooks or course syllabi, they are typically saved for the end of the semester or as one of the last book chapters. For LGBTQ people, specifically, it can be quite common for psychologists-in-training to receive very little formal training on how to work effectively with LGBTQ people, let alone LGBTQ people with other marginalized identities. In fact, the first time that some clinicians ever learn about LGBTQ issues is during their first contact with a queer or trans client or patient. In this way, they may not only be inept in providing services, but they could ethically cause harm in their work with individuals from a collective group with a history of being significantly harmed by psychologists in the past.

Further, because many scholars in the field of LGBTQ psychology have historically taken a colorblind or umbrella approach, the unique experiences of LGBTQ people of color, LGBTQ people with disabilities, LGBTQ immigrants, or transgender or gender nonconforming people have continued to be omitted or erased in the field (Nadal, 2013, 2020). Models have been theorized and normalized on white, cisgender, educated, or higher socioeconomic status values, with the presumption that they would fit or be generalizable for all LGBTQ people. It was not even until recently that professional organizations of psychologists have recognized the ways that racial, gendered, and sexualized hierarchies have persisted—suggesting that even though LGBTQ people of all backgrounds may undergo discrimination due to their sexual orientations or gender identities, many LGBTQ people with historically privileged identities have the capacity to discriminate or hold biases against others, maintain status quos, and even perpetuate false narratives of a universal LGBTQ experience. Accordingly, we approach this work with an intersectional lens—understanding the influence of multiple systems of oppression (e.g., cissexism, heterosexism, racism, sexism, xenophobia, ableism, classism, etc.) and making intentional efforts to center the experiences of those who have been historically been erased or silenced.

We also wrote this book, with the intention of including as many facets of psychology as possible—from clinical work to research methodology to health psychology and forensic psychology. We acknowledge that specific subfields of psychology may omit LGBTQ issues altogether, or that they may present stereotypical or outdated stereotypes of LGBTQ people as their only inclusion. As an example, in forensic psychology, the study of LGBTQ people is generally nonexistent; and when LGBTQ people are presented, they are done so in criminalized ways via such tropes as "homosexual" serial killers or child predators (Nadal, 2020). Similarly, when LGBTQ people are discussed in health, medicine, and health psychology, they are often referred to only by their disparities and problematic behaviors, without fully acknowledging the roles of systemic oppression on these disparities, or the resilience of LGBTQ people who navigate or overcome those disparities (Gahagan & Colpitts, 2017). In this way, we wanted to change the ways that scholars approach LGBTQ people in general. Instead of focusing on pathologies and deficits, we aim to focus on strengths and resilience.

We also wanted to create a space that would provide as much up-to-date information on the growing world of LGBTQ people, highlighting the diverse identities and perspectives of people who may identify as LGBTQ. Though we know that this umbrella term exists, we celebrate that there are so many new and emerging terms that are used to describe people's experiences. In this way, we know there isn't one LGBTQ community, but that there are several LGBTQ communities.

Finally, we also wrote this book intentionally as scholars of color who navigate racism, transphobia, heterosexism, sexism, xenophobia, ableism, and other forms of oppression across various aspects of our lives. In this way, intersectional identities and lenses are personally and critically important for us. Our ethnic identities—as descendants of people from the Philippines and Puerto Rico—have impacted the historical trauma that our families and communities have experienced through colonialism, racism, and classism. Our intersectionalities have impacted the ways that we navigate our teachings as professors within the City University of New York— one of the largest public university systems in the world—particularly as we recognize we are among the few BIPOC tenured Full Professors in our institutions, in which BIPOC students are the majority population. Our intersectionalities have influenced our memberships in professional settings, including more general psychology organizations (American Psychological Association), racial/ethnic organizations (Asian American Psychological Association or National Latinx Psychological Association), and LGBTQ organizations (Center for LGBTQ Studies). Our intersectionalities have even encouraged our participation in the creation of new spaces for us to celebrate our authentic selves (LGBTQ Scholars of Color National Network). While discussing one's own positionalities is something that is often excluded from academic scholarship, it is important to name these experiences— not just as a way of "queering" psychology, but also as a way for readers to understand why this book (and this work) is so important for us.

5   What This Book Covers

This book covers 16 additional chapters—each written by a unique author or group of authors. In an attempt to "queer" our approaches, we encouraged our authors to utilize the methods and styles that they believed would be most effective in approaching their topics. We encourage them to cover various topics and theoretical approaches and to use their positionalities to determine their best approaches to the topic they were assigned (a topic that all would be considered experts in). The one commonality for each chapter is that each includes an intersectional case study, in order to demonstrate how LGBTQ people would navigate some of the concepts presented, in their everyday lives.

One of the aspects that we were intentional about was that we wanted our authors to represent the diverse spectrum of our communities. In perusing authors' names you'll notice that every chapter will have at least one author of color and that most will have scholars of color as the first author. You'll also notice that our authors represent a diverse range of geographic locations, racial backgrounds, ethnicities, ages, and psychology subfields. Our authors include clinicians and practitioners, professors and researchers, administrative leaders, and students. Our authors identify as queer, trans, bisexual, lesbian, gay, and other identities. We even encourage authors to use their own terminology when describing queer and trans people, as we understand that labels and identity differ greatly across spaces and positionalities. So, although traditional scholarship relies on standards and consistencies, we honor diversity and complexities.

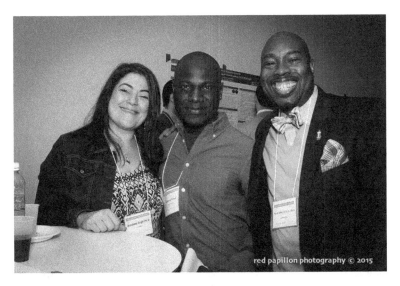

Fig. 3 Drs. Annelise Singh, Sulaimon Giwa, and David Julius Ford at the LGBTQ Scholars of Color National Network Conference in 2015. Photo Courtesy of Riya Ortiz/Red Papillon Photography

In this way, we also recognize that we may not be able to cover every single identity—at least not in depth as each identity or community deserves. For example, while we aim to include to people of various marginalized identities (and provide case examples in which people's intersectional identities are considered), we recognize that there is so much more work can be written about certain groups. As an example, we will not be able to include all of the nuances or experiences of every single racial or ethnic group, nor can we possibly cover all gender identities, abilities, religious groups, or the intersection them all. Instead, we hope that our overviews and our attempts can encourage future authors and scholars to examine these nuanced experiences and identities as well.

As you read these pages, we hope you feel compelled to ingest the information that is presented, while creating space to critique and challenge your previous learnings of the topics. We hope you disrupt systems that have perpetuated power and oppression towards queer and trans people (as well as people of all marginalized groups). We also hope that you take what you learn and share it with others. If we really want to change the status quo—especially in psychology—we need to approach it from several angles. People in power need to change policies, trainings, standards, ethical guidelines. People with less power need to pressure those in power. People across the entire system need to do their individual parts to educate and disseminate accurate and LGBTQ-affirming information. In all working individually and collective, we all do our parts to queer psychology. And in doing so, marginalized voices are heard; power is reconsidered; and perhaps, change, equities, and social justice will become realities (Fig. 3).

References

American Psychological Association. (2012). Guidelines for psychological practice with lesbian, gay, and bisexual clients. *American Psychologist, 67*(1), 10–42.

American Psychological Association. (2015). Guidelines for psychological practice with transgender and gender nonconforming people. *American Psychologist, 70*(9), 832–864.

Brim, M., & Ghaziani, A. (2016). Introduction: Queer methods. *Women's Studies Quarterly, 44*(3/4), 14–27.

Brown, J. B. (1997). *Two spirit people: American Indian, lesbian women and gay men*. New York: Psychology Press.

Burnes, T. R., Singh, A. A., & Witherspoon, R. G. (2017). Sex positivity and counseling psychology: An introduction to the major contribution. *The Counseling Psychologist, 45*(4), 470–486.

Butler, J. (2011). *Gender trouble: Feminism and the subversion of identity*. New York: Routledge.

Chung, Y. B., & Singh, A. A. (2009). Lesbian, gay, bisexual, and transgender Asian Americans. In N. Tewari & A. N. Alvarez (Eds.), *Asian American psychology: Current perspectives* (pp. 233–246). New York: Routledge.

Cyrus, K. (2017). Multiple minorities as multiply marginalized: Applying the minority stress theory to LGBTQ people of color. *Journal of Gay & Lesbian Mental Health, 21*(3), 194–202.

Gahagan, J., & Colpitts, E. (2017). Understanding and measuring LGBTQ pathways to health: A scoping review of strengths-based health promotion approaches in LGBTQ health research. *Journal of Homosexuality, 64*(1), 95–121.

Greene, B. (1994). Ethnic-minority lesbians and gay men: Mental health and treatment issues. *Journal of Consulting and Clinical Psychology, 62*(2), 243–251.

Greene, B. (Ed.). (1997). *Psychological perspectives on lesbian and gay issues: Ethnic and cultural diversity among lesbians and gay men*. Newbury Park: Sage.

Herek, G. M. (2007). Confronting sexual stigma and prejudice: Theory and practice. *Journal of Social Issues, 63*(4), 905–925.

Hooker, E. (1993). Reflections of a 40-year exploration: A scientific view on homosexuality. *American Psychologist, 48*(4), 450–453.

Kafer, A. (2013). *Feminist, queer, crip*. Bloomington, IN: Indiana University Press.

Kimmel, D. C., & Browning, C. (1999). A history of Division 44 (Society for the psychological study of lesbian, gay, and bisexual issues). In D. A. Dewsbury (Ed.), *Unification through division: Histories of the divisions of the American Psychological Association* (Vol. 4, pp. 129–150). Washington, DC: American Psychological Association.

Mayo, C. (2007). Queering foundations: Queer and lesbian, gay, bisexual, and transgender educational research. *Review of Research in Education, 31*, 78–94.

Miller, R. A., Wynn, R. D., & Webb, K. W. (2019). "This really interesting juggling act": How university students manage disability/queer identity disclosure and visibility. *Journal of Diversity in Higher Education, 12*(4), 307–318.

Morales, E. (2013). Latino lesbian, gay, bisexual, and transgender immigrants in the United States. *Journal of LGBT Issues in Counseling, 7*(2), 172–184.

Nadal, K. L. (2013). *That's so gay! Microaggressions and the lesbian, gay, bisexual, and transgender community*. Washington, DC: American Psychological Association.

Nadal, K. L. (2017). "Let's get in formation": On becoming a psychologist–activist in the 21st century. *American Psychologist, 72*(9), 935–946.

Nadal, K. L. (2020). *Queering law and order: lesbian, gay, bisexual, transgender and queer people and the criminal justice system*. Lexington Books/Rowman & Little.

Stein, M. (2019). *The stonewall riots: A documentary history*. New York: NYU Press.

Stryker, S. (2008). *Transgender history*. Berkeley, CA: Seal Press.

Williams, J. L. (2019). Disability as an intersectional diversity variable in the psychology curriculum. In J. A. Mena & K. Quina (Eds.), *Integrating multiculturalism and intersectionality into the psychology curriculum: Strategies for instructors* (pp. 157–168). Washington, DC: American Psychological Association.

Intersectional Approaches to Queer Psychology

Angela Ferguson

1 Introduction

The realities and voices of White, cisgender, heterosexual, English-speaking, young, middle-class, able-bodied, Christian men have been centered in the social and behavioral sciences as preeminent in discourses of "normalcy", power, and privilege. What has resulted are epistemologies that have become standard within social science research and theories; "elite white males' perspectives are hegemonized, playing a regulatory role in scientific discourses and practices" (Pereira, 2015, p. 2330). Scientific discourses hierarchically position "elite White male" perspectives, values, beliefs, and uninterrogated power and privilege, thereby suppressing and invalidating the perspectives of all others who do not identify with or who are not included in this group. Consequently, hegemonic epistemologies maintain and normalize domination by an elite few, subordinating and marginalizing all others outside of this "elite" group. Categories such as race, gender, sexuality, and class have been constructed and defined using Eurocentric ideologies, values and beliefs, hegemonic theories and then positioning them as having hierarchical power and privilege while all others are positioned as the "Other". Therefore, scholarly discussions of social identities "replicate rather than interrogate social hierarchies; "academic discourses can serve as potent mechanisms of dominance, infusing the reading situation with strategies of subordination that go unremarked because they are authorized by scholarly norms and traditions" (Tomlinson, 2013, p. 255) (Fig. 1).

The original version of this chapter was revised. The correction to this chapter is available at https://doi.org/10.1007/978-3-030-74146-4_18

A. Ferguson (✉)
Howard University, School of Education, Washington, DC, USA
e-mail: adferguson@howard.edu

15

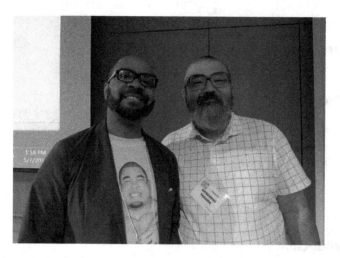

Fig. 1 Professor Andre Carrington and artist Gengoroh Tagame at the queers and comics conference in 2015. Photo courtesy of Center for LGBTQ Studies

When we review the long history of scientific research and literature in the field of psychology, "the implicit equation of minorities and pathology is a common theme" (Sue & Sue, 2003, p. 52). Moreover, because our scientific epistemologies have centered the "elite male" perspective in research and theories, consideration of "the others" have not been centered, and therefore have not been included in guiding our understanding of human behavior and psychological functioning. Consequently, much of the psychological literature has legitimized deficit-based research for members of minority and marginalized group members. Another consequence of hegemonic epistemologies is that they perpetuate the belief that all human behavior is universal, which again marginalizes individuals who are not part of an elite male paradigm. Although some researchers focused on marginalized and minority individuals, it wasn't until the 1970's when "social scientists … argued that cultural differences [were] not synonymous with deviance or deprivation, a view that formed the basis for the cultural and social difference paradigm" (Carter, 1995, p. 43). Several psychologists, theorists and researchers emerged focusing on investigations of behavior that included the way in which race, ethnicity, gender, family, religion, sexuality, socioeconomic status, and a host of contextual factors affected and shaped behavior (Reid, 2002), as well as identity. Each of these "construct[s] emanate from its own set of unique sociopolitical contexts and historical underpinnings ..... [and] represent significant social group experiences whose membership incorporates critical psychological processes and consequences" (Miville & Ferguson 2014, p. 3).

A number of social identity theorists and researchers introduced theoretical perspectives and models that brought attention and visibility to distinct marginalized social groups (Atkinson et al., 1979; Carter, 1995; Casas & Pytluk, 1995; Cass, 1979; Cross Jr., 1971, 1995; Downing & Roush, 1985; Helms, 1984, 1995; Sue & Sue, 1977). Social identity models provided a contextual understanding of how sociopolitical and sociocultural worldviews significantly influenced an individual's psychological development and well-being (Cross Jr., 1971, 1991, 1995; Phinney,

1996) as well as membership in marginalized social groups (Tafjel, 1974). This line of research and theorizing not only challenged decades long of misinformation and stereotypes about members of marginalized groups, but also revealed the ways in which structural oppression and privilege negatively affected social group identity, interpersonal relationships, and personal self-esteem. These models also provided some of the first glimpses of how "social structures and institutions create, shape and maintain social identities" (Dottolo & Stewart, 2008, p. 350), introducing the field to concepts and processes that had previously been overlooked.

Early sexual orientation models (Cass, 1979, 1984; Coleman, 1982; Troiden, 1989) were among the first to introduce the concept of sexuality as a way of framing how an individual made meaning of same-gendered sexuality as an identity formation process (Broido, 2000). These discourses and models focused on the developmental tasks required to form a positive gay or lesbian identity. Moreover, "gay identity theory represented an important shift in emphasis in developmental theory, ways from the concern of etiology and psychopathology characteristic of the illness model toward articulation of the factors involved in the formation of positive gay and lesbian identities (Fox, 1995, p. 53). However, inasmuch as these models and theories were groundbreaking, they primarily centered White middle-class cisgender men in both the conceptualization and in the samples. Consequently, other identity factors (e.g., gender identity, race, social class, immigration status) were not integrated in these models and therefore did not reflect the experiences of people outside of dominant hegemonic groups (i.e., White, male, cisgender). Subsequent research has found that the integration of multiple group memberships such as race and ethnicity (Fukuyama & Ferguson, 2000; Harper et al., 2004; Herek et al., 2009), class (Frable 1997; Liu et al. 2004), gender (Diamond & Butterworth 2008), age (Woolf, 1998; Cahill et al., 2000; Floyd & Bakeman, 2006), and (dis)ability (Gill 1997) can result in unique psychological stressors related to negotiating affiliations with multiple cultural group memberships, as well as negotiating multiple forms of oppression and discrimination (Ferguson et al., 2014).

2 LBGTQ+ Community (and Communities)

The term "LGBTQ+" is generally used to be inclusive of a broad, diverse spectrum of all nonheterosexual and noncisgender gender and sexual minorities (e.g., lesbian, gay, bisexual, transgender, queer; American Psychological Association, 2015; Morandini et al., 2017). In many ways, it is an imprecise construct to describe the many unique, specific characteristics and concerns of individuals generally included under this umbrella term. The term is imprecise for many reasons, one of them being that we live in a world in which gender and sexuality are socially constructed based on a Eurocentric heteronormative perspective. Consequently, individuals who either do not ascribe to, identify with, are nonconforming to binary gender roles or do not live their lives within heteronormative ideals and definitions have not been included in self-defining what it means to be a non-heterosexual, non-gender conforming individual. The structural oppression is framed in dual binaries: gender (e.g., male/female) and sexuality/gender expression (e.g., heterosexual/non-heterosexual). As a result, individuals are left to define and frame their gender and sexuality either within or in juxtaposition of these binaries, which may feel limiting and constraining to an individual's true sense of self. Very little research has examined the ways in which LGBTQ+ individuals perceive and self-define their own identities that are most relevant to how they see themselves.

The term is also imprecise because it is uncertain who is being centered in the discourse and/or analyses. Much of the literature in the psychological and behavioral sciences has focused on the long history of discrimination (e.g., homophobia and heterosexism) and the negative psychological and physical consequences of discrimination LGBTQ+ people in the United States have experienced (see Casey et al., 2019). However, because singular frameworks of analyses are used, we have only a partial understanding of how discrimination affects individuals who identify as LGBTQ+ and how various social identities are situated within systems of oppression. Moreover, singular frameworks of analyses limit an exploration of how multiple forms of oppression impact not only the individual, but the communities in which the individual lives. For example, when exploring homophobia with a sample of LGBTQ+ communities as a sole form of oppression, this unit of analysis provides a limited understanding of how oppression impacts members of this group. Moreover, it perpetuates the belief that only one form of oppression can occur at one time with one group of people, and that sources of discrimination are experienced in the same way for all individuals within a respective social group. Other forms of oppression (e.g., racism, transphobia, biphobia, xenophobia) may also be significant sources of oppression but ignored due to the single framework of analysis. This framework also overlooks the relative status, prestige, power and privilege that may exist for "marginalized" populations. In this way, one must consider if there indeed is an LGBTQ community, or if it would be more accurate to use the label "LGBTQ communities".

Although marginalized group members share similar experiences of discrimination and oppression, forms of oppression vary based on a variety of systemic and individual factors such as: a) similarity or distance from Whiteness, White cultural values, and/or the "elite White male" norm(s); b) respective racial and cultural social histories in the United States; c) gendered social histories and identities; and d) level of sexual minority identity development. Scholars should take into consideration the interrelated factors that create complex patterns of discrimination that affect social identities, as well as the variations of oppression within as well as between social identity categories.

3 Intersectionality

Social identity researchers and theorists brought much needed attention to the psychological development and experiences of minority individuals. Moreover, their efforts to isolate and describe the psychological effects of structural discrimination, prejudice, and institutional forms of oppression on the formation of a healthy identity for marginalized group members was groundbreaking. However, one-dimensional, identity-based models often center and/or prioritize the relative importance of one social identity, thereby concentrating their analysis of identity formation and experiences of oppression to one dimension of an individual's social location. Consequently, these discourses fail to capture how individuals in multiple marginalized identity groups navigate and intersect social identities such as race, gender, class, sexual orientation, and disability at the micro level, as well as navigate multiple and interlocking structural systems of oppression (e.g., racism sexism, heterosexism) at the macro level (Collins, 1990; Crenshaw, 1989, 1991), as well as at the micro level.

Although many single-identity researchers provided much of the foundational theories that examined the ways in which discrimination and prejudice impacted marginalized individuals' identity development, they oversimplified the complex experiences of individuals who held several marginalized social identities simultaneously (Fattoracci et al., 2020), and privileged the "elite White male" perspectives (Dovidio & Gaertner, 2004). Since the development of these early theories, psychologists have recognized the need to adopt an intersectional approach to better capture how social identities work together to influence people's experiences (Cole, 2009). In this way, traditional thinking about sexual orientation and gender expression is expanded beyond a one-dimensional, homogenous category and instead looks at the range and dimensions of sexual minority identities that includes gender, race/ethnicity, (dis)ability, socioeconomic status, and age.

Though single-axis analyses can seem intuitive given that the scientific method requires that a variable be deconstructed into singular units of analysis in order to be understood, discussing only one social identity in isolation of other intersected identities perpetuates a perspective that social groups are homogenous and that as a member of a respective marginalized group (e.g., race, gender, sexual identity), all members experience forms of oppression equally, and in the same way(s). These discourses have lead researchers, practitioners, academics, and theorists to think of identity from a single, monolithic dimension, "speak[ing] as if race is something Blacks have, sexual orientation is something gays and lesbiaxns have, gender is something women have, ethnicity is something so called 'ethnics' have" (Gates, 1996, p. 3) which serves to negate and disregard individuals who have multiple, marginalized social identities, thereby obscuring. One-dimensional identity models also "conflates or ignores intra-group differences" (Crenshaw, 1991, p. 1241).

As a way of understanding and analyzing the complexity of the ways in which individuals navigate multiple marginalized group memberships and multiple forms of oppression, intersectionality research helps analyze how people are located in terms of social structures that capture the power relationship implied by those structures (Stewart & McDermott, 2004). In her 1989 landmark legal paper "Demarginalizing the Intersection of Race and Sex," Kimberlé Crenshaw introduced the term intersectionality, which asserts that individuals experience disadvantage and oppression not from a singular factor such as sexual identity or race, but from the interaction of multiple factors that are necessarily inextricable (Crenshaw,

1991; Collins, 1995; Hooks, 1989). "This approach analyzes the mutually constitutive relations among hierarchical social identities such as those based on gender and race. The fundamental idea behind this approach is that any individual occupies different positions in different hierarchical systems" (Gianettoni & Roux, 2010). Intersectionality theory highlights the nuanced relationships between social identities and the social environment, and emphasizes how power and privilege uniquely influences social locations and identities (Mahalingam, 2007; Whitfield et al., 2014). In her interview with Steinmetz, (2020),

> basically, a lens, a prism, for seeing the way in which various forms of inequality often operate together and exacerbate each other. We tend to talk about race inequality as separate from inequality based on gender, class, sexuality or immigrant status. What's often missing is how some people are subject to all of these, and the experience is not just the sum of its parts (Steinmetz, 2020, p. 82).

The term "intersectionality" is rooted in Black feminist activism and scholarship. Originally, the concept challenged the marginalization of Black women, particularly in mainstream feminist discourses and activism. Crenshaw argued that Black women experienced discrimination (e.g., racism and sexism) because of both their race and gender. She further asserted that due to the social structures of power and privilege, Black men had male privilege and were centered in discourses of antiracism; White women had White privilege and were centered in discourses of gender and sexism. Yet, Black women's unique experience of oppression is often marginalized and sometimes invisible in discourses and scholarly research pertaining to racism *and* sexism. In this regard, Black women's voices and concerns are silenced.

While intersectionality was initially centered on the marginalization of Black women it has been expanded to include other women of color (e.g., Combahee River Collective, 1982; Moräga, 1983; Moräga & Anzáldua, 1983) who were prompted to voice their subordinated positionalities. Hill Collins, (1990) went on to apply the principles of intersectionality to include class, and later sexual orientation. Further, intersectionality also consider[s] the conflux not only of multiple identities, but also of various oppressions (systemic and internalized values of domination based on one's social location), privileges (access to resources and opportunities), history (the lineage and the collaboration of policies and laws that reinscribe values of domination that either maintain groups' susceptibility or providing opportunity (Ferguson et al., 2014).

Membership in multiple marginalized social groups poses challenges relative to navigating intersected, social identities. The intersections of race, ethnicity, gender, sexual orientation/gender identity, class, (dis)ability, sexuality, religion, immigration status are experienced as a coherent identity at the individual level and shapes the way an individual makes meaning of their sense of self, formulates their personal and interpersonal presentation, enters into intimate relationships, interacts within and outside of respective social groups, and interact with family. One identity cannot be extracted (e.g., gender) to assert its primacy among other identities (e.g., race, class, immigrant stats), and one form of oppression cannot be extracted (e.g., sexism, cissexism, racism) to assert its primacy among other oppressions.

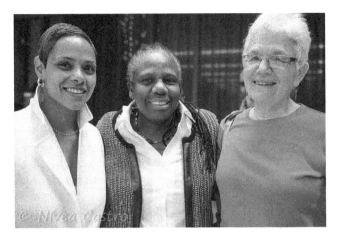

Fig. 2 Three LGBTQ community leaders (Marta Esquilin, Denise Hinds, Julie Schwartzburg) at an event hosted by the Center for LGBTQ Studies. Photo by Nivea Castro

Intersectionality asserts that the interaction of multiple identity factors is interdependent, as well as the structural forms of oppressions in which they live. Intersectionality asserts that advantage and disadvantage are conferred not from a singular factor such as sexual identity, but from the interaction of multiple factors that are interlocking and inextricable (Crenshaw, 1989; Collins, 1995; hooks, 1989). Advantage and disadvantage are contingent on context and the systems in which the individual is interacting (Fig. 2).

> "At its core, intersectionality is the embodiment in theory of the real-world fact that systems of inequality, from the experiential to the structural, are interdependent. The upshot of this for psychologists is that social identities cannot be studied independently of one another, nor separately from the processes that maintain inequality (be it racism, sexism, classism, ableism, or heterosexism)" (Warner & Shields, 2013 p. 804).

4   LGBTQ+ and Intersectionality

The Stonewall Uprisings (June 28, 1969) were a defining historical event for the LGBTQ+ community. It served as a catalyst for the visibility of LGBTQ+ individuals and foundation of LGBTQ+ activism and civil rights. Much of the narrative concerning this event has centered on one social category (sexual orientation/gender identity) and only one form of structural oppression (homophobia). However, fractures along myriad points of identity (e.g., race, gender, sexuality, gender identity, religion, class) were also present. At this same time period, other social/political movements were occurring (e.g., Black activism and women's activism), and while social/political collectives are important to push a political agenda, they can also marginalize members within those collectives. Therefore, activism and civil rights may have been different for a gay cisgender White male and for a Latinx transgender woman. In this example, the intersectionality of race, gender, sexual orientation/ gender identity can cut across each other in various combinations; the individual's experience of oppression, power and privilege may vary depending on setting and context.

As noted earlier in the chapter, the epistemologies that have become standard within social and behavioral science research and theories have emerged from the "elite white male" perspective. Consequently, most research that has been conducted uses a dominant group population as the default population under study unless otherwise noted. Individuals belonging to and/or identifying as non-members of the "elite male group" are often subordinated, marginalized, or are minimally included in the sample population. As a result, research paradigms that compare dominant group members (e.g., White, able-bodied men) to marginalized group members (e.g., White, able-bodied women) perpetuate the inherent power and privilege individuals with dominant social identities enjoy and the disparities that are experienced by individuals with non-majority social identities. Therefore, most research focused on discrimination often discusses the negative effects of not only the experience of discrimination but also the effects of social structures that prevent the marginalized individual/group from enjoying the many privileges of society (Helms & Cook, 1999, p. 28).

Discrimination against LGBTQ+ individuals has received a great deal of attention from researchers during the past several years (Herek, 2007). However, much less research has attended to the complexity of LGBTQ+ identities by including the multidimensional and dynamic interactions between race, gender, sexuality, class, (dis)ability, and religion. These identities help define individual and group identity; they impact respective within group cultural assumptions and influence many of the activities and personal spaces of an LGBTQ+ person. "The confluence of one's multiple marginalized and privileged identities is an interaction that creates a unique experience" (Museus & Griffin, 2001, p. 8). Although LGBTQ+ individuals may experience similar discriminatory oppressions (homophobia, heterosexism), key differences are experienced by individuals depending on their social categories. Consequently, gaps exist about the psychosocial costs and benefits of LGBTQ+ individuals' experiences at the intersections of their social identities. Purdie-Vaughns and Eibach (2008) asserted that individuals with multiple stigmatized or marginalized identities are placed in a position of subordination within at least two majority/minority social groups (e.g., racial minority/sexual minority). However, individuals with multiple stigmatized or marginalized identities may hold several concurrent majority and minority identities (e.g., cisgender Latinx male, transgender African American woman, cisgender White female; cisgender White bisexual) and may experience multiple, simultaneous forms of oppression.

The United States has seen many advances with regard to social justice issues, however despite these advances, systemic injustices, inequities and oppressions still remain with regard to race, gender, sexuality, religion (dis)ability and age, "widening the gap of disparities in economics, health care, employment, housing, education, and …. overall quality of life" (Woody, 2014, p. 146). Additionally, despite the advances that have been made examining marginalized populations, social group experiences continue to be discussed within the framework of structural oppression. "Categories such as race, gender, social class, and sexuality do not simply describe groups that may be different or similar; they encapsulate historical and continuing relations of political, material, and social inequality and stigma" (Cole, 2009, p. 173). Health outcomes, psychological health, economic and education disparities are all implicitly or explicitly framed around the structural ways in which power and privilege are afforded to just an elite few. More specifically, structural inequality influences contact between and within marginalized communities primarily due to their relationship to the "elite White male" paradigm.

4.1   Race

Carter (1995) asserted that "the role and influence of race have been debated in the [social sciences] for many decades" (p. 48). It is a significant identifier, particularly within Western society, and although it has no consensual biological or physiological definition, most researchers' conceptions of race are often correlated with phenotypic attributes (Helms & Cook, 1999). Race has long been a silent construct within social and behavioral research unless the focus has been on non-White racial/ ethnic groups or if the research compared White group members with non-White group members; primarily because "many Whites do not think of themselves in racial terms" (Carter, 1995). However, despite the fact that Whiteness is often not explicitly stated/addressed in discussions of race, it is implicitly centered by default. As a result, Whiteness has not been interrogated in a way as to explore the implicit and explicit power and privilege that it bestows upon its group members, and its discussion in research perpetuates "a 'deficit model paradigm' in our methodologies, continuing the ideology that Whiteness [is] superior to …… non-White racial and ethnic groups" (Ferguson et al., 2014, p. 50). Much of the research focused on LGBTQ+ individuals also center White, cisgender males, and generally addresses one form of oppression (e.g., homophobia), but does not address the privilege and power of belonging to a majority racial social group. Researchers have often defined homophobia from this lens, and erroneously concluded that all LGBTQ+ members experience homophobia, and experience it in the same way. The idea that homophobia may also be gendered or racialized has yet to be researched and discussed within the layered and intersected ways that oppression may be experienced.

4.2   Gender

For most societies and cultures around the world, gender has been conceptualized as a binary construct (being either "male" or "female") largely determined by biological anatomy (genetic and hormonal), and considered absolute and stable across the lifespan. Moreover, some scholars have asserted how heteronormative ideology (Hegarty, Pratto, & Lemieux, 2004) and heterosexual masculinity (Herek, 1986) "serve as a social force that maintains dominant group members' status" (Ray & Parkhill, 2021, p. 49), which privileges and normalizes the experiences and identities of White, cisgender, hetersexual men. Black feminist scholars have criticized White feminist scholars for centering White, cisgender women in discourses pertaining to gender as well. "In the United States, the normative form of hegemonic masculinity is defined by race (White), sexual orientation (heterosexual), socioeconomic status (middle class) and the possession of certain traits: assertiveness, dominance, control, physical strength, and emotional restraint" (Griffith et al., 2012, p. S187). Consequently, the fluidity and complexity of the diverse ways in which individuals experience their biological sex, gender, and sexuality are marginalized, and the "experiences of men and women of color ..... are missing, overlooked, or generalized within the experiences of White individuals, thereby constricting the scope of the discourse related to multiple or diverse forms of gender, sexual identity and sexuality" (Ferguson et al., 2014 p. 49). Additionally, individuals who do not fully uphold and/or adhere to hegemonic ideals of masculinity (e.g., cisgender women, gender nonconforming people, non-heterosexual men, transgender people) are often marginalized and not centered in discourses of gender in positive, privileged ways.

4.3 Age

Much of the aging literature is based on the assumption that older adults are a homogeneous group; the "traditional focus in the aging population has been centered on older, White, middle class women. Thus, much of the theory, research, and perceptions of those over age 65, as well as health care practices, have routinely targeted this demographic group" (Vacha-Haase et al., 2014, p. 66). Consequently, individuals who hold other identities are not centered in the discourses of aging. Despite there being no official census count available of the number of LGBT senior adults living in the United States (Choi and Meyer, 2016), it is estimated that there are approximately 2.7 million LGBTQ+ senior adults 50+ in the United States (Fredriksen-Goldsen et al., 2016).

Older adults share similar age-related experiences, regardless of characteristics such as gender, sexual orientation, race/ethnicity, socioeconomic status, religion and (dis)ability. Many experience physical, biological/neurological, cognitive, and social support challenges due to an aging body and a changing social environment with regard to family, friendship groups, and housing. However, several differences exist within this group due to structural oppression that pose barriers such as access to adequate health care and social services, or availability of suitable living alternatives. For example, structural oppressions are located differently in social contexts such that a White cisgender male may have privilege and face less discrimination in accessing health care than an Asian transgender male or a cisgender Latinx person with a (dis)ability.

4.4 Socioeconomic Status

Socioeconomic status (SES) is pervasive in and affects all aspects of individuals'
lives (e.g., psychological and physical well-being and health, personal, social, and
environmental, and material resources) and includes broad dimensions (e.g., education, income, occupation, material resources).

Although social scientists continue to disagree about how best to operation-
alize SES,

> which indicators are the most valid (e.g., occupation vs. education vs. neighborhood), and
> the translation of different combinations of these indicators into class groupings (e.g., col-
> lege degree plus corporate position equals "middle class"), the fundamental conceptualiza-
> tion involves access to resources" (APA, 2007, p. 5).

Additionally, the distribution of resources and the extent of economic inequality
is tied to the axes of structural oppression, which is connected to the social demo-
graphics within that society. Researchers have found that many individuals who
have minority or marginalized social identities (e.g., culture, race, ethnicity, gender,
age, disability status, and sexuality) often experience overall lower SES, are unin-
sured or underinsured, experience a greater proportion of concentrated poverty,
have lower overall incomes even when they have the same levels of education and
occupation as their peers, constitute a disproportionate percentage of the unemployed and underemployed, and/or live below the poverty line (APA, 2007; Gay and
Lesbian Medical Association, 2001; Massey, 1990; Shapiro, 2004). This is not to
say that all individuals with minority/marginalized identities experience inequality
in the distribution of wealth, and/or access to material resources; however, multiple
axes of oppression often shape any one dimension of SES and can determine relative status, power, privilege, ultimately resulting in varying access to resources,
(e.g., health and mental health access, housing). Additionally, some aspects of SES
may result in more or less advantages for people of color, older adults, people living
with a dis(ability) and LGBTQ+ individuals. For example, a transgender Latinx
female may not have the same job opportunities as a White cisgender gay male,
despite both individuals having the same level of education and/or social class. Due
to existing structural oppressions, past and ongoing forms of discrimination (e.g.,
racism, heterosexism, ableism, ageism), poverty rates, employment, health and
mental health access will continue to have an effect on individuals' ability to attain
material and economic resources as well as determine relative status, power,
privilege.

5 Case Study

Andrea is a 57-year old cisgender Black lesbian-identified woman. She has a master's degree in business, has attended church all of her life, and has had few dating
relationships during her lifetime. She remembers being attracted to women all of her

life, but she did not discuss her feelings with anyone in her family or with her friends. The high school she attended was predominantly White, but students of various racial/ethnic groups were also present. Although Andrea was very involved in high school activities (e.g., band, student clubs, drama club) and was well liked, she never felt that she fit in and always felt somewhat isolated and separate from many of the students. In her current job, she is also well liked and respected however, she has been denied promotion in her organization for the past 3 years, despite receiving high evaluations from her supervisors and being well qualified for the promotion.

Andrea's identities locate her in unique ways relative to the structural oppressions that exist in any one context, thus she may be experiencing many proximal (internalized) and distal (external) forms of oppression. She is an African American cisgender lesbian woman in a society and organization in which social structures of racism, sexism, heterosexism, and ageism converge.

Her Christian religion, being cisgender and having an advanced education are areas of privilege for Andrea, however she has also experienced overt "isms" and microaggressions all of her life. As a young girl, her awareness of herself as a Black person was very clear to her. Her family members were Black and she resided in a community in which she felt the strong presence of Black people in her life. Andrea felt very connected to her Black Church, however as she emerged into her teenage years, she began feeling somewhat separated from members of the congregation and awkward when engaged in conversations pertaining to dating and romantic interests.

Within the context of her family, community and church, Andrea felt very centered and empowered relative to her racial identity. Race was one of the first identifiable aspects of Andrea's identity; her family, community and church's racial socialization helped her develop strategies for managing racism in her life. However, she felt disempowered relative to her sexual orientation, and the overt/covert oppression of sexism and heterosexism within these contexts. Andrea grew up in a family, and attended a church in which dominant heteronormative beliefs regarding biological sex and gender prevailed; that is, men and women were expected to ascribe to cisgender masculine and feminine roles, respectively and were presumed to engage in "traditional" heterosexual relationships and sexual behavior (Harbath, 2014; Ray and Parkhill, 2021). Andrea's gender and sexual orientation identities did not locate her as centered in heteronormative privilege; her feelings of disempowerment often led her to remain silent.

Throughout childhood, Andrea heard many messages that reflected heterosexual, homophobic and sexist beliefs such as: (a) When will you get married (e.g., what is his name)? (b) When will you have children (e.g., biological children with a male); You don't want children when you're old? (c) What's wrong with those people (LGBTQ); why can't they just be normal? (d) They've sinned against God; he will punish them; (e) Don't be too ambitious dear; you don't want to make more money than your husband. All of these messages conveyed structural forms of oppression that existed both in-and-outside of Andrea's home. Although messages related to Andrea's racial identity were not expressed inside her home, however she certainly heard many racial slurs in her school, in the media, and from some community members. Her identities related to gender and sexual orientation were spouted throughout her childhood and internalized as ways in which she wasn't "normal" and in indirect ways, she was "othered".

As Andrea achieved advanced educational degrees, she found that they allowed her to compete for jobs in a variety of employment and career areas that others with less educational degrees did not. She also thought that her advanced education would place her in higher level positions in organizations. Education located her in a position of potential socioeconomic advantage, access to health insurance, and housing choices. "However, women still continue to face workplace hardships such as fewer promotions, less support and implicit bias. Additionally, on average women are paid 80 centers less for every dollar a man earns—a trend that's expected to continue through the 23rd century. Latinas earn $1,135,440 less than men, and Black women receive $946,120 less over the course of a 40-year career" (Brown, 2019). The structural oppressions that exist in the workplace are complex and are embedded in the traditional so-called "boy's club". In this context, Andrea's gender, race, sexual orientation, and age locate her in disadvantaged positions within the workplace, despite her level of education, years of experience, and workplace performance. Moreover, although Andrea was not explicitly "excluded" from the workplace, her opportunities for advancement and other career benefits (e.g., promotion, pay equity) may likely be systemically stifled.

Andrea also may have been exposed to the threat of ageism in her workplace. Implicit bias about her cognitive functioning, her skill in the use of technology, her perceived inflexibility, and potential health problems may have existed in the structural oppressions in the workplace, leading to negative stereotypes of her. Andrea considered leaving her current organization and applying to other organizations locally and out-of-state, however she feared that her potential employers might perceive her as "too old" to hire her. Ageism is based on opinions that older people are slow, resistant to change, crotchety, do not know and cannot learn about technology, have multiple health problems, and are simply behind the times (Nelson, 2005). Although ADEA (Age Discrimination in Employment Act) was signed into law in 1967, it did not provide age-based protections to employees similar to the way in which Title VII of the Civil Rights Act provided protections related to race, gender or religion. Consequently, many "older" people experience age discrimination in their workplaces, with little recourse. Under the law, Andrea's social identities are treated as separate because forms of discrimination (e.g., race; gender; age; and sexual orientation) are viewed as independent of one another, as each form of oppression is connected to a separate statute. The legal system fails to protect against cases involving intersectional forms of oppression, all of which serve as potential barriers to workplace opportunities.

Andrea has experienced a great deal of advantage regarding her religious practices, as she belongs to a Christian faith. She enjoys the freedom of openly talking about her faith in God and does not worry about discrimination based on her Christian affiliation. However, like many churches, her church has conservative religious views, is opposed to same-sex marriage, and views homosexuality as sinful. Although her church is tolerant of LGB individuals, they are not as tolerant of transgender congregants, and Andrea does not openly express her sexual orientation in church or at church activities/events. This lack of acceptance and the homophobia that exists in the church has a negative impact on her religious spirit.

Andrea's life as a cisgender, Black lesbian is not only shaped by heterosexism and homophobia, but by multiple forms of oppression throughout her life. These axes of oppression impact her personal, social, employment, religious and environmental experiences. In order to understand Andrea, it is important to not view her as simply having three separate identities (e.g., race, gender, sexual orientation), but to view her identities as intersected in her everyday life. Collins (2000) asserted that people can locate themselves within a primary system of oppression, but are challenged so see how their thoughts and behaviors contribute to another person's subordination (see also Windsong, 2018). In this way, it is important to not only understand oppression at the micro level (e.g. individual attitudes and behaviors), but also at the macro level (e.g., individual privilege and disadvantage).

6 Summary

Intersectionality is a unique way of viewing and conceptualizing individuals who have multiple, social identities. That individual's identity "produces altogether new forms of subjective experiences that are unique, nonadditive, and not reducible to the original identities that went into them" (Diamond & Butterworth, 2008, p. 366). Single dimensional identity models center one aspect of an individual's identity and "conflates or ignores intra-group differences" (Crenshaw, 1991, p. 1241). It is important that researchers, practitioners, and theorists consider that multiple social identities, as well as multiple forms of oppression are intersected with and shape all of an individual's identities and that facets of psychological health and well-being reflect combinations of identities (Fig. 3).

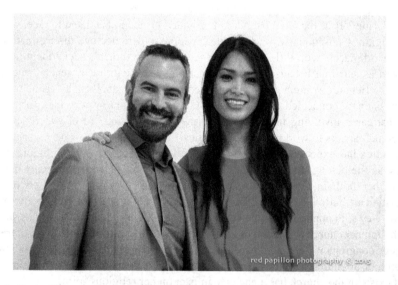

Fig. 3 Dr. Axel Monroig (clinical psychologist) and Geena Rocero (model/activist) at the LGBTQ scholars of color national conference in 2015. Photo courtesy of Riya Ortiz/Red Papillon photography

References

American Psychological Association. (2015). *Definitions related to sexual orientation and gender diversity in APA documents*. Retrieved from https://www.apa.org/pi/lgbt/resources/sexuality-definitions.pdf

American Psychological Association, Task Force on Socioeconomic Status. (2007). *Report of the APA task force on socioeconomic status*. Washington, DC: American Psychological Association.

Atkinson, D. R., Morten, G., & Sue, D. W. (1979). *Counseling American minorities: A cross-cultural perspective*. Dubuque, IA: Brown.

Broido, E. M. (2000). Constructing identity: The nature and meaning of lesbian, gay, and bixsexual identities. In R. M. Perez, K. A. DeBord, & K. J. Bieschke (Eds.), *Handbook of counseling and psychotherapy with lesbian, gay, and bisexual clients* (pp. 13–33). Washington, DC: American Psychological Association.

Brown, D. (2019). *Equal pay day 2019: Women still earn lower salaries, fewer promotions*. USA Today Published April 2, 2019.

Cahill, S., South, K., & Spade, J. (2000). *Outing age: Public policy issues affecting gay, lesbian, bisexual and transgender elders*. Washington, DC: National Gay and Lesbian Task Force Policy Institute. Retrieved from http://www.lgbthealth.net/downloads/research/NGLTFoutingage.pdf.

Carter, R. T. (1995). *The influence of race and racial identity in psychotherapy*. New York: Wiley & Sons.

Casas, J. M., & Pytluk, S. D. (1995). Hispanic identity development. In J. G. Ponterotto, J. M. Casas, L. A. Suzuki, & C. M. Alexander (Eds.), *Handbook of multicultural counseling* (pp. 155–180). Thousand Oaks, CA: Sage.

Casey, L. S., Reisner, S. L., Findling, M. G., Blendon, R. J., Benson, J. M., Sayde, J. M., & Miller, C. (2019). Discrimination in the United States: Experiences of lesbian, gay, bisexual, transgender, and queer Americans. *Health Services Research, 54*, 1454–1466. https://doi.org/10.1111/1475-6773.13229.

Cass, V. C. (1979). Homosexual identity formation: A theoretical model. *Journal of Homosexuality, 4*, 219–235.

Cass, V. C. (1984). Homosexual identity formation: Testing a theoretical model. *Journal of Sex Research, 20*(2), 143–167. https://doi.org/10.1080/00224498409551214.

Choi, S. K., & Meyer, I. H. (2016). *LGBT aging: A review of research findings, needs, and policy implications*. Los Angeles: The Williams Institute.

Cole, E. R. (2009). Intersectionality and research in psychology. *American Psychologist, 64*(3), 170–180. https://doi.org/10.1037/a0014564.

Coleman, E. (1982). Developmental stages of the coming out process. *Journal of Homosexuality, 7*, 31–43.

Collective, C. R. (1982). A black feminist statement: The Combahee River collective. In G. T. Hull, P. Bell-Scott, & B. Smith (Eds.), *All the women are white, all the blacks are men, but some of us are brave: Black women's studies* (pp. 13–22). New York, NY: The Feminist Press at CUNY.

Collins, P. H. (1990). *Black feminist thought: Knowledge, consciousness and the politics of empowerment*. New York: Routledge.

Collins, P. H. (1995). The social construction of black feminist thought. In B. Guy-Sheftall (Ed.), *Words of fire: An anthology of African American feminist thought* (pp. 337–357). New York: The New Press.

Collins, P. H. (2000). *Black feminist thought* (2nd ed). New York: Routledge.

Crenshaw, K. (1989). Demarginalizing the intersection of race and sex: A black feminist critique of antidiscrimination doctrine, feminist theory, and antiracist politics. *University of Chicago Legal Forum, 14*, 139–167.

Crenshaw, K. (1991). Mapping the margins: Intersectionality, identity politics, and violence against women of color. *Stanford Law Review, 43*, 1241–1299.

Cross, W. E., Jr. (1971). The negro-to-black conversion experience: Towards a psychology of black liberation. *Black World, 20*, 13–27.

Cross, W. E., Jr. (1991). *Shades of black: Diversity in African American identity*. Philadelphia, PA: Temple University Press.

Cross, W. E., Jr. (1995). The psychology of Nigrescence: Revisiting the Cross model. In J. G. Ponterotto, J. M. Casas, L. A. Suzuki, & C. M. Alexander (Eds.), *Handbook of multicultural counseling* (pp. 93–122). Thousand Oaks, CA: Sage.

Diamond, L. M., & Butterworth, M. (2008). Questioning gender and sexual identity: Dynamic links over time. *Sex Roles, 59*, 365,376. https://doi.org/10.1007/s1199-008-9425-3.

Dottolo, A., & Stewart, A. (2008). "Don't ever forget now, you're a black man in America": Intersections of race, class and gender in encounters with the police. *Sex Roles, 59*(5–6), 350–364. https://doi.org/10.1007/s11199-007-9387-x.

Dovidio, J. F., & Gaertner, S. L. (2004). Aversive racism. *Advances in Experimental Social Psychology, 36*, 1–52. https://doi.org/10.1016/S0065-2601(04)36001-6.

Downing, N. E., & Roush, K. L. (1985). From passive acceptant to active commitment: A model of feminist identity development for women. *The Counseling Psychologist, 13*(4), 695–709. https://doi.org/10.1177/0011000085134013.

Fattoracci, E. S. M., Revels-Macalinao, M., & Huynh, Q.-L. (2020). Greater than the sum of racism and heterosexism: Intersectional microaggressions toward racial/ethnic and sexual minority group members. *Cultural Diversity and Ethnic Minority Psychology*. Advance online publication. https://doi.org/10.1037/cdp0000329.

Ferguson, A. D., Carr, G., & Snitman, A. (2014). Intersections of race/ethnicity, gender and sexual minority communities. In M. L. Miville & A. D. Ferguson (Eds.), *Handbook of race-ethnicity and gender in psychology* (pp. 45–63). New York: Springer.

Floyd, F. J., & Bakeman, R. (2006). Coming-out across the life course: Implications of age and historical context. *Archives of Sexual Behavior, 35*, 287–296. https://doi.org/10.1007/s10508-006-9022-x.

Fox, R. C. (1995). Bisexual identities. In A. R. D'Augelli & C. J. Patterson (Eds.), *Lesbian, gay, and bisexual identities over the lifespan: Psychological perspectives* (pp. 48–86). New York, NY: Oxford University Press.

Frable, D. E. S. (1997). Gender, racial, ethnic, sexual, and class identities. *Annual Review of Psychology, 48*, 139–162.

Fredriksen-Goldsen, K. I., Kim, H.-J., Goldsen, J., Shiu, C., & Emlet, C. A. (2016). *Addressing social, economic, and health disparities of LGBT older adults & best practices in data collection*. Seattle, WA: LGBT+ National Aging Research Center, University of Washington. Retrieved from http://caringandaging.org/wordpress/wp-content/uploads/2016/05/2016-Disparities-Factsheet-Final-Final.pdf.

Fukuyama, M. A., & Ferguson, A. D. (2000). Lesbian, gay, and bisexual people of color: Understanding cultural complexity and managing multiple oppressions. In R. M. Perez, K. A. Debord, & K. J. Bieschke (Eds.), *Handbook of counseling and psychotherapy with lesbian, gay, and bisexual clients* (pp. 81–105). Washington, DC: American Psychological Association.

Gates, H. L. (1996). The ethics of identity. *Pathways, 20*(3), 3–4.

Gay and Lesbian Medical Association (GLMA). (2001, April). *Healthy people 2010: Companion document for lesbian, gay, bisexual, and transgender (LGBY) health*. Retrieved May, 2006, from www.glma.org/_data/n_0001/resources/live/HealthyCompanionDoc3.pdf.

Gianettoni, L., & Roux, P. (2010). Interconnecting race and gender relations: Racism, sexism and the attribution of sexism to the racialized other. *Sex Roles, 62*, 374–386. https://doi.org/10.1007/s11199-010-9755-9.

Gill, C. J. (1997). Four types of integration in disability identity development. *Journal of Vocational Rehabilitation, 9*, 39–46. https://doi.org/10.1016/S1052-2263(97)00020-2.

Griffith, D. M., Gunter, K., & Watkins, D. C. (2012). Measuring masculinity in research on men of color: Findings and future directions. *American Journal of Public Health, 102*(S2), S187–S194.

Habarth, J. M. (2014). Development of the heteronormative attitudes and beliefs scale. *Psychology and Sexuality, 6*, 166–188. https://doi.org/10.1080/19419899.2013.876444.

Harper, G. W., Jernewall, N., & Zea, M. C. (2004). Giving voice to emerging science and theory for lesbian, gay and bisexual people of color. *Cultural Diversity and Ethnic Minority Psychology, 10*(3), 187–199. https://doi.org/10.1037/1099-9809.10.3.187.

Hegarty, P., Pratto, F., & Lemieux, A. F. (2004). Heterosexual ambivalence and heterocentric norms: Drinking in intergroup discomfort. *Group Processes & Intergroup Relations, 7*, 119–130. https://doi.org/10.1177/1368430204041399.

Helms, J. E. (1984). Toward a theoretical explanation of the effects of race on counseling: A black and white model. *The Counseling Psychologist, 12*, 153–165.

Helms, J. E. (1995). An update of Helms's white and people of color racial identity models. In J. G. Ponterotto, J. M. Casas, L. A. Suzuki, & C. M. Alexander (Eds.), *Handbook of multicultural counseling* (pp. 181–191). Thousand Oaks, CA: Sage.

Helms, J. E., & Cook, D. A. (1999). *Using race and culture in counseling and psychotherapy: Theory and process.* Needham Heights, MA: Allyn and Bacon.

Herek, G. M. (1986). On heterosexual masculinity: Some psychical consequences of the social construction of gender and sexuality. *The American Behavioral Scientist, 29*, 563–577. https://doi.org/10.1177/000276486029005005.

Herek, G. M. (2007). Confronting sexual stigma and prejudice: Theory and practice. *Journal of Social Issues, 63*, 905–925. https://doi.org/10.1111/j.1540-4560.2007.00544.x.

Herek, G. M., Gillis, J. R., & Cogan, J. C. (2009). Internalized stigma among sexual minority adults: Insights from a social psychological perspective. *Journal of Counseling Psychology, 56*, 32–43. https://doi.org/10.1037/a0014672.

hooks, B. (1989). *Talking back: Talking feminist, talking Black.* Boston: South End Press.

Liu, W. M., Ali, S. R., Soleck, G., Hopps, J., Dunston, K., & Pickett, T., Jr. (2004). Using social-class in counseling psychology research. *Journal of Counseling Psychology, 51*, 3–18.

Mahalingam, R. (2007). Culture, power and psychology of marginality. In A. Fuligni (Ed.), *Contesting stereotypes and creating identities: Social categories, social identities, and educational participation* (pp. 42–65). New York: Sage.

Massey, D. S. (1990). American apartheid: Segregation and the making of the underclass. *American Journal of Sociology, 96*, 329–357.

Miville, M. L., & Ferguson, A. D. (2014). Intersections of race-ethnicity and gender on identity development and social roles. In M. L. Miville & A. D. Ferguson (Eds.), *Handbook of race-ethnicity and gender in psychology* (pp. 3–21). New York: Springer.

Morága, C. (1983). *Loving in the war years.* Cambridge, MA: South End Press.

Morága, C., & Anzáldua, G. (1983). *This bridge called my back: Writings by radical women of color.* New York, NY: Kitchen Table, Women of Color Press.

Morandini, J. S., Blaszczynski, A., & Dar-Nimrod, I. (2017). Who adopts queer and pansexual sexual identities? *Journal of Sex Research, 54*, 911–922. https://doi.org/10.1080/00224499.2016.1249332.

Museus, S.D., & Griffin, K.A. (2011). Mapping the margins in higher education: On the promise of intersectionality frameworks in research and discourse. *New Directions for Institutional Research, 2011*(151), 5–13. https://doi.org/10.1002/ir.395.

Nelson, T. D. (2005). Ageism: Prejudice against our feared future self. *Journal of Social Issues, 61*(2), 207–221.

Pereira, A. C. (2015). Power, knowledge and black feminist thought's enduring contribution towards social justice. *Racial and Ethnic Studies, 38*(13), 2329–2333. https://doi.org/10.1080/01419870.2015.1058494.

Phinney, J. (1996). When we talk about American ethnic groups, what do we mean? *American Psychologist, 51*(9), 918–927.

Purdie-Vaughns, V., & Eibach, R. P. (2008). Intersectional invisibility: The distinctive advantages and disadvantages of multiple subordinate group identities. *Sex Roles, 59*, 377–391.

Ray, T.N. & Parkhill, M.R. (2021). Heteronormatvitiy, disgust sensitivity, and hostile attitudes toward gay men: Potential mechanisms to maintain social hierarchies. *Sex Roles, 84*(1/2), 49–60. https://doi.org/10.1007/s11199-020-01146-w.

Reid, P. T. (2002). Multicultural psychology: Bringing together gender and ethnicity. *Cultural Diversity and Ethnic Minority Psychology, 8,* 103–114. https://doi.org/10.1037//1099-9809.8.2.103.

Shapiro, T. (2004). *The hidden cost of being African-American: How wealth perpetuates inequality.* New York: Oxford University Press.

Steinmetz, K. (2020). Q & A: Kimberlé Crenshaw. *TIME Magazine, 195*(7/8), 82.

Stewart, A. J., & McDermott, C. (2004). Gender psychology. *Annual Review of Psychology, 55,* 519–544.

Sue, D. W., & Sue, D. (1977). Barriers to effective cross-cultural counseling. *Journal of Counseling Psychology, 24,* 420–429.

Sue, D. W., & Sue, D. (2003). *Counseling the culturally different: Theory and practice* (4th ed.). New York: John Wiley & Sons.

Tafjel, H. (1974). Social identity and intergroup behavior. *Social Science Information, 13,* 65–93.

Tomlinson, B. (2013). Colonizing intersectionality: Replicating racial hierarchy in feminist academic arguments. *Social Identities, 19*(2), 254–272. https://doi.org/10.1080/1350463 0.2013.789613.

Troiden, R. R. (1989). The formation of homosexual identities. *The Journal of Homosexuality, 17*(1/2), 43–73.

Vacha-Haase, T., Donaldson, W., & Foster, A. (2014). Race-ethnicity and gender in older adults. In M. L. Miville & A. D. Ferguson (Eds.), *Handbook of race-ethnicity and gender in psychology* (pp. 65–83). New York: Springer.

Warner, L., & Shields, S. (2013). The intersections of sexuality, gender, and race: Identity research at the crossroads. *Sex Roles, 68*(11–12), 803–810. https://doi.org/10.1007/s11199-013-0281-4.

Whitfield, D. L., Walls, N. E., Langenderfer-Magruder, L., & Clark, B. (2014). Queer is the new black? Not so much: Racial disparities in anti-LGBTQ discrimination. *Journal of Gay & Lesbian Social Services, 26,* 426–440. https://doi.org/10.1080/10538720.2014.955556.

Windsong, E. A. (2018). Incorporating intersectionality into research design: An example using qualitative interviews. *International Journal of Social Research Methodology, 21*(2), 135–147. https://doi.org/10.1080/13645579.2016.1268361.

Woody, I. (2014). Aging out: A qualitative exploration of ageism and heterosexism among aging African American lesbians and gay men. *Journal of Homosexuality, 61*(1), 145–165. https://doi.org/10.1080/00918369.2013.835603.

Woolf, L. (1998). *Gay and lesbian aging.* Webster Groves, MO: Webster University.

Gender Identity as a Social Developmental Process

Angelica Puzio and Alexis Forbes

1 Introduction

The process of establishing a gender identity, or the gender group that an individual identifies with, is one of the most ubiquitous psychological processes observed across cultures. Members of nearly all societies report a sense of belonging to specific gender groups, despite cross-cultural differences in languages, histories, and ideologies (Wood & Eagly, 2009). The field's understanding of the concept has evolved significantly in the last 20 years (e.g., Singh, 2016; American Psychological Association, 2015). Gender identity has long been thought of as a developmental process in which children come to understand their identity as a "boy" or "girl," and subsequently view gender as permanent. More recently, social psychologists have challenged this notion by arguing that children's identification with gender identities on the transgender spectrum is developmentally normative (e.g., Olson & Gülgöz, 2018; Tate et al., 2014.) Advances in social psychology have shown gender to be both a developmental phenomenon (meaning that there are periods of stability and change over time), and also a social one, meaning that the process of knowing and experiencing one's gender is intertwined with "interpersonal relationships, interpersonal attitudes, and social signaling" (Tate et al., 2014, p. 304). Public and academic sensitivity towards the experiences of people whose gender identities lie outside of the binary conception of man and woman has increased by large margins

---

The original version of this chapter was revised. The correction to this chapter is available at
https://doi.org/10.1007/978-3-030-74146-4_18

A. Puzio (✉)
Department of Applied Psychology, New York University, New York, NY, USA
e-mail: angelicapuzio@nyu.edu

A. Forbes
Bonora Rountree, Trial Consulting and Research, San Francisco, CA, USA

K. L. Nadal and M. R. Scharrón-del Río (ed.), *Queer Psychology*,
https://doi.org/10.1007/978-3-030-74146-4_3

(Bowers & Whitley, 2020). These shifts require psychologists to integrate new advances into research and practice in order to more fully characterize the way gender is experienced and expressed among diverse populations (Fig. 1).

Gender identity development research has a homogenous past. White cisgender scholars from the United States and Europe have largely focused on the experiences of white cisgender children in the United States and Europe, and the science reflects this narrowly centered viewpoint. As Tadishi Dozono (2017) notes, the approach taken in this chapter is to "not end in a place where one thinks, 'how strange the past was' or 'how strange those other genders are,' but rather to think about how strange and particular one's own contexts and assumptions are, amidst a vast array of interpretations of reality" (p. 426). By pointing out perspectives outside of the mainstream, such as gender structures within indigenous cultures, dominant theories tend to lose their strong grip on the field's narrow and deeply westernized conceptualization of the concept. Until very recently, the experiences of transgender and gender non-conforming individuals were absent from mainstream psychological theories about how gender develops, although there is a long history of social scientists' documentation of (and often pathologization of) gender non-conforming people (e.g., Garfinkel, 1967; Stoller, 1968). To the degree possible, we rely on non-Eurocentric and indigenous perspectives whenever possible throughout the chapter.

The purpose of this chapter is to integrate scientific advances in gender identity development research with perspectives on gender that are typically marginalized. We argue that when viewed holistically, the process of identifying with a gender group is most accurately described as a social developmental process that is bound by individuals' unique cultural contexts. Although experiences of discrimination and minority stress often come along with gender identities outside of man and woman, we do not explicitly focus on describing experiences of prejudice and

Fig. 1 Dominique Jackson (actress) poses with Cecilia Gentili (trans activist and community organizer). Photo Courtesy of Cecilia Gentili

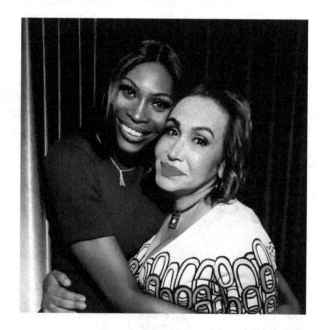

violence faced by individuals in marginalized gender groups (but readers should see Grant et al., 2011). Rather, we concentrate on advances in the field's intersectional understanding of gender identity as a persisting psychological phenomenon and the implications this has for policy and practice. Before we turn our focus to these contributions, we define some common terms that will be used throughout the chapter, as previously described by Best and Puzio (2019), unless otherwise noted.

- *Gender identity* refers to self-identification with a specific gender category (e.g., man, woman, or non-binary).
- *Sex* refers to anatomical and physiological differences between individuals that are typically described as male and female. Although commonly thought of as two dimorphic categories, an individual's sex can be expressed non-dimorphically across a range of factors, some of which include reproductive organs, genitals, and hormones. People who exhibit variation from male and female sex categories are typically described as *intersex* or as having *disorders of sexual development* (DSD),[1] which occur in roughly 1 out of 100 infants (Brown et al., 2020).
- *Cisgender* describes individuals whose birth-assigned sex category aligns with their gender identity (e.g., a person who was assigned as "female" at birth and has the gender identity of "woman").
- *Transgender* or *transgender spectrum* describes individuals whose birth assigned sex categories do not align with their gender identity (e.g., a person who was assigned "male" at birth and has the gender identity of "woman").
- *Gender role ideology* is the degree to which traditional social roles that gender groups are thought to occupy with differential frequency are accepted or endorsed (e.g., "Women should put effort into their appearance"). Gender role ideologies are typically described as varying on a continuum anchored at "traditional" and increasing towards "progressive" or "egalitarian" ideology. Gender role ideologies can be expressed by individuals, groups, or larger systems such as schools or governments.
- *Genderqueer, queer, gender non-conforming, and non-binary (sometimes "enby" for short)* are used to describe gender identites that exist between or beyond the gender binary. These terms can describe a multitude of identities that reject or do not conform to the gender binary.
- *The gender binary* is the notion that human beings and their behavior are categorizable into two mutually exclusive gender categories of man/masculine and woman/feminine, of which there is no in between or overlap (Drescher, 2010).

2   Self-Identification and Labels

Gender identity measurement has become more varied with the advent of research with transgender and gender non-conforming (TGNC) populations. It is common for researchers who specialize in TGNC research to allow respondents to write-in

---

[1] There is considerable debate around the appropriate term. Some individuals and activists believe that DSD is the most appropriate term to bring about informed medical treatment. Others find this term stigmatizing and prefer "intersex" or "hermaphrodite." (Drescher, 2010).

their self-identifying gender identity label. One reason for this is that past measures have been microaggressive toward TGNC people; therefore, giving the respondent the option to label themselves resolves that issue. Unfortunately, in order to make broader recommendations for the mental and physical health of TGNC communities, researchers need a way to group individuals who are likely to have similar experiences. Sometimes, self-identification precludes grouping, as individuals who have similar life experiences may not use the same label for their gender identity. Though the body of research with TGNC populations is growing, it is important to be able to aggregate across datasets for a clearer picture of the common experiences or problems these individuals face. Nonidentical self-identification labels can sometimes complicate that endeavor.

In the 2010s, more diverse terminology and labels for gender identity became more widely recognized (e.g., Harrison et al., 2012). For instance, non-cisgender people might identify as two-spirit, bigender, agender, genderqueer, gender non-binary, gender fluid, gender variant, or transgender. Having a more diverse vocabulary for non-cisgender identities has multiple benefits. First, awareness of more appropriate terms helps to prevent microaggressions and microinvalidations on the part of researchers, healthcare providers, mental health professionals, and educators. Second, having a broader set of terminology increases the likelihood that people will find a term that conveys how they identify their gender. In other words, people who may have struggled to conceptualize their gender within the boundaries of a cisgender context have access to terms that are becoming more commonly understood. Finally, as terms are more popularized, it is more feasible for researchers to make informed judgements about people who identify with a specific term. For instance, understanding how the experiences of people who identify as gender fluid differ from those who identify as genderqueer could have implications for research on self-esteem and mental health. As the spectrum model of gender identity becomes more widely accepted, the collection of new labels and self-identifying terminology will continue to grow (Fig. 2).

3   History of Gender Identity in Social Science

Discussions of *dominant* theories of gender identity development should begin with an acknowledgement of the larger assumptions that these ideas rest upon. In this section, we will discuss several ways that previous theorists have described how and why humans come to understand themselves as gendered beings. Most of these perspectives describe processes in which individuals typically come to think of themselves as cisgender by using information available within their social environments. In other words, these theories often assume that becoming cisgender is a natural and ultimately adaptive process of human development. We wish to point out that these processes are only "natural" to the extent that prevailing ideological structures of gender present in our society are "natural." Stage theories, or theories that describe human development as a sequential process, such as learning how to crawl or form words, often presume there is a correct and natural course of human

Fig. 2 Noam Parness—a genderqueer community organizer and art curator poses at an event hosted by the Center for LGBTQ Studies. Photo Courtesy of Nivea Castro

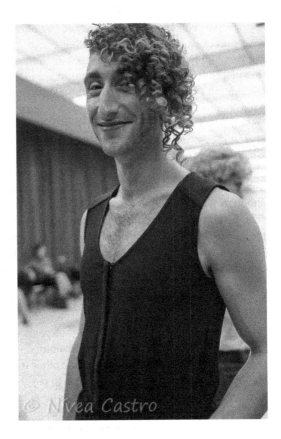

development. The flaw in logic, then, is that dominant gender identity theories are often *teleological*, meaning they implicitly argue for a destiny or grand design to society's gender structure when in fact many individuals do not adhere to that structure. This issue is precisely why dominant theories fail to propose mechanisms for when humans develop gender identities outside of woman and man. It should be clear that the processes we describe in this section may indeed be typical, but typical is not synonymous with "adaptive" or "natural."

Until recently, psychologists have largely accepted two dominant definitions of gender identity that date back to the 1960s and 1970s. The first widely acknowledged definition, which refers to gender identity as little more than a psychological experience of categorizing one's gentials, was derived from Robert Stoller's *Sex and Gender*. Stoller (1968) proposed the concept of *core gender identity*, the idea that identification with a gender group comes from three sources: (1) a sense of awareness of one's genitals, (2) the acknowledgement of one's gender from members of the home environment, and (3) a "biological force" (p. 40). This definition characterizes gender identity as an awareness of the social meaning that is ascribed to one's genitals, which contemporary theorists see as problematic and in conflict with intersex and transgender children's experiences. Although Freud had earlier claimed that sex and gender could diverge (see Freud, 1905, 1925, 1932), Stoller's (1968) case studies explicitly instantiated that sex and gender could exist as separate and not "inevitably bound" (p. vi) into the canon of clinical psychology. His documentation of TGNC individuals was revolutionary in its time, but with it came the explicit declaration that deviation from complete alignment between sex and gender was pathological. This notion of gender deviance or pathology has pervaded psychiatry and clinical psychology since, which we discuss at length later in the chapter.

The second dominant perspective, which defines gender identity as the degree to which a person endorses certain traits that society has deemed masculine or feminine, originates from Sandra Bem's gender schema theory (Bem, 1974, 1981). Similar to Stoller, Bem's conceptualizing of gender identity has occupied a strong, although less clinically widespread, place in the field's understanding of the concept. She drew from cognitive schema theories in her understanding of gender identity, or the idea that individuals organize information into mental templates (e.g., "buses that take children to school are yellow") from which they can then easily and quickly understand new information (e.g., "that particular bus is yellow, so it must be taking children to school"). According to gender schema theory, each individual has a "gender schema" in which they organize gender-related information, including information about the self. Thus, one could infer gender identity from examining the set of traits associated with male and female gender groups, which Bem measured with the "Bem Sex Role Inventory" (BSRI, see the *Measuring Gender Identity* section later in this chapter for other trait measures). Bem endorsed "psychological androgyny" as advantageous to psychological adjustment, such that individuals should aim to endorse both masculine and feminine traits.

The field's understanding of gender has expanded beyond a trait based perspective in recent years and now considers Bem's notion of traits to be culturally masculinized or feminized rather than characteristics that are essential to men and women. It seems unlikely, as Egan and Perry (2001) have noted, that individuals' report of personality traits at a given moment could reflect the complete psychological experience of self-identifying with a particular gender group. Despite these limitations, perceptions of "fit" within the traits associated with a given gender may still be at play in constituting gender identity as one piece of a larger puzzle. The core feature of Bem's contribution is the proposition that gender identity development takes place in a social context. The idea that individuals perceive and then integrate information about gender into their developing self-concept, rather than simply learn to acknowledge physiology, has had lasting value in the field.

Both Bem and Stoller's ideas of gender identity represent early thinking within the field of psychology. Current perspectives would describe the process of establishing a gender identity as "developmentally acquiring self-knowledge that translates into self-categorization as female, male, or some other gender identity" (Tate, 2014, p. 8), but we review these advances later in the section titled *Current Perspectives on Gender Identity*. However, the idea that establishing a gender identity is a developmental process has largely been credited to the stage theories of Jean Piaget (1983), Lawrence Kohlberg (1966), and Walter Mischel (1966), three highly influential thinkers within mainstream psychology. Their theories are often referred to as cognitive developmental theories of gender development because of their focus on children's cognitive labeling or gradual recognition of themselves as cisgender.

Similar to Piaget's descriptions of children's gradual development of object permanence, or the understanding that objects exist even when we cannot see them, Kohlberg (1966) proposed that children come to understand gender in a similar, stage-like manner. Near the age of three, he proposed that children come to label themselves according to the gender label that others use to describe them (see also Slaby and Frey 1975). Then, between the ages of three and seven, children acquire what he calls gender constancy, or the internal sense that gender is fixed and immutable. For example, a child may use information available in their social environment to determine that "I am a boy. I'm a boy no matter what. Because I'm a boy, I like to do things that I see other boys do." However, Mischel (1966) used a behaviorist approach that is now referred to as a social-learning theory of gender development. Through this perspective, children's sense of gender is derived through social rewards (e.g.., "People say I'm a boy. People like when I do boy things. Therefore, I must be a boy").

Both Kohlberg and Mischel put emphasis on the role of others in facilitating the child's recognition of their gender, but the proposed mechanisms differ between theories. Kohlberg proposed that reaching the cognitive stage of gender constancy motivates gender norm adherence, whereas Mischel proposed that being rewarded for adhering to gender norms leads the child to make the inference that one is, indeed, the gender that others have determined them to be. These theories captured a great deal of attention among social and developmental psychologists who study gender, but they have since been questioned and challenged for two major reasons. First, they cannot account for gender variance in childhood. In other words, social learning and cognitive developmental theories do not explain children who develop gender identities outside of boy and girl, and they adequately explain children who resist their gender socialization (e.g., "People say I'm a boy. People like when I do boy things. But I like doing girl things instead"). Second, as we point out in the beginning of this section, both approaches implicitly argue for a teleological or "grand design" logic to the way gender operates. As Pascoe and Bridges (2016) point out, this logic collapses when an element of society's gender structure changes. For example, when more girls enroll in school sports compared to 40 years ago, social-learning and cognitive developmental theorists have no mechanism to describe why such a change took place. This is because both of these theoretical stances assume that individuals adhere to a naturally imposed gender binary, when in fact many people–including children–resist a binary conceptualization of gender.

Before shifting our attention to some of the more modern theories about gender development, let's highlight three components of the early theories that are still relevant to today's gender theories. From Stoller (1968) and Freud (1905, 1925), we learn that gender and sex do not always align. From Bem (1974, Bem 1981), we learn that establishing a gender identity is a dynamic interaction where individuals use cognitive structures of categorization to make sense of information in their social environments. And finally, from early developmental theorists Kohlberg and

Mischel (Kohlberg, 1966; Mischel, 1966) we learn that gender identity is developed over time and likely in dynamic interaction with an individuals' social context.[2] In turn, there are many components of these earlier theories that should be firmly opposed: the notion that gender identities outside of or beyond the gender binary are indicative of mental disorder, the idea that individuals select their gender identities based solely on a myriad of traits, and that gender is immutable after a certain developmental stage.

4 Gender Today: A Social Developmental Process

4.1 Two Major Models of Gender

Contemporary theorists propose gender identity development as a multidimensional process that considers the possibility of resistance *or* adherence to the gender binary, meaning that these theories take into account gender variance beyond the cisgender gender identity. They also separate aspects of gender that are felt internally or privately and the aspects that exist in the social world (e.g., gender categorization from others, such as being told "you're a girl," vs. a personally felt "I am a girl"). We first focus on Egan and Perry (2001), who propose a five-dimension model of gender identity. These dimensions are (1) knowledge of membership to a gender category, (2) gender typicality or degree to which one feels they are similar or different from members of the gender group, (3) felt pressure to conform to social expectations for the gender group, (4) felt contentment with belonging to this group, and (5) a sense of favoritism or superiority towards one's own group in relation to other gender groups.

The second major perspective we review, written by Tate and her colleagues (Tate et al., 2014; Tate, 2014), updated Egan and Perry's model to consist of five different facets. These are: (a) "birth-assignment to a gender category by a cultural authority," (b) "one's self-categorization into a gender group," (c) "one's recognition of and possible adherence to stereotypes and expectations associated with their own and other gender groups," (d) "one's expression of gender as embodied by the use of names and accouterments associated with gender groups," and (e) "one's attitudinal and cognitive evaluation of members of one's gender ingroup" (Tate et al., 2014; p. 303). The model presented by Egan and Perry is particularly geared toward children and adolescents, whereas Tate and colleagues' is more suited for adults and more fully integrates the experiences of transgender and gender nonconforming individuals. We position gender identity as a social developmental process by assessing the points of overlap and contrast in these perspectives.

---

[2] Freud also argued the point that gender developed over time, although more implicitly than Kohlberg and Mischel.

4.2   Dimension 1: Membership Knowledge

Egan and Perry (2001) suggested that a more dimensional model of gender identity could expand the reach of cognitive developmental, social learning, and trait-based theories and improve on their limitations. They refined and aggregated elements of these perspectives to create a multidimensional construct, starting with their first proposed dimension of "knowledge of membership in a gender category" (p. 451). Three-year-old Children's ability to respond to the question "Are you a boy or a girl?" suggests to Egan and Perry that gender identity involves a knowledge of gender that reaches "constancy" by age six or seven. The field has little idea of what is meant by gender "knowledge" in the first years of life, however. For example, does a three-year-old's response of "I'm a girl" reflect an embodied identification with girlhood or a learned response of giving the "correct" answer to an adult? This point is unclear. However, children's insistence on belonging to a gender group is seen widely across children who are raised in cultures that ask this question, and is seen in both transgender and cisgender children (Olson & Gülgöz 2018). Researchers have, however, documented differences in transgender and cisgender children's beliefs about gender constancy, as transgender children are more likely to believe that gender can change over the course of the lifespan (Ruble et al., 2007). Recognizing the near ubiquity of children's self-labeling, Egan and Perry theorized that the cognitive developmental process of early gender group knowledge is a fundamental component of gender identity.

4.3   Dimensions 2 & 3: Gender Typicality and Felt Pressure

Egan and Perry (2001) also drew from trait based perspectives, but with an important update to include not only how much a child engages in gendered behavior but also their experience of pressure to do so. They note that Bem's (1981) perspective was limited in that most individuals only show a moderate degree of gender-stereotyped behaviors, yet tend to clearly identify with a gender group. For example, a man may be unconflicted about his gender identity but also endorses traits culturally deemed feminine, such as nurturance for his children and putting effort into his physical appearance. However, the process of inferring gender identity from behavior may be slightly different for children. Drawing from Maccoby's (1998) research, Egan and Perry (2001) conclude that "self-observation of concrete, easily observable aspects of sex typing, such as activity choices and playmate preferences, may be especially important for feeling that one is a good fit with one's gender" (p. 453). Of course, children's sex typing is not a fully endogenous beahvior. Children are influenced by their familial and social contexts, which led to a separate dimension that takes into account the pressure to conform to expectations for their assigned gender.

4.4   Dimensions 4 & 5: Gender Compatibility and Outgroup Favoritism

Egan and Perry argue that children experience a felt sense of compatibility or lack of compatibility with their gender group after establishing membership knowledge (Dimension 1). This can be described as an experience of belonging to their gender, which some children experience in the negative sense of dissatisfaction or lack of belonging. They draw on social psychologists' work on group membership to argue that a sense of belonging to a gender typically fosters a sense of superiority, favoritism, or preference for that group (e.g., Tajfel & Turner 1979). These behaviors are typically observed in children's same-gender play and favorable descriptions of their own gender group, and are argued to be a dimension of gender identity at least during childhood.

Broadly, Egan and Perry's model made the contribution that children's gender identity is constructed over time through a multifaceted evaluation of how they are perceived by others, but also how it feels to be their gender and not another gender. Using these five dimensions as sources from which to make an inference, children arrive at their gender identity. According to this model, a child who has a solidified sense of their cisgender identity would (1) know that they are perceived as a boy, (2) behave in ways that are culturally expected for boys, (3) feel pressure to conform to gender expectations for boys, (4) feel compatible with the male gender group, and (5) experience a sense of favoritism towards boys as opposed to girls or another gender. This model leaves some limited room for gender variant identities, such as a child who has knowledge of the gender they are perceived to be but feels belonging, contentment, and a sense of gender group superiority when engaging in activities and traits associated with another gender, like Rey in our case study example at the end of this chapter. However, as Tate and others will argue, Egan and Perry's model can be expanded to fully encapsulate and normalize transgender and gender variant experiences.

5   The Gender Bundle: Tate and Colleagues

Social and personality psychologists have called for an updated understanding of gender identity that can integrate the experiences of trans and gender non-conforming people. Egan and Perry's model is concerned primarily with the child's developing understanding of gender *after* identification has taken place, particularly their felt compatibility with the gender assignment given to them by others. This assumes that the child will internalize the label put forward by adults, which we discuss in earlier sections as a teleological approach (assumes a "grand design") that does not capture a large portion of children. For example, some transgender girls "may have never experienced their self-categorization as male—even when treated in a social manner based on this category by family and close others" (Tate et al., 2014, p. 307). If a child does not identify with the gender label that others ascribe to them, the rest of the model, which focuses on compatibility with this label, becomes difficult to apply. In fact, some children identify with being both male and female, and sometimes neither. Some estimates suggest that 1.3% of youth identify as transgender by the time they reach middle school (Shields et al., 2013), and this number is thought to increase to about 2.4% by adulthood (Tate et al., 2013). These individuals' experiences can guide psychologists to new understandings of gender, as Tate suggests by noting that "genderqueer/non-binary experiences invite theorists and researchers to consider the possibility that gender self categorization is a process of identifying to some degree with all available gender categories within one's culture" (Tate et al., 2014, p. 309).

Acknowledging ways in which the field was limited in its ability to describe identities on the transgender spectrum, Tate et al. (2014) developed the gender bundle (Fig. 3). This approach considers the components of gender to be a bundle, much like "separate objects that are bundled together in one package" (p. 304). By viewing it's components separately and not as interrelated dimensions, it becomes more possible to integrate the experiences of all children–transgender, gendernon-confirming, and cisgender–under it's umbrella. Importantly, Tate and colleagues intentionally do not comment on how the components of the bundle are interrelated or distinguishable from one another, as the purpose of the model is descriptive rather than predictive. It is not intended to infer one aspect of gender by simply knowing another. Gender is exceedingly complex, and this model allows for that complexity.

5.1 Gender Bundle: Facets A & B

Egan and Perry (2001) use the term "membership knowledge" to label the process of one's self-categorization into a gender group. Tate and colleagues separate this category into the membership group that one is assigned at birth (Facet A) and an

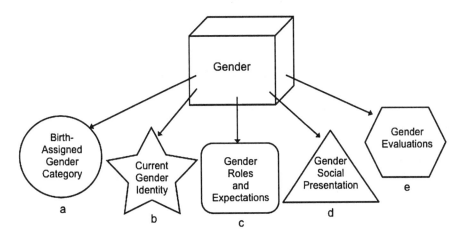

Fig. 3 The gender bundle. Tate et al. (2014)

individual's current self-identified gender label (Facet B). This broadens the reach of the concept of group "membership," explicitly acknowledging that membership can be experienced differently from an internal and external perspective. For example, although Rey (the person described in our case study) has a clear knowledge of being labeled male at birth, they understand that they internally are "just not a boy." By emphasizing Facet B as "current" gender identity, the gender bundle approach is able to consider that gender is not bound by age–it can change and sometimes does. Differentiating between sex assignment and current gender identity eliminates the need to focus so much on "awareness" of one's assigned gender category, a component that is better suited in understanding gender in children rather than adults.

5.2   Gender Bundle: Facets C, D, & E

The last components of the model require the individual to know Facets A (*Birth-Assigned Gender Category*) and B (*Current Gender Identity)* so that they might have reference points of their gender "ingroups" and "outgroups." Using the descriptions of Dimensions 2–5 in Egan and Perry's model, Facets C, D, and E (*Gender Roles and Expectations, Gender Social Presentation*, and *Gender Evaluations,* respectively) are largely self-explanatory and primarily concern how a person experiences gender in the social world and how their own gender is evaluated by others. Facet D, the social presentation of gender, is particularly new to gender identity models in psychology. This facet acknowledges that despite how an individual may vary on Facets A, B, C, and E, their presentation of gender to the world can be similar or altogether different from how others (or even themselves) understand their gender. For example, a transgender woman who is not "out" to her community may have a social presentation as a man despite an internal knowledge that she is a woman. These complexities were previously uncaptured by Egan and Perry's (2001) multidimensional model. Tate and colleagues' approach serves psychologists greatly in showing all possible combinations and idiosyncrasies within the gender bundle to be valid and within the range of healthy development.

6   Indigenous, Historical, & Cross-Cultural Perspectives

Scholars from indigenous and non-Western cultures have commented on how dominant theories do not capture how gender is and can be experienced within their societies. Indigenous peoples are those who, among other factors identified by Corntassel (2003), "are ancestrally related and identify themselves, based on oral/written histories, as the descendants of the original ancestral homelands" (p. 92). While writing this chapter, we found that there were few primary resources about gender development from indigenous communities themselves, but we rely on the voices of these scholars when it is possible. As a White and Black scholar describing these traditions, we recognize that we are not adequate narrators about indigenous and cross cultural experiences. We direct readers to Driskill et al. (2011), Mirandé (2017), Tikuna and Picq (2016), for some exceptional research that speaks about indigenous and cross cultural gender minorities from scholars who are part of or deeply embedded in these communities).

Cultures with third gender practices have received much focus from gender scholars, so much so that their existence has been exoticized and "othered" in order to teach about gender diversity (Dozono, 2017). Our point here is not to do that, but rather to highlight the ways that gender is embedded in social life beyond self-identification and outward expression in ways that even the gender bundle model does not capture. In their ethnographic work with the *Muxes* of Juchitán, a third gender group in Oaxaca, Mexico, Mirandé (2017) describes the ways that gender identity can be experienced as a way of retaining cultural practices and traditions. Muxes are "biological males who also manifest feminine identities in their dress and attire, but they are not transsexual nor are they seeking to become women" (385). The muxes embody qualities that Western cultures associate with both men and women, and their gender is described not as between the gender binary but rather beyond it altogether. The notion of a gender identity that goes beyond the concept of gender itself is similar to the *hijra* third gender group of India (see Reddy, 2005). Many other indigenous cultures have non-binary gender systems, including the Two Spirit gender identity within many Native American cultures, the Metis of Nepal, and the Mashoga of Kenya (Driskill et al., 2011). These individuals and their communities cannot be understood with the blunt theoretical tool of a teleological perspective; their identities transcend what dominant models have described. Importantly, the communities described here show that gender cannot be easily encapsulated into clean components and reveal the many ways that gender development is articulated by the cultures in which children are reared. Importantly, indigenous gender systems show that the lines between gender and other social structures, such as religion and cultural traditions, can be complex and multilayered.

Historical perspectives challenge the concept of gender permanence, one of the most dominant gender identity concepts in psychology. In Albania, *burrnesha* or "sworn virgins," take on a vow of chastity and embody the social role of men in situations of economic hardship when males are absent from families. For *burrneshas*, the transition to manhood is motivated less by an internal desire to live as a man and more by economic necessity in a highly patriarchal system. Something similar, although motivated by different reasons, is seen in Iran where gender reassignment surgeries are sometimes performed as an alternative to homosexuality. Some experts suggest that over 150,000 transgender individuals live in Iran, and that many of these transitions take place in order for gay individuals to engage in relationships that can be socially deemed as heterosexual (Drescher, 2007). These practices reflect that gender can transform in response to certain cultural and economic contexts, especially those that are oppressive (Young, 2000). This shows the gender bundle model in action, particularly Facet D (the social presentation of one's gender identity) as a component of gender that can change as a response to one's context. The multidimensional model of gender identity development from Egan and Perry

(2001) is limited in this aspect, as these practices challenge the concept of reaching a fixed sense of "membership knowledge" and "compatibility" with binary gender groups.

Psychological theories about gender, such as those reviewed in the beginning of this chapter, are meant to capture what they propose as universal human processes. The universality of these theories is exposed as troublesome when set against the information that gender development can and does occur in incredibly diverse ways across human cultures. However, models like the gender bundle may be a step in a direction to more fully capture the many facets of gender and how they are contextually and culturally bound. When indigenous and cross-cultural perspectives are incorporated into the cannon of gender identity theory, psychologists using mainstream frameworks might begin to interrogate "how exotic, strange, limited, and narrow our dominant categories of gender are" (Dozono, 2017, p. 430).

7 Measuring Gender Identity

In the past, psychologists' measurement relied more on a schema of gendered traits and ideologies (i.e., trait theories) than on the individual's self-identification (for a review, see Forbes, 2017). However, gender ideologies continue to shift throughout time. These shifts affect the construct validity of trait and ideology measures, requiring social scientists to reevaluate how gender identity should be measured. There are some differences in how gender identity was originally measured, and how psychologists, sociologists, and other research and advocacy groups have revised the definitions and measurement of gender identity (Fig. 4).

7.1 Measuring Gender Identity in the Past: A Brief Review

The change in measurement of gender identity has happened incrementally over the course of numerous research endeavors and survey projects. The early research on gender measured the presence of certain "traits," or personality characteristics, that were deemed feminine or masculine (which we discuss conceptually under our section titled "History of Gender Identity in Social Science").

One of the most well-known measures is the Bem Sex Role Inventory (BSRI). Developed by Sandra Bem (Bem 1974), the BSRI provides a list of traits thought to be, at that time, associated with women (feminine) or associated with men (masculine). Feminine traits were characteristics like "warm," "affectionate," "loyal," and "likes children," and some of the masculine traits were "forceful," "analytical," "leadership ability," and "self-sufficient." The BSRI is a self-report measure on a likert-type scale for each of the gendered or androgynous traits. Bem's goal was to demonstrate that gendered traits exist on more than just a binary plane. Specifically, the participant's score on the measure would result in one of four labels that were

Fig. 4 A model's artistic interpretations of the complexities of gender binaries. Photo Courtesy of Dean Shim

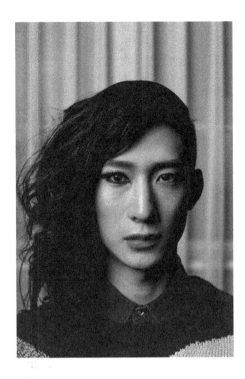

not tied to the sex that the individual was assigned at birth: masculine, feminine, androgynous, and undifferentiated personalities.

Boldizar (1991) created the Child Sex Role Inventory (CSRI), a measure that was intended to be "conceptually equivalent" to the Bem Sex Role Inventory. Instead of offering a selection of traits associated with gender identity in adults, the CSRI used words or phrases that are more relevant to children. On the CSRI, children reported their level of identification with characteristics articulating their self-worth, athletic competence, cognitive performance, and toy or activity preferences. Subsequent studies have used the CSRI for investigating the relationship between gender-role identity (i.e., level of masculinity and femininity) with brain volume (Priess et al., 2009), mental health (Belfi et al., 2014), self-esteem (Indhumathi, 2019), and career aspirations (Indhumathi, 2019). Other commonly used trait based measures developed during the seventies and eighties include the Personal Attributes Questionnaire (PAQ) (Spence et al., 1975) and Children's Personal Attributes Questionnaire (CPAQ) (Hall & Halberstadt, 1980).

Another method of measuring gender identity has been through a respondent's endorsement of sets of traditional "ideals" for cisgender men and women. The Adolescent Masculinity in Relationships Scale (AMRIS) (Chu et al., 2005), along with the Male Role Norms Scale (MRNS) (Thompson Jr. & Pleck, 1986), and the Male Role Attitudes Scale (MRAS) (Pleck et al., 1993) require participants to identify with descriptive phrases and traditional stereotypes about how boys or men should behave interpersonally, including a focus on agency and assertiveness.

Likewise, the Adolescent Femininity Ideology Scale (AFIS) (Tolman & Porche, 2000), the Conformity to Feminine Norms Inventory (CFNI) (Mahalik et al. 2005), and the Feminine Ideology Scale (FIS) (Levant et al., 2007) measure the extent to which one endorses traditional stereotypes about how girls or women should behave, with an emphasis on physical attractiveness and emotionality. Measuring gender identity in this way would be in line with a trait based perspective, which we describe as problematic and outdated in the above sections. Such measures are better described as estimates of gender ideology.

7.2 Changes in Gender Identity Measurement

Gender identity measurement research has evolved over time. The trait based measures use gendered stereotypes that are outdated and, in some cases, negative. Due to an increasing endorsement of egalitarian gender ideologies among the public and academics, researchers have begun to think of new ways to measure one's identification with gender norms. Another shift in American culture that has promoted changes in how gender identity is discussed and measured is the increase of research on gender nonconformity, and on people who have non-cisgender or non-binary gender identities. Additionally, the diversity of gendered behavior for people who have same-sex romantic relationships has led researchers to reduce reliance on cisgender, heterosexualist gender norms with regard to gender identity measurement. Taken together, these cultural acknowledgments and increased cultural competency regarding gender identity have perpetuated the transition from binary classifications to spectrum-oriented measures.

The process of creating a questionnaire that measures all gender identities requires a multifaceted approach. The Williams Institute (The GenIUSS Group, 2013) recommends that researchers use at least a two-step method when measuring gender identity. Research questionnaires must include an item regarding an individual's current gender identity (i.e., male, non-binary, transgender female, etc.). Additionally, for the purposes of context, the questionnaires should also include an item about the respondent's birth-assigned sex (i.e., female, male, intersex). Researchers' understanding of the experience of people's gender identity is incomplete without information regarding one's socially-perceived, or socially-assigned gender identity; that is, the gender that others evaluate them to be. This is especially relevant for research purposed with furthering the understanding of the experience of people who identify as transgender or gender nonconforming (TGNC). Thus, gender identity measures should include items that inform researchers about non-binary gender identities.

Wylie et al. (2010) used a multi-step approach to measure gender identity and nonconformity. This approach included the two steps recommended by the Williams Institute, along with two other items to measure gender presentation. One item read: "A person's appearance, style, or dress may affect the way people think of them. On average, how do you think people would describe your appearance, style, or dress?"

Another item read: "A person's mannerisms (such as the way they walk or talk) may affect the way people think of them. On average, how do you think people would describe your mannerisms?" Participants were given the following seven options: "very feminine," "mostly feminine," "somewhat feminine," "equally masculine and feminine," "somewhat masculine," "mostly masculine," and "very masculine". One disadvantage of gender identity measures that use masculinity and gender nonconformity is that they do not account for the extent to which a person who identifies as transgender might appear gender conforming according to their gender identity.

8 Towards a Non-Pathological Model of Gender Identity

Those wishing to understand their gender identity or cope with stigmatization, particularly within cultures and contexts that do not outwardly accept gender variance, may seek the help of a psychologist or medical doctor. These professionals play a critical role in supporting the health and wellness of those on the transgender or genderqueer spectrum (Drescher, 2010). Thus, it is important that professional doctrine and training matches the needs of gender variant individuals. Historically, however, the psychological and medical establishment have been hostile, and often harmful, to gender variant people. Dominant theories of gender development sometimes consider gender identities beyond man and woman, but typically view transgender and gender-nonconforming individuals as pathological or mentally disordered. The American Psychological Association has revamped its official stance on gender variance and has identified several areas for improvement in terms of specialized training guidelines for community health experts (APA, 2015). Still, transgender actvists argue that the field is far from reaching an intersectional, nonpathologized understanding of how to care for individuals outside of the gender binary.

A pathological focus on gender variance was prevalent within the American Psychological Association's Diagnostic Statistical Manual (DSM) until 2013 and in the International Classification of Diseases (ICD) until 2015 (See Fig. 5) (Drescher, 2013). Categorizing non-binary gender identities as mental disorders appeared in the DSM formally in 1980 under two separate "Gender Identity Disorder in Childhood" (GIDC) and "Transsexualism" (intended for adolescents and adults). These two definitions were later revised to include "Non-Transsexual Type Gender Dysphoria in Adolescents [Adults]" (designated by "by life stage" in the figure), and then were re-revised to collapse these definitions together in a catch-all diagnosis of "Gender Identity Disorder" or GID, with specifications for the diagnosis in children and adults (Drescher, 2013).

Remnants of a pathological focus are present, but fading, within psychiatry and clinical psychology. Today, the most recent edition of the DSM uses the Gender Dysphoria diagnosis to refer to those who experience distress as a result of a felt incongruence between their sexed anatomy and gender identity (APA, 2013). The inclusion of this condition is debated—however, some argue that its existence can help people receive treatment and care in situations of distress, or possibly help transgender children receive gender affirming treatment earlier (Scharrón-del Río et al., 2014). Access to affirming interventions/therapies is critical to people who are experiencing stress in a non-affirming society (e.g., Olson et al., 2016; Singh, 2016; Scharrón-del Río et al., 2014).

While the APA and medical professionals have sought to abandon classifications defined by pathology, most health insurance institutions, including Medicare and Medicaid, require that these standard gender affirming therapies are deemed "medically necessary" (Mallory & Tentindo, 2019). These therapeutic interventions, including hormone therapy, are prohibitively expensive without sufficient health insurance coverage. Even people with federal and state-sponsored health insurance plans (Medicaid and Medicare) have difficulty accessing care depending on the regulations governing the rights of people who identify as transgender in their home states. For these individuals, as with others, obtaining their gender affirming therapies depends heavily on the therapies being deemed medically necessary, a fraught threshold that can preclude TGNC people from receiving care.

Despite lack of agreement about the status and persistence of Gender Dysphoria, the American Psychological Association is beginning to more intentionally address the concerns of the TGNC community. The APA's task force on Gender Identity and Gender Variance has identified major areas for improving their professional training and guidelines for community health providers and experts (APA, 2015). The task force's first goal is to educate all psychologists on gender as a non-binary construct that exists independently from sex assigned at birth, and other goals within the report address the various biases that providers commonly hold against TGNC individuals. This education is intended to have a strong emphasis on socioeconomic status and race, which greatly inform the lived experience of discrimination, stigmatization, and violence towards transgeder people. A full summary of the training components can be found in the report.

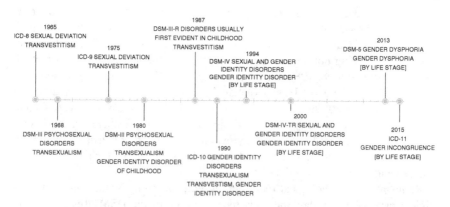

Fig. 5 Historical timeline of transgender identity in the Diagnostic Statistical Manual (DSM) & International Classification of Diseases (ICD)

9 Case Study

The subject of our case study is Rey–a 30-year-old African American living in Los Angeles. Because of disabilities, Rey has never been employed and relies on government aid. Rey currently identifies as gender non-binary and was assigned male sex at birth. Rey prefers the pronouns "they," "their," and "them." Rey's gender identity categorization has varied on a spectrum between male and non-binary/gender fluid throughout their life. To Rey, it does not make sense to define their gender identity. Rey feels freer without labels and the constraints that come with connotations and schemas of gendered behavior. Rey recognized early in life that they did not identify with, nor were they fond of engaging with the social norms associated with their birth-assigned gender. When asked about Rey's gender identity, Rey emphasized that their conception of their gender identity is filtered first through the lens of race and racism.

10 Rey in Early Childhood

Rey was raised as male with two cisgender parents who identified as a woman and man, respectively. He also had a twin brother and a cisgender older sister. Their household was moderately religious and middle-class. They went to church as a family almost every Sunday. The family was not fully dependent upon public assistance but received food stamps when Rey was a child. Though Rey's mother was a feminist, gender nonconformity by Rey or Rey's brother was discouraged. However, when Rey was a toddler and preschooler, Rey and their brother would take their older sister's toys—specifically dolls—and play contently with them. They were more interested in dolls than in any of their other toys. Their mother got them their own Cabbage Patch Kids and Barbie dolls for Christmas when Rey was five. She was reluctant to violate that norm at the time but she told their sister that it was to help them "get it out of their system." Rey remembers that their mother also painted Rey's brother's toenails after repeated requests. Rey's memories regarding gender as a young child were such that Rey did not glean joy from the activities that boys were "supposed to do." Rey was aware that they were physically a boy at that time. But, not wanting to engage in boys' activities, as was expected by Rey's extended family and broader community, felt odd and disjointed to Rey, even in early childhood.

11   Rey in Middle Childhood

When Rey was in elementary school, their mother encouraged them to play basketball. Rey says that this period of time stuck out to them because they had a strong
feeling that they did not want to participate, for two reasons. First, Rey was not very
good at it, and second, Rey "did not want to hang out with a bunch of dudes." At the
time, Rey did not understand why, but they knew that they did not have the same
motivation as Rey's teammates, nor did Rey feel like part of that team or the culture
of that community. Rey felt out of place, confused, and frustrated that they were
required to participate. It was at that time that Rey became exposed to traditional
male gender norms of showing physical strength, aggression, and competition.
Simultaneously, Rey noticed that their family and community expected Rey to conform, happily and naturally, to those norms.

One part of Rey's identity that did feel true and natural at that time was their
identity as a Black person. At that age, Rey lived in Black neighborhoods, went to
an African Methodist Episcopal Church, and went to predominantly Black schools.
The music their family listened to, the food they ate, the shows they watched, and
the jokes they made appealed to Rey, bringing an unconscious sense of belonging.
At the same time, homophobia, heterosexism, distaste for gender nonconformity
was commonplace in their Black community. Even though Rey was young, there
seemed to be a lot of things Rey liked doing that "might be okay for those white
people, but Black boys just can't be doing stuff like that."

The difference between girls' play and boys' play was starker in elementary
school than it was when Rey was a preschooler or toddler. Rey did not like boys'
play, interests, or attitudes. It was not just about lacking an interest in sports: to Rey,
masculine clothes were ugly, and the thought of engaging in competitive physical
activity was unappealing. Rey embraced glamour and was interested in design and
fashion but "did not identify with being a girl; just not a boy." Still, Rey regrets that
they did not advocate for engaging in their traditionally feminine interests as a child
and wonders if the social anxiety and self-doubt Rey often experiences as an adult
would be better if they had been more validating and expressive with their true self.

Rey talked of the time when Rey "accidentally came out" to their mother. They
were in the car, looking through a clothing catalog when Rey thought to themselves,
aloud, "Oh, he's cute!" Rey got a look from their mother in the rearview mirror and
immediately regretted momentarily forgetting to manage their growing romantic
interest in, and attraction to, boys.

12   Rey in Late Adolescence

High school was a remarkable time of identity formation for Rey. During high
school, Rey's gender, racial, and sexual orientation identities became clearer. Rey
remembers being generally unhappy in high school. Their parents divorced when

Rey was in elementary school and, at the time of high school, lived in two different states hundreds of miles away from each other. Rey attended high school in the two states and hated both. For a period of time, Rey and their brother lived with their father in the northeast, the predominantly Black community that Rey grew up in. For another period of time, Rey and their brother lived with their mother in the South. They lived in a county that was upper-middle class, predominantly white, and, even in the mid-2000's, riddled with racism.

In the predominantly Black high school, Rey and Rey's brother were not two of the "cool kids." The community in general was very materialistic and having the latest sneakers or wearing expensive clothing brands was the primary form of achieving high status for adolescents. Rey's father could not afford to buy them the latest sneakers, nor did they have expensive clothing. To Rey, their clothes were disappointing, non-affirming, and "hideous." Their father only bought them traditionally masculine clothes which came from a bargain store which lacked creativity and glamour, from Rey's perspective. Additionally, there might have been a few openly nonconforming male students but otherwise, most of the students were supremely homophobic. In animosity, the male students called each other slurs like "faggot" and "pussy," deriding any deviations from aggressive masculinity. Similar to Rey's experience of being on the basketball team, Rey remembers disconnecting from all aspects of that high school culture and sometimes missed class to avoid judgment or bullying from their fellow students.

Rey says that they were relieved to leave that school when they went to go live with their mother in the South. Unfortunately, that relief was short-lived. Rey says that the homophobia and aggressive anti-gay behaviors were not as blatant at the new school. However, subtle racism and racial microaggressions were unavoidable. Out of 150 students, there were only four African Americans at Rey's new high school. Rey says that the racism was not explicit, it was more about exclusivity, devaluing the experience of African Americans and prioritizing the world of whiteness. Again, Rey felt so disconnected from the students that they did not engage or participate in school. Rey remembers their romantic attraction to boys being more prominent at the new high school. Rey found other boys who were attracted to them and those were the first validating experiences Rey had that were related to sexual orientation. In elementary school and throughout high school, Rey identified as a boy. Eventually, in high school and shortly after, Rey identified as a "gay boy." Rey emphasizes, however, that they were "way more focused on being a Black kid in a white school than on being gay."

13   Rey in Early-Adulthood

Rey spent their late-teens and early-20s identifying as a gay man living in Los Angeles. Rey used mobile phone apps like Grindr and Adam for Adam—apps known in the gay community for meeting other gay men and prompting sexual relationships. Rey says that Rey learned a lot about Rey's identity according to their experiences on those social networking "hookup" apps. Primarily, Rey observed rampant racism on the dating apps for gay men (See Hutson et al., 2018). Often, users are sorting by race, eliminating people of color from their search results and feeds, to communicate only with white users. Additionally, in many white and non-white users' profiles, they include comments like "No Blacks," or "No Asians." When Rey would attempt to contact some of these users they would "auto-block" Rey after Rey said "hello." Or, they would ignore several of Rey's messages until Rey wrote, "Just say you're not into Black guys." Rey said that the user would then respond with long paragraphs explaining how they are not racist. To Rey, it felt very racist.

The process of engaging in social contact validating one aspect of Rey's identity was interrupted and ruined with the reminder of how they were devalued because they are African American. Rey became resentful of the apps and of the racist behaviors and microaggressions that seemed so common among its users. Over time, Rey drifted away from identifying as a gay man, as that did not quite fit Rey's understanding of themself. One thing that Rey was able to benefit from on the apps was meeting and interacting with people of non-binary or transgender gender identities. Rey says that they used to think that non-cisgender people were "weird." Rey emphasizes that the dislike for those identities at that time was not rooted in any self-hate or denial of Rey's own non-binary gender identity. Rey believes that they were ignorant of the concept of a non-binary gender identity and the "rules" that did or did not come with that identity. Rey would read profiles for non-binary users and identify with their philosophies or approaches to life and dating.

After spending years of identifying as a gay man, Rey began to think about themselves as a pansexual, gender non-binary person. Rey slowly allowed themselves to imagine the feeling of wearing high-heeled shoes, beautiful dresses, and having long, flowing hair. Rey said that so much more of their life made sense after finding the "non-binary" and spectrum-oriented concept for their persistent gender identity and removing the idea that they were "sick" for wanting to live that life.

Rey continues to identify as non-binary and does not label their sexual orientation. Rey is often perceived as a cisgender male in their clothing and personal grooming, but they have confided in some of their closest family members that they want to be glamorous in feminine fashion and wear makeup. Rey clarifies that they do not want to live as a woman and does not identify as transgender. However, Rey wishes that they had disposable income to spend on glamorous, inspired clothing and shoes. Rey believes that if they had more money, their wardrobe would have a wide selection of clothing that is traditionally associated with women. Rey remarks that validating that aspect of their identity would involve money for laser hair removal, hair weaves or wigs, men's-sized high-heeled shoes, different types of feminine attire. Rey also says that it would take courage to "put myself out there like that" and dreams about exploring that part of their identity as they get older.

14 Conclusion

In the beginning of this chapter, we asked readers to consider Dozono's perspective of arriving in a place of thinking about gender as "how strange and particular one's own contexts and assumptions are, amidst a vast array of interpretations of reality" (2017, p. 426). We hope it is clear from this reading that there are a vast number of interpretations of gender that are wholly valid and healthy–to think of one or another experience of gender as "correct" is to ignore the expansive diversity of how human life can be lived and *is already lived* in many cultures. The consequences of ignoring these realities have violent repercutions for transgender and gender non-conforming people. The field's gradual transition to incorporating the experiences of those who live outside of and beyond the gender binary is a step in the right direction. However, as readers will note, the disruption of dominant theories and the proliferation of more expansive gender theories leaves many questions open for empirical debate. For example, we know little about how the psychological experience of gender is instantiated in the brain or the exact mechanisms through which gender identity becomes established in the human psyche. Although we understand that culture informs how people arrive at their own gender labels, the biological, environmental, and epigenetic reasons why certain individuals and not others resist their socialization is a nascent field.

The evidence presented in this chapter documents the slow changing tide of how gender is understood by social scientists. We emphasize how the field has grown primarily through the work of queer scholars of color who point out that gender identity develops over time within a social context, particularly the culturally specific ideologies and hierarchies in which people live. As awareness of gender variance grows in the social sciences, we hope to see the field grow in rigor and breadth by doing away with theories that reflect only a tightly circumscribed range of possibilities of what gender can be. Integrating the perspectives of queer, trans, and non-genderconforming people of color into the canon of gender identity theory will be central to this pursuit.

References

American Psychiatric Association. (2013). *Diagnostic and statistical manual of mental disorders (DSM–5)*. Washington, DC: American Psychiatric Publishing.
American Psychological Association. (2015). *Guidelines for psychological practice with transgender and gender nonconforming people*. Washington, DC: APA.
Bem, S. L. (1974). The measurement of psychological androgyny. *Journal of Consulting and Clinical Psychology, 42*, 155–162.
Bem, S. L. (1981). Gender schema theory: A cognitive account of sex typing. *Psychological Review, 88*, 354–364.
Best, D. L., & Puzio, A. (2019). Gender and culture. In D. Matsumoto (Ed.), *The Oxford handbook of culture and psychology* (pp. 235–291). New York: NY: Oxford University Press.
Boldizar, J. P. (1991). Assessing sex typing and androgyny in children: The Children's Sex Role Inventory. *Developmental Psychology, 27*, 505–515.

Bowers, M. M., & Whitley, C. T. (2020). What drives support for transgender rights? Assessing the effects of biological attribution on US public opinion of transgender rights. *Sex Roles*, 1–13.

Brown, C., Biefeld, S., & Tam, M. (2020). *Gender in childhood*. Cambridge, UK: Cambridge University Press.

Chu, J. Y., Porche, M. V., & Tolman, D. L. (2005). The adolescent masculinity ideology in relationships scale: Development and validation of a new measure for boys. *Men and Masculinities, 8*, 93–115.

Corntassel, J. (2003). Who is indigenous? 'Peoplehood' and ethnonationalist approaches to rearticulating indigenous identity. *Nationalism and Ethnic Politics, 9*(1), 75–100.

Dozono, T. (2017). Teaching alternative and indegenous gender systems in world history: A queer approach. *The History Teacher, 50*(3), 425–447.

Drescher, J. (2007). From bisexuality to intersexuality: Rethinking gender categories. *Contemporary Psychoanalysis, 43*, 204–228.

Drescher, J. (2010). Queer diagnoses: Parallels and contrasts in the history of homosexuality, gender variance, and the Diagnostic and Statistical Manual. *Archives of Sexual Behavior, 38*, 427–460.

Drescher, J. (2013). Gender identity diagnoses: History and controversies. In B. P. C. Kreukels, T. D. Steensma, & A. L. C. deVries (Eds.), *Gender dysphoria and disorders of sex development, progress in care and knowledge* (pp. 137–150). New York, NY: Springer.

Driskill, Q. L., Finley, C., Gilley, B. J., & Morgensen, S. L. (2011). Introduction. In Q. L. Driskill, C. Finley, B. J. Gilley, & S. L. Morgensen (Eds.), *Queer indigenous studies: Critical interventions in theory, politics, and literature*. Tucson, AZ: University of Arizona Press.

Egan, S. K., & Perry, D. G. (2001). Gender identity: A multidimensional analysis with implications for psychosocial adjustment. *Developmental Psychology, 37*, 451–463.

Eagly, A. H., Beall, A. L., & Sternberg, R. J. (2004). *The psychology of gender* (2nd ed.). New York, NY: Guilford Press.

Forbes, A. (2017). Measuring gender identity. In K. Nadal (Ed.), *The SAGE encyclopedia of psychology and gender* (pp. 1133–1136). Thousand Oaks, CA: SAGE Publications, Inc.

Freud, S. (1905). *Three essays on the theory of sexuality* (p. 2000). New York: Basic Books.

Freud, S. (1925). *Some psychical consequences of the anatomical distinction between the sexes. Standard Edition, 18* (pp. 145–172). London: Hogarth Press, 1955.

Garfinkel, H. (1967). *Studies in ethnomethodology*. Englewood Cliffs, NJ: Prentice-Hall.

Gower, A. L., Rider, N., Coleman, E., Brown, C., McMorris, B. J., & Eisenberg, M. E. (2018). Perceived gender presentation among transgender and gender diverse youth: Approaches to analysis and associations with bully victimization and emotional distress. *LGBT Health, 5*, 312–319.

Grant, J. M., Mottet, L. A., Tanis, J., Harrison, J., Herman, J. L., & Keisling, M. (2011). *Injustice at every turn: A report of the national transgender discrimination survey*. Washington, DC: National Center for Transgender Equality and National Gay and Lesbian Task Force.

Hall, J. A., & Halberstadt, A. G. (1980). Masculinity and femininity in children: Development of the children's personal attributes questionnaire. *Developmental Psychology, 16*(4), 270–280.

Harrison, J., Grant, J., & Herman, J. L. (2012). A gender not listed here: Genderqueers, gender rebels, and otherwise in the National Transgender Discrimination Survey. *LGBTQ Public Policy Journal, 2*(1), 13–24.

Hutson, J., Taft, J. G., Barocas, S., & Levy, K. (2018). Debiasing desire: Addressing bias & discrimination on intimate platforms. *Proceedings on the Association for Computer Machinery (ACM) Human-Computer Interaction, 2*(Article 73), 1–18. https://doi.org/10.1145/3274342.

Indhumathi, R. (2019). The influence of sex role perception on career aspirations and self-esteem in children with a preference for Disney movies. *The International Journal of Indian Psychology, 7*, 183–195. https://doi.org/10.25215/0701.020.

Kohlberg, L. (1966). A cognitive-developmental analysis of children's sex-role concepts and attitudes. In E. E. Maccoby (Ed.), *The development of sex differences* (pp. 82–173). Stanford, CA: Stanford University Press.

Levant, R., Richmond, K., Cook, S., House, A. T., & Aupont, M. (2007). The femininity ideology scale: Factor structure, reliability, convergent and discriminant validity, and social contextual variation. *Sex Roles, 57*, 373–383.

Mahalik, J. R., Morray, E. B., Coonerty-Femiano, A., Ludlow, L. H., Slattery, S. M., & Smiler, A. (2005). Development of the conformity to feminine norms inventory. *Sex Roles, 52*, 417–433.

Mallory, C., & Tentindo, W. (2019). *Medicaid coverage for gender-affirming care*. Williams Institute (UCLA School of Law).

Mirandé, A. (2017). *Behind the mask: Gender hybridity in a Zapotec community*. Tucson, AZ: University of Arizona Press.

Mischel, W. (1966). A social learning view of sex differences in behavior. In E. Maccoby (Ed.), *The development of sex differences* (pp. 57–81). Stanford: Stanford University Press.

Olson, K. R., Durwood, L., DeMeules, M., & McLaughlin, K. A. (2016). Mental health of transgender children who are supported in their identities. *Pediatrics, 137*(3), 1–8.

Olson, K. R., & Gülgöz, S. (2018). Early findings from the transyouth project: Gender development in transgender children. *Child Development Perspectives, 12*(2), 93–97.

Pascoe, C. J., & Bridges, T. (2016). *Exploring masculinities: Identity, inequality, continuity and change*. New York: Oxford University Press.

Piaget, J. (1983). Piaget's theory. In P. H. Mussen (Series Ed.) & W. Kesson (Vol. Ed.), *Handbook of child psychology: History, theory, and methods* (4th ed., pp. 104–128). New York: Wiley.

Pleck, J. H., Sonenstein, F. L., & Ku, L. C. (1993). Masculine ideology: Its impact on adolescent males' heterosexual relationships. *Journal of Social Issues, 49*, 11–29.

Reddy, G. (2005). *With respect to sex: Negotiating Hijra identity in South India*. Chicago: University of Chicago Press.

Ruble, D. N., Taylor, L. J., Cyphers, L., Greulich, F. K., Lurye, L. E., & Shrout, P. E. (2007). The role of gender constancy in early gender development. *Child Development, 78*, 1121–1136.

Scharrón-del Río, M. R., Dragowski, E. A., & Phillips, J. J. (2014). Therapeutic work with gender variant children: What school psychologists need to know. *School Psychology Forum, 8*(1), 38–55.

Shields, J. P., Cohen, R., Glassman, J. R., Whitaker, K., Franks, H., & Bertolini, I. (2013). Estimating population size and demographic characteristics of lesbian, gay, bisexual, and transgender youth in middle school. *Journal of Adolescent Health, 52*(2), 248–250.

Singh, A. A. (2016). Moving from affirmation to liberation in psychological practice with transgender and gender nonconforming clients. *American Psychologist, 71*(8), 755–762.

Slaby, & Frey. (1975). Development of gender constancy and selective attention to same-sex models. *Child Development, 46*, 849–856.

Spence, J. T., Helmreich, R., & Stapp, J. (1975). Ratings of self and peers on sex role attributes and their relation to self-esteem and conceptions of masculinity and femininity. *Journal of Personality and Social Psychology, 32*(1), 29–39.

Stoller, R. J. (1968). *Sex and gender: Volume I the development of masculinity and femininity*. Palo Alto, CA: Stanford University Press.

Tajfel, H., & Turner, J. (1979). An integrative theory of intergroup conflict. In W. G. Austin & S. Worchel (Eds.), *The social psychology of intergroup relations* (pp. 33–47). Monterey, CA: Brooks/Cole.

Tate, C. C. (2014). Gender identity as a personality process. In B. Miller (Ed.), *Gender identity: Disorders, developmental perspectives and social implications* (pp. 1–22). Hauppauge, NY: Nova Science Publishers.

Tate, C. C., Ledbetter, J. N., & Youssef, C. P. (2013). A two-question method for assessing gender categories in the social and medical sciences. *Journal of Sex Research, 50*(8), 767–776.

Tate, C. C., Youssef, C. P., & Bettergarcia, J. N. (2014). Integrating the study of transgender spectrum and cisgender experiences of self-categorization from a personality perspective. *Review of General Psychology, 18*(4), 302–312.

The GenIUSS Group: The Williams Institute. (2013). *Gender-related measures overview.* University of California Los Angeles School of Law. Retrieved from https://williamsinstitute. law.ucla.edu/wp-content/uploads/Gender-Related-Measures-Overview-Feb-2013.pdf

Thompson, E. H., Jr., & Pleck, J. H. (1986). The structure of male role norms. *American Behavioral Scientist, 29,* 531–543.

Tikuna, J., & Picq, M. (2016). Queering Amazonia: Homo-affective relations among Tikuna society. In M. Aguirre, M. Garzon, M. A. Viteri, & M. L. Picq (Eds.), *Queering paradigms V: Queering narratives of modernity* (pp. 113–134). Peter Lang: Bern, Switzerland.

Tolman, D. L., & Porche, M. V. (2000). The adolescent femininity ideology scale: Development and validation of a new measure for girls. *Psychology of Women Quarterly, 24,* 365–376.

Wood, W., & Eagly, A. H. (2009). Gender. In S. T. Fiske, D. T. Gilbert, & G. Lindzey (Eds.), *Handbook of social psychology* (Vol. 1, 5th ed., pp. 629–667). Hoboken, NJ: Wiley.

Wylie, S. A., Corliss, H. L., Boulanger, V., Prokop, L. A., & Austin, S. B. (2010). Socially assigned gender nonconformity: A brief measure for use in surveillance and investigation of health disparities. *Sex Roles, 63,* 264–B1276.

Reclaiming All of Me:
The Racial Queer Identity Framework

Hector Y. Adames and Nayeli Y. Chavez-Dueñas

There is something powerful in the way we sustain and thrive in face of multiple forms of oppression ... this becomes part of who we are.

You are born, you develop, you are shaped, and in the process, you begin to understand who you are. The process of becoming and claiming all of who we are is one of the most central yet complex tasks of human development—it requires us to grapple with, explore, and make decisions that fundamentally impact our lives. To borrow from our mentor, Dr. Joseph L. White, understanding who you are involves answering challenging but crucial questions: Who do you say you are? Who is the you that others see? Who is the you that you allow others to see and why? Who is the you that nobody knows?

Social scientists have attempted to provide answers to these four critical questions through various theories of identity. In psychology, identity theories predominantly focus on describing and explaining how individuals make sense of who they are. One of the most influential psychology theorists, Erik Erikson, proposed a theory of identity that depicts how people define and integrate various aspects of the self (e.g., intrapersonal, social) while synthesizing biological, psychological, and societal demands (Erikson, 1980; Lerner, 2002). Although less prominent, Erikson's work also emphasized development in context, underscoring how people's identities are influenced by the broader structures in society where individuals are embedded (see Syed & Fish, 2018). Oppression, both past and present, shapes the identity of people who are members of various structurally minoritized groups (e.g., Black, Indigenous, women, queer). Thus, in psychology, personal identity refers to the adaptation of specific personal attitudes, feelings, characteristics, and behaviors about the self within a social context (Erikson, 1980; Lerner, 2002).

H. Y. Adames (*) · N. Y. Chavez-Dueñas
Department of Counseling Psychology, The Chicago School of Professional Psychology, Chicago, IL, USA
e-mail: hadames@thechicagoschool.edu; nchavez@thechicagoschool.edu

© The Author(s), under exclusive license to Springer Nature Switzerland AG 2021
K. L. Nadal and M. R. Scharrón-del Río (ed.), *Queer Psychology*,
https://doi.org/10.1007/978-3-030-74146-4_4

Similarly, social theory describes identity as the process of connecting with a larger group of people with similar values, characteristics, world views, beliefs, and practices (i.e., social identity theory). Expressed differently a focus on the collective, rather than the individual falls within the realm of sociology. From this perspective, social identity is shaped by how individuals connect, disconnect, identify, or not identify with various social group categories (e.g., race, ethnicity, gender, sexual orientation) in which society structurally places them (e.g., Asian, African American, Indigenous, lesbian, gay, bisexual, transgender). In other words, a person's ideologies, feelings, and behaviors are also shaped by their social group membership and the structural power that these groups have within a given society.

While psychological and sociological theories provide frameworks for us to understand identity, the emphasis on structural inequities and the complex relationship between privilege and oppression among minoritized people is seldom emphasized in identity models (Adames & Chavez-Dueñas, 2017). In response to this underdeveloped area in identity studies, this chapter introduces the *Racial Queer Identity Framework* (RQI) which explicitly focuses on how racism, heterosexism, and cissexism[1] overlap and interlock to uniquely impact identity development among Queer People of Color (QPOC). The framework is grounded on theories of intersectionality, racial identity development, and collective history of oppression and resistance.

1 Queerness, Race, and Gender: Language Is Limited and Bound by History

Communicating our subjectivities with others confronts us with both intra and interpersonal questions to consider. As curiosity about our experiences begins to surface, we become inquisitive about our existence, what we are feeling, and whether to share our subjectivities with others. We use language to make sense of our intrapersonal world. We also consider the possible interpersonal dynamics and outcomes when we share who we are with others. In many ways, language can liberate us and connect us to others, but it can also limit us since language is bound by politics, context, and epistemology (Adames & Chavez-Dueñas, 2017). For QPOC, the language we speak reminds us of the history of oppression, exploitation, and abuse that our communities have experienced. The words we use to describe ourselves and our subjectivities are often myopic and come from the people who enslaved, colonized, and exploited our Communities of Color. Words undoubtedly shape our collective and individual consciousness and ultimately how we answer the question of "Who do I say I am?"

---

[1] These three terms describe ideologies and systems of oppression that dehumanize, disparage, and stigmatize (a) Black, Indigenous, and People of Color (racism) and (b) any nonheterosexual (heterosexism) and cisnormative (cissexism) form of behavior, identity, relationship, or community.

1.1 Naming Myopic Language

Academic definitions of commonly used constructs such as gender, sex, and sexuality have often been described in simplistic and narrow ways. To illustrate, sex has been used to describe the "(a) chromosomal composition, (b) reproductive apparatus, (c) secondary characteristics that are usually associated with these chromosomal differences, (d) the intrapersonal characteristics presumed to be possessed by males and females, and (e) in the case of sex roles, any and all behaviors differentially expected for and appropriate to people on the basis of membership in these various sexual categories" (Unger, 1979, p. 1085–1086). From this perspective, the term sex is understood to be binary, which fails to capture human variations in sex differences including individuals who are intersex (e.g., 46 XX Intersex, 46 XY Intersex, True Gonadal Intersex, Complex or Undetermined Intersex). Moreover, studies focused on sex differences often resort to using surface and dichotomous interpretations about men and women based on biological differences without considering the role of history, culture, and context. Given these pitfalls, Unger (1979) proposed using the term *gender* to define the social construct used to describe the sets of behaviors, traits, and expectations that a given culture assigns as men or women. However, Unger's perspective was not well received by scholars in the late 1970s (see Maccoby, 1988). Instead, opponents to Unger's framing argued that there is no difference between the concepts of sex and gender since the biological and social aspects of these two constructs are not entirely exclusive (e.g., Maccoby, 1988). These early arguments continue to reverberate today. For instance, we can observe how media continues to use sex and gender interchangeably impacting how we think about these concepts. Nonetheless, similar to sex, gender was initially defined within a binary framework.

Psychology has adopted a definition of gender similar to Unger (1979). According to the American Psychological Association (APA) *Guidelines for Psychological Practice with Lesbian, Gay, and Bisexual Clients,* gender includes "the attitudes, feelings, and behaviors that a given culture associates with a person's biological sex" (APA, 2012, p. 11). From this lens, culture is understood to influence gender, including: (a) *gender norms* or the behaviors that are aligned with cultural expectations or (b) *gender nonconformity,* which underscores incongruence between cultural expectations and a person's gender. APA and Unger's definitions are complementary as they both conceptualize gender as a verb. Despite the importance of understanding gender from a behavioral lens, this perspective fails to explicitly capture people's subtle and subjective sense of what gender means to them. As a result, *gender identity* is used to connote an individual's internal sense of a gendered-self (e.g., man, woman, male, female, womxn, agender, gender non-conforming). APA (2015) describes gender identity as "a person's deeply felt, inherent sense of being a girl, woman, or female; a boy, a man, or male; a blend of male or female; or an alternative gender" (p. 834). For individuals whose gender identity is aligned with their sex assigned at birth, the term *cisgender* is used (APA, 2015; Tate et al., 2014). Lastly, the term *gender expression* describes the way society interprets how an individual conveys who they are through clothing, communication patterns (e.g., nonverbal communication, voice intonation), and other actions or interests. Hence, a person's gender expression may or may not be consistent with socially prescribed gender roles and may or may not reflect the person's gender and gender identity (APA, 2008, p. 28).

1.2   Interplay Between Sex, Gender, Gender Expression, and Sexual and Affectional Orientation

Sexuality is an influential and complex aspect of human development. Beyond the heteronormative realm of reproduction, sexuality also refers to how we see ourselves and relate to others. An important aspect of sexuality is sexual orientation, typically described by social scientists as "the sex of those to whom one is sexually and romantically attracted" (APA, 2012, p. 11). Several taxonomies are used to categorize people into different sexual orientations, including: gay and lesbian for individuals who are attracted to members of their same sex, heterosexual for individuals who are attracted to people of a different sex from their own, and bisexual for people attracted to both sexes (APA, 2012; Garnets & Kimmel, 2003). While these categories begin to provide language to describe the intricacies of sexual orientation, a categorical approach fails to capture how sexual orientation exists on a continuum (Kinsey et al., 1953) and may be fluid for some people, particularly individuals who identify as women (Diamond, 2007; Peplau & Garnets, 2000).

While there has been an increasing understanding and appreciation for sexual orientation existing on a continuum, most of the literature continues to be saturated with reductionistic concepts that fail to capture the diverse lived experience of people. For instance, sexual orientation is often discussed in relation to attraction (e.g., same sex attraction, same sex marriage) based on people's sex (see APA, 2012). Similarly, albeit less common, Shively and De Cecco (1977) defined sexual orientation as a person's sexual and/or emotional attraction to another person. Theoretically, Shively and De Cecco's definition allows space for gender also to be considered when discussing attraction instead of solely sex (see also Battle & Harris, 2013; Parks, 2001). More recently, the American Psychological Association Guidelines for Psychological Practice with Transgender and Gender Nonconforming People (2015) describes attraction in terms of gender (e.g., same gender loving relationships). Nonetheless, these notions of sexual orientation continue to be myopic. For instance, what exactly are we attracted to in others? Are we attracted to people's sex? Is it their gender? Gender expression? Is it the way that they talk, walk, dress, and communicate that romantically or emotionally draws us to others? Or can it be other aspects of the person's self that are appealing to us? Is attraction at first sight real?

1.3   **What's Neuroscience Got to Do With It?**

Using real-time, brain scans, neuroscience research provides insight that helps us theorize about the interplay between sex, gender, gender expression, and sexual orientation. For instance, a study by Contreras et al., (2013) revealed that the first characteristics that people process when meeting others include their physiognomy (e.g., skin color, facial features) and perceived sex (Contreras et al., 2013). They describe how the brain simultaneously processes people's physiognomy and perceived sex before the person adds meaning to what they are observing. Building on this line of empirical work, we argue that when an individual comes in contact with others, they classify the person into a specific sex and make generalizations about the person's gender. However, such classification may or may not align with the person's biological sex and/or how they identify their gender. Instead, we posit that what the brain is processing is a person's gender expression which we are socialized to interpret as a person's sex and gender identity, but this may or may not be accurate. Continuing with this thinking, we propose that people are attracted to people's gender expression, and not exclusively the person's sex or gender identity since these aspects of the self are not immediately evident to us when we encounter others. Regrettably, we are rarely encouraged to pause, think, and consider the interplay between sex, gender, gender expression, and sexual orientation—when we do, we may feel confused, conflicted, and at times scared given that we are born and socialized in a world that is structured and fueled by White, heterosexist, patriarchal, cissexist, and binary norms and values.

People who do not fit into the binary ways in which society is structured have always existed. For example, throughout history we have always had people (e.g., *muxe/muxhe, hijras, fa'afafine*[2]) who are intersex, transgender, gender expansive, or would otherwise not use binary pronouns (he, she). Unfortunately, the linguistic limitations of many languages prevent people from describing themselves in ways that accurately capture their internal experiences of sex and gender. However, not all languages are limiting. There are many languages throughout the world that are not gendered. For instance, many Latin American Indigenous languages allow for an expansive description and understanding of sex and gender (e.g., *Nahuatl*; see Bowles, 2019).

---

[2] *Muxe*, also spelled as *muxhe*, is a third gender or non-binary person among the Indigenous Zapotec Oaxacan People in Mexico (see Stephen 2002). Similarly, *hijras*, are non-binary people from India who have a recorded history of over 4000 years (see Kumar 2019). *Fa'afafine* are the third gender people from Samoa and the Samoan diaspora (see Schmidt 2010). For additional international queer perspectives and experiences see Nakamura, and Logie, C. H. (Eds.). (2020).

2 People of Color and Sexual and Affectional Orientation

Although research shows that people's brains simultaneously process the physiognomy and perceived sex of others, the literature often neglects the unique ways that sex, gender, and race overlap to create a unique gendered-sexuality experience that is simultaneously racialized. To illustrate, many of the concepts used to study sex, gender, gender identity, and gender expression do not consider race which may have different connotations for people depending on their racialized lives. For this reason, gender and sexual minoritized People of Color have created ways to better capture their racialized experiences. *Queerness* is one of the terms gaining popularity among many sexual minorities, given that the concept aims to capture all social parts of people, including their race and ethnicity.

2.1 Revisiting Queerness

Historically, the concept of queerness has been used as a pejorative term, with younger generations reclaiming queer as both a political stance and an umbrella term to describe sexual orientation and gender non-conforming folx. With regards to sexual orientation, queer is often used as a collective term by individuals who identify and/or are socially categorized as lesbian, gay, bisexual, gender expansive, and transgender (Mosley et al., 2019b; Newsweek Staff, 1991). Politically, queerness aims to disrupt binary thinking and socialization (e.g., men-women; gay-heterosexual; masculine-feminine) by centering and embracing the fluidity of gender, sexual orientation, behaviors, affection, and desires that come from such expansion. More recently, the concept of queerness has been embraced by many POC to communicate their racialized experiences as individuals with membership in multiple minoritized social groups. Milan and Katrin Milan (2016) powerfully capture the concept of queerness as lived, experienced, and described by many Queer People of Color. They explain, "Not queer like gay; queer like escaping definition. Queer like some sort of fluidity and limitlessness all at once. Queer like a freedom too strange to be conquered. Queer like the fearlessness to imagine what love can look like, and to pursue it" (para 18).

2.2 Queer People of Color and Racial-Gendered-Heterosexism

While QPOC share many of the experiences and concerns of Queer White People (QWP; heterosexism, cissexism) they also face the toxicity of racism and ethnocentrism. Building on the tradition of Black Women and Black Queer Women (e.g., Collins, 2009; Combahee River Collective, 1977/1995; Crenshaw, 1989, 1991) we are introducing the concept of *racial-gendered-heterosexism* to capture the unique and interlocking ways that QPOC are systemically dehumanized and oppressed. To illustrate, QPOC in the United States (U.S.) are more likely to live in poverty and have poorer health outcomes when compared to QWP in general (Budge et al., 2016; Badgett et al., 2019). In addition, QPOC are impacted by the murders of Black, Indigenous, and People of Color, the criminalization of immigrants, and the increasing attacks on civil rights including voting suppression (see Adames et al., 2018; Cerezo et al., 2014; Cerezo, 2016; Mosley et al., 2019a). When we use frameworks that capture the distinct ways that QPOC are concurrently impacted by racism, heterosexism, sexism, and cissexism, we can better identify, name, and address the problems that uniquely affect this community. For instance, while 72% of victims of anti-LGBT homicide were transgender women, 67% percent were transgender Women of Color (National Coalition of Anti-Violence Programs, 2014). QPOC are also negatively impacted by racism within the queer community. To demonstrate, when Proposition-8, a California ballot proposition and a state constitutional amendment that proposed to eliminate the rights of "same-sex" couples to marry was adopted, leaders of LGBT organizations vilified and blamed the African American community (see Kaufman, 2011; Kiesling, 2017). However, the reality is that African Americans voted for progressive Pro-LGBT candidates (Kaufman, 2011; Kiesling, 2017). There is also a history of QPOC being erased and excluded by the White Queer Community. To illustrate, while the *2009 Hate Crimes Prevention Act*,[3] which expanded the federal definition of a hate crime, was motivated by the murders of Matthew Shepard (White gay male) and James Byrd Jr. (Black heterosexual male), the legislation is commonly referred to as *The Matthew Shepard Act* instead of its official name, *The Matthew Shepard and James Byrd Jr. Hate Crimes Prevention Act*. This practice decenters race and the lynching of James Byrd Jr. while only centering the White gay male experience (Kiesling, 2017). The experiences of Women of Color and Queer Women of Color are further relegated to the margins. As an example, the Women's March has been criticized for excluding and silencing their voices (Kiesling, 2017). Put succinctly, the experience of QPOC is not the same as their White queer siblings.

2.3   The Gay Liberation Movement and QPOC

The exclusion of QPOCs by QWP stands in direct contrast with the achievements made by the *Gay Liberation Movement*. As a result, the Queer Community of Color has not fully benefited from the progress made by the *Gay Liberation Movement*,

---

[3] The *2009 Hate Crimes Prevention Act* expanded "the federal definition of hate crimes, enhancing the legal toolkit available to prosecutors, and increasing the ability of federal law enforcement to support our state and local partners. This law removed the existing jurisdictional obstacles to prosecutions of certain race- and religion-motivated violence and added new federal protections against crimes based on gender, disability, gender identity, or sexual orientation" (U.S. Department of Justice, 2019, para. 2).

including advances in civil and human rights such as the increase in the percentage of people reporting being more accepting of LGBT people (Pew Research Center, 2013) and the landmark U.S. Supreme Court decision of Obergefell v. Hodges that guaranteed same-sex couples the right to marry (History, 2020). To this end, QWP have disproportionately benefited from the *Gay Liberation Movement* despite the fact that QPOC spearheaded the *Gay Liberation Movement* including Stormé DeLarverie, Sylvia Rivera, Marsha P. Johnson, and Miss Major Griffin-Gracy among others (Cruikshank, 1992; Tran, 2018). Sadly, the work of these revolutionary Queer Siblings of Color who organized and led the Cooper Do-nuts in Los Angeles in 1959, the Compton's Cafeteria in San Francisco in 1966, and the historic Stonewall protests in New York in 1969 (James, 2019) is often ignored and not acknowledged. In other words, QWP have erased the contributions of QPOC despite benefiting from their sacrifice, brilliance, and resistance.

Overall, the lack of an intersectional discourse separates race-from-gender-from-sexuality and consequently extrapolates racism from sexism, from heterosexism, which erroneously suggests that QPOC cannot possibly experience all these forms of oppression simultaneously as illustrated by the theory of intersectionality introduced by Black Feminist and Black Queer Women scholars and activists (see Combahee River Collective, 1977/1995; Crenshaw, 1989). This fragmentation of the self, and how QPOC are uniquely oppressed, leaves many individuals of this community often feeling like they can only, and "should only", focus on one aspect of their identity at a time while negating other aspects of who they are. This framing and pattern are mirrored in the literature, where identity is predominantly described and studied in silos.

3   Models of Queer and Racial Identity Development

In the past half a century, several fundamental theories describing the identity development process for Queer People and People of Color have been developed. Below we briefly present and review some of the most well-known and widely used identity models. While each model describes the development of queer *or* racial identity, they all fail to capture how different aspects of the self develop simultaneously albeit in different ways (e.g., pace, direction).

3.1   *Queer Identity*

One of the most notable and referenced psychological models of identity for queer people is the *Cass Model of Gay/Lesbian Identity Development,* created in the late 1970s. Like other frameworks, the *Cass Model* is based on the assumption that people go through a process where they develop an awareness about being different from others (Cass, 1979). In this case, the difference is based on being attracted to people in non-heteronormative ways. Following some level of awareness, folx then begin to consider and explore what it means to be a member of a sexual minoritized and stigmatized social group. People may start to wonder what being part of the queer community might be like—and what it would mean if they acted upon their feelings and attraction. People may then rationalize their new awareness and deny what they are feeling (e.g., telling themselves that they are just going through a phase), which is often followed by some level of resolution and eventual acceptance where the person integrates their sexual orientation with other parts of the self (Cass, 1979). Table 1 provides the six stages of the *Cass Model* of identity along with ideologies that accompany each stage. Another well referenced model of queer identity is the *Inclusive Model of Sexual Minority Identity* (IMSMI; Fassinger & Miller, 1997; McCarn & Fassinger 1996). Similar to the *Cass Model*, the IMSMI describes a process of identity development for queer people. However, the IMSMI considers two levels where a queer development takes place, including: (a) at the personal level where individuals have an internal awareness and acceptance of self (psychological/intrapersonal), and (b) at the group membership level, which describes the extent to which an individual connects and relates with the queer community (social identity). Of note, neither models consider or address race or ethnicity in the identity development of Queer People of Color.

3.2   Racial and Ethnic Identity

Developed by Atkinson et al. (1989), The Racial/Cultural Identity Development (R/ CID) model was designed to describe experiences of discrimination among individuals from minoritized racial and ethnic groups in the United States (e.g., African Americans, Asian Americans, Latinxs, Native Americans, and American Arab, Middle Eastern, and North Africans). This conceptual framework seeks to outline the process that Black, Indigenous, and People of Color go through as they develop an understanding of their cultural heritage, the dominant culture, and the relationship between both. The R/CID is made up of five stages including: (a) conformity, (b) dissonance, (c) resistance and immersion, (d) introspection, (e) integrative

Table 1 The Cass model of queer identity

Stages		Relevant ideologies
Stage 1	Identity confusion	Who am I
Stage 2	Identity comparison	I am the only one like this
Stage 3	Identity tolerance	I probably am
Stage 4	Identity acceptance	I know who I am and where I belong
Stage 5	Identity pride	This is my community and I like it
Stage 6	Identity synthesis	I am many things

Note. The stages were developed by Cass (1979). The relevant ideologies were created by the authors awareness. In the *Conformity* stage, individuals prefer the values of the dominant group and may view members of their own racial, ethnic, and cultural group with disdain. Oftentimes, individuals in this stage have internalized the negative biases about their group and view their own group membership as unimportant. In the *Dissonance* stage, individuals experience an event that leads to questioning the beliefs, attitudes, and values held in the previous stage. In the *Resistance and Immersion* stage "there is an unequivocal all-encompassing endorsement of their racial and cultural groups' attitudes and values along with an overall rejection of the values held by the dominant group" (Adames & Chavez-Dueñas, 2017, p. 147). In the fourth stage, called *Introspection,* people develop an understanding of themselves as members of their racial, ethnic, and cultural group. In this stage, people can differentiate between their perspectives and those of their group. They also no longer hold an idealized view of their racial and cultural groups. Lastly, the final stage is *Integrative Awareness* which is characterized by people being able to see both positive and negative aspects of different cultures and a commitment to ending all forms of oppression.

One note to keep in mind is how the concepts of race, ethnicity, and culture are used interchangeably in the R/CID model. Framing the three concepts synonymously has been critiqued since the consensus among scholars in the social sciences posit that race, ethnicity, and culture are distinct albeit closely intertwined constructs (Alvarez et al., 2016; Helms & Cook 1999). To illustrate, culture is described as the "complex constellation of [learned] mores, values, customs, traditions, and practices that guide and influence people's cognitive, affective, and behavioral response to life circumstances" (Parham et al., 1999, p. 14). In other words, culture is what we do (Adames & Chavez-Dueñas, 2017). Ethnicity describes an individual's national, regional, or tribal lineage (Adames & Chavez-Dueñas, 2017). Ethnicity is where we come from. Generally, race is described as a social construct (made up classification system) that groups and ranks people into superior and inferior categories according to their shared physical characteristics (e.g., skin color, facial features, hair texture) which then has social, political, and economic implications (Helms & Cook, 1999; Jones, 1997). Hence, race refers to how others perceive us and how society categorizes us based on our phenotype which has consequences (e.g., privilege). Several other identity models specifically focus on (a) the development of racial identity (see Cross's Racial Identity Model; Cross Jr. & Vandiver, 2001; People of Color Racial Identity Attitude Scale, Helms, 1995), (d) ethnic identity (see Nadal, 2011; Phinney, 1992), and (c) both racial and ethnic identity while also considering the role of skin-color gradient (see The Centering Racial and Ethnic Identity for Latinxs Framework [C-REIL], Adames & Chavez-Dueñas, 2017). Although all of the identity development models presented in this section focus on different aspects of the self (i.e., race, culture, and/or ethnicity), they describe a similar process that results from three predominate phases including: (1) crisis/awakening, (2) exploration and experimentation, and (3) commitment or incorporation of culture, ethnicity, race and into the self. Similar to the queer models of identity, models of racial, cultural, and ethnic identity also fall short—that is, they do not consider or address the role of sexuality for People of Color.

4 The Racial Queer Identity Framework (RQI)

As described in the previous section, most existing models on racial/ethnic and queer identity are unidimensional and discount (a) how various aspects of people's identity develop simultaneously and (b) how overlapping and interlocking systems of oppression add meaning to the self. To stimulate a nuanced and multidimensional description of identity development among QPOC we present the *Racial Queer Identity Framework* (RQI) in Fig. 1. Accordingly, the RQI framework consists of three parts that include: intersectionality (Part-I), affirming vs. non-affirming messages about queerness and race that people receive (Part-II), and four possible overlapping and interlocking *racial queer schemas* (RQS; Part-III), which are described below.

Overall, the RQI framework aims to evoke answers to the list of questions proposed at the beginning of the chapter: Who do you say you are? Who is the you that others see? Who is the you that you allow others to see and why? Who is the you that nobody knows?

4.1 Part-I: Intersectionality

Intersectionality theory, an analytical framework introduced by Black Queer Women and Black feminist social justice activists and scholars (Collins, 2009; Combahee River Collective, 1977/1995; Crenshaw, 1989, 1991), was created to specifically name and illustrate how systems of oppression uniquely impact Black Women (e.g., gendered-racism; Collins, 2009; Crenshaw, 1989, 1991; Essed, 1991; Lewis & Neville, 2015). Since then, Intersectionality theory has been applied to other groups of people who also experience multiple forms of oppression (e.g., nativism, heterosexism, cissexism; see Adames et al., 2020; Chavez-Dueñas et al., 2019). A classification system, introduced by Dill and Kohlman (2011), divides intersectionality into either (a) *weak,* which focuses on multiple identities or (b) *strong,* that centers and underscores how systems of inequity and oppression impact people who hold membership in different minoritized social groups. Traditionally, the study of social identities has predominantly focused on either the intrapersonal processes of identity development (e.g., psychology) or the process of acquiring a sense of collective group membership. (e.g., sociology), however, the interplay between both, and the role of overlapping forms of oppression, is rarely considered. Hence, to better capture and describe the identity development of QPOC, we need to consider (a) the individuals' internal subjective processes, (b) their social group membership, and (c) how historical and systemic forces (e.g., policies, institutional oppression) uniquely collide to shape a person's identity (see Adames et al., 2018; Chavez-Dueñas & Adames, 2020; Grzanka, 2020). Part-I of the RQI framework depicts all three. A queer person's internal subjectivity about their social group membership is illustrated by the constructs in the overlapping inner circles (i.e., sexual orientation,

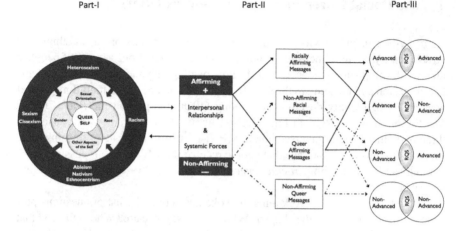

Fig. 1 The Racial Queer Identity (RQI) Framework. Note. *RQS* Racial queer schemas

race, gender, other aspects of the self). The external layer portrays the historical and current systemic forces (e.g., policies, laws, practices) that create, maintain, and fuel oppression (e.g., heterosexism, racism, sexism, cissexism, ableism, nativism, ethnocentrism). These systemic forces of oppression also impact and add meaning to the development of a queer self, as illustrated by the arrows pointing back to the overlapping circles (i.e., internal subjective processes). The use of intersectionality theory in the RQI framework allows us to generate an expansive and multidimensional understanding of QPOC using an analytical stance that synchronously considers an inside-out and an outside-in perspective. In addition, the RQI framework requires us to consider the affirming and non-affirming messages that QPOC receive from not only those they interact with (e.g., interpersonal relationships such as family, caregivers, peers) but also the narratives supported and reinforced by institutions (e.g., systemic forces such as laws, policies, media, educational and health systems). Part II of the RQI framework underscores the importance of these messages.

4.2   Part-II: Affirming Vs. Non-Affirming Messages About Queerness and Race

Socialization, the process through which children are introduced to their own culture's expectations, norms, and customs, is a fundamental aspect of human development. Contained within the process of socialization are implicit and explicit messages about the rules, beliefs, and expectations associated with (a) specific gender roles, sexual behaviors, and sexuality, a process known as *gendered sexual socialization* (Gansen, 2017), and (b) race and racism (Neblett Jr. et al., 2008). From a very early age, children hear, learn, and internalize heteronormative and cis-gendered-racial messages. For instance, children are taught and expected to behave in accordance with the sex they were assigned at birth (Bos et al., 2012). In the U.S., children assigned female at birth are taught and reinforced to be more passive, quiet, obedient, cooperative, and caring. Alternatively, children assigned male at birth are socialized and encouraged to be more active, outspoken, aggressive, and are reinforced for not expressing what are typically considered vulnerable emotions such as sadness and fear (Wienclaw, 2011). In addition to gender-role socialization, children also "begin to make sense of heteronormativity and rules associated with sexuality through interactions with their teachers and peers in preschool" (Gansen, 2017, p. 255). Similarly, children hear, learn, and internalize negative messages about their racial group membership (Lesane-Brown, 2006) and witness how groups are treated differently. However, Children of Color can also learn and internalize positive racial messages from caregivers through verbal and nonverbal communication about racialized experiences, a process known as *racial socialization* (Lesane-Brown, 2006). While the first agents of socialization are typically primary caregivers, other individuals, groups (e.g., extended family, teachers, peers), and institutions (e.g., media, judicial, educational and health systems) also serve an influential role in this process. Hughes et al. (2006) describe four components of racial-ethnic socialization including: (a) instilling cultural pride, (b) preparation for bias, (c) promotion of mistrust, and (d) egalitarianism. Overall, Part-II of the RQI framework considers both the affirming and non-affirming messages that QPOC receive throughout their lives about race and gender from both systemic forces and their interpersonal relationships. These messages are depicted by the boxes labeled racially and queer affirming and non-affirming messages in Fig. 1.

4.3   Part-III: Four Racial Queer Schemas (RQS)

While the empirical literature on *gendered sexual socialization* and *racial socialization* is robust and growing, both processes are rarely described, discussed, and studied simultaneously. To this end, we use Helms' (1990, 1994) description of racial schemas, which are the cognitive and affective "filters" that impact how people perceive and respond to racism, in the RQI framework. In Fig. 1, we illustrate and describe how QPOC interpret the world through one of four unique racial queer lenses. Each racial queer schemas (RQS) influence an individual's ability to recognize, minimize, or deny experiences of *racial-gendered-heterosexism*, which ultimately impacts the self. In the following sections, we describe each of the four racial queer schemas.

4.3.1   Advanced—Advanced RQS: Reclaiming All of Me

The first schema of the RQI framework is *advanced—advanced*. This schema is characterized by QPOC who consciously think of themselves as racial queer—not just a Person of Color or a Queer Person, but a person who is grounded and comfortable with the uniqueness of their whole self (advanced—advanced). QPOC using this schema have a nuanced understanding of who they are as a racial queer being and what that means in a white-supremacy- heteronormative culture. Despite the overlapping ways QPOC are oppressed, people using this schema seek to belong and create communities where their whole selves are welcomed and celebrated. They view their social group memberships as a source of pride despite being dehumanized and impacted by multiple forms of oppression. They reject negative messages about their racial queerness and are able to counter these messages with a firm understanding of the unique strengths and qualities of their racial queer community. Individuals using an *advanced—advanced* schema also demonstrate a commitment to ending all forms of oppression by recommitting oneself daily to refuse and resist the invitation to use the norms and narratives created by white supremacy culture, patriarchy, and heterosexism to define oneself and one's community.

4.3.2   Advanced—Non-Advanced RQS: Reclaiming Race and Compartmentalizing Queerness

The second schema of the RQI framework is *advanced—non-advanced*. This schema is characterized by QPOC that compartmentalize their race and queerness to minimize or avoid discomfort and anxiety associated with conflicting values, cognitions, emotions, and beliefs about being or questioning their sexuality. People using this schema consciously think of themselves as a racial or racialized being (advanced) but not a queer being (non-advanced). Similarly, they are comfortable with their racial group membership, Still, they may question their sexuality, experience attraction to people of the same gender, yet deny these aspects of themselves or believe that they are the only ones having these experiences. They have internalized negative and heteronormative messages about queerness, such as the idea that queerness does not exist in Communities of Color, queerness is a mental illness, follow the "love the sinner, hate the sin" ethos, and the like. While individuals using this schema have internalized messages about their queerness they can counter negative messages about their racial group with pride and understanding of the unique strengths of their racial community. They demonstrate a commitment to ending racism, but do not challenge heterosexism, cissexism, nor see how QPOC are uniquely impacted by racialized heterosexism. Instead, they may blame the oppression QPOC experience only on their queerness.

4.3.3   Non-Advanced—Advanced RQS: Reclaiming Queerness and Compartmentalizing Race

The third schema of the RQI framework is *non-advanced—advanced*. Individuals who use this schema attach low salience to racial issues (non-advanced) but are grounded and comfortable with their queerness (advanced). People using this schema are able to understand and identify heterosexism and heteronormativity; however, they deny or rationalize the impact of racism on their lives and those of their racial group. In turn, they internalize negative stereotypes about their own racial group, experience self-rejection, and harbor prejudice towards members of their own racial group. They feel connected to the gay community and proud of their queerness. They are likely to identify with White people and believe that White people are superior to People of Color. Individuals using this schema may also see QWP as leaders in the gay liberation movement, believing that QWP are exemplary because they can "freely" be queer while simultaneously viewing Communities of Color as misguided or pathologized for not accepting their queerness. In turn, this dynamic could further strengthen a non-advanced racial identity.

4.3.4 Non-Advanced—Non-Advanced RQS: Rejecting All of Me

The fourth schema of the RQI framework is *non-advanced—non-advanced*. This schema is characterized by individuals who do not consciously think about themselves as a Person of Color (non-advanced), nor a Queer person (non-advanced), and let alone as a unique racialized queer person. QPOC using this schema may be questioning their sexuality, experiencing attraction to people of the same gender, yet denying it or believing that they are the only ones in the world having these experiences. Concurrently, they often do not see themselves as racial beings and understand themselves and the world through a color-blind paradigm. They are more likely to identify with White people, express preference for White people's values and norms, and internalize negative messages about members of their own racial group. People using this schema may also deny or rationalize the impact of racism on their lives. Hence, they walk around with filters that cloud their ability to see and understand the multiple and complex ways in which white supremacy culture, patriarchy, and heterosexism are working in tandem to impact their existence and how they are answering the fundamental question of "who am I?"

4.4 Dominant Society Response

While QPOC may use different RQS to view themselves and interpret the world, the dominant society in the U.S. has historically reinforced and upheld white supremacy culture, patriarchy, and heterosexism—a structural practice that continues to prevail today. Put differently, the dominant U.S. society has never welcomed racial queer individuals, especially those who challenge the power structures and resist oppression. Hence, the RQI framework assumes that there is a bidirectional relationship between the affirming and non-affirming messages that QPOC receive from (a) their interpersonal relationships, (b) the systemic forces in the society (e.g., school, media), and (c) the schemas that QPOC develop. In turn, the RQS that individuals develop will impact whether a QPOC challenges both interpersonal and systemic forces in society. For instance, a QPOC who uses an *advanced— advanced* schema will understand how racism, ethnocentrism, heterosexism,

sexism, and cissexism uniquely overlap and impact their lives. As a result, they will work to challenge these oppressive forces instead of internalizing their inter-locking forms of subjugation. Conversely, a QPOC that is using a *non-advanced—non-advanced* schema will have difficulty recognizing societal messages that are invalidating. Consequently, they will have difficulty understanding how toxic, pathologizing, and harmful societal messages, policies, and practices affect them. Moreover, QPOC using this schema fail to challenge racism, heterosexism, and cissexism. Instead, they are more likely to blame themselves for how society is structured to oppress their existence. Overall, understanding people's identity requires us to acknowledge and center the connection between systems of oppression and how we give meaning to our intrapersonal world.

5   Applying the Racial Queer Identity Framework: The Case of Yari and Angelica

Yari is a 23-year-old dark-skin Peruvian immigrant cis-woman who uses she/her/ella pronouns and identifies as a lesbian. She is completing her associate degree at a community college. Yari comes from a traditional Peruvian family who is very proud of their Indigenous Quechua roots. Although they speak Spanish at home, their values and traditions are closely connected to their Indigenous heritage. Yari loves her family but at times feels that they are "too strict *y cerrados* [closed minded]." However, she considers herself "one of the lucky ones" since her family is okay with her dating women, although they rarely talk much about her sexuality. Yari's gender expression can be described as what society would classify as "masculine." She often uses self-deprecating humor with her queer friends, who are pre-dominately White, as a way of connecting with them. She says, "Yeah, my parents knew I was gay the minute they saw me, look at me!" Yari often feels ashamed of her family. She wishes they were more like the parents of her White peers who just let them live their life. Instead, her parents are "*muy metiches* [nosy]." They call her daily to find out what she is up to and when she is coming over to visit. Yari feels that most of the difficulties she has experienced in life are due to her being queer. But she reports being proud of who she is and often wears queer affirmative emblems (e.g., rainbow flags). When asked about her race, Yari says she doesn't think much about being Peruvian and reports she is "not really experiencing racism." She pro-claims, "The only race I see is the human race."

For the past five years, Yari has worked as a barista at a coffee shop where she met Angelica, a 24-year-old Mexican American cis-woman co-worker. Initially, Yari was annoyed by how Angelica would often talk about how People of Color are treated in this country and how the U.S. cages undocumented children at the border. Yari would usually roll her eyes when Angelica talked about politics, government, and White people. They would often get into heated conversations, although lately, they have turned into playful banters. Despite these differences, Yari and Angelica began to spend time outside of work and developed a close friendship over time. In the last few months, Yari feels that her relationship with Angelica is deeper than a friendship. She is beginning to feel "some type of way." At times, Yari thinks she is growing romantic feelings for Angelica and believes that Angelica may feel the same way about her. Yari wants to tell Angelica how she feels but worries that Angelica would reject her as Angelica has never dated a woman before. When Yari finally reveals her feelings to Angelica, she is surprised to hear Angelica say, "You're dope. I really like spending time with you too, Yari, but I don't want to make things complicated, but yeah, I cannot stop thinking about you. It's all very confusing. I need to figure this out ... these feelings are somewhat uncomfortable."

The case of Yari and Angelica illustrates how two Queer Latinx women can belong to similar social groups (e.g., gender, sex, ethnicity, sexual orientation), be impacted by similar overlapping forms of oppression (e.g., sexism, nativism, racism), and yet still use different schemas to make sense of the world and their racial-gendered-queer identity or emerging identity (e.g., Angelica's queerness). Using the RQI framework, we can begin to think of the affirming and non-affirming messages that Yari and Angelica have received from their interpersonal relationships and the systemic forces that add meaning to how they view themselves as racial queer women. Based on the RQI framework, we can see that Yari is using the *non-advanced—advanced RQS*. As described in the case, Yari feels disconnected from her Peruvian roots and her family. Her friendships are predominantly with QWP, race has a low salience in her life, and she does not seem to understand racial oppression and how it has affected her life. However, she is deeply connected with the Queer community and acknowledges the negative impact heterosexism has had on her. She internalizes being rejected likely due to racism, ethnocentrism, and nativism. Alternatively, Angelica is using an *advanced—non-advanced schema* to view herself and the world. Angelica is proud of her heritage can recognize how racial oppression impacts People of Color; however, when it comes to her sexuality, Angelica feels very confused about the feelings she has for Yari.

6 Conclusion

In closing, we welcome all of the Yaris, Angelicas, and QPOC throughout the world to reclaim all of who you are. Yes, nurture all of you. Reflect on how systemic oppression impacts your livelihood and well-being. Resist the toxic invitation from White supremacy culture, patriarchy, and heterosexism to internalize and embody their colonizing ideologies and practices. Together we can build and strengthen our communities by focusing on developing healthy identities and, equally important, by sustaining our collective struggle against structural oppression. Our resistance is an antidote to the poison in the harmful messages QPOC receive from society and its laws, policies, and institutions. Our resistance provides us with a sense of belonging and a pathway for building a healthy, meaningful view of ourselves. Only then can we materialize "a world where I can be, without having to cease being me, where you can be, without having to cease being you, and where neither you nor I will force one another to be like either me or you" (Marcos, 2001, p. 169). We can, we must, and we will build healthy and viable worlds for all of our Queer Siblings of Color.

References

Adames, H. Y., & Chavez-Dueñas, N. Y. (2017). Cultural foundations and interventions in Latino/a mental health: History, theory, and within group differences. Routledge Press.
Adames, H. Y., Chavez-Dueñas, N. Y., Salas, S. P., & Manley, C. R. (2020). Intersectionality as a practice of dementia care for sexual and gender minoritized Latinxs. In H. Y. Adames & Y. N. Tazeau (Eds.), *Caring for Latinxs with dementia in a globalized world*. New York: Springer. https://doi.org/10.1007/978-1-0716-0132-7_12
Adames, H. Y., Chavez-Dueñas, N. Y., Sharma, S., & La Roche, M. J. (2018). Intersectionality in psychotherapy: The experiences of an AfroLatinx queer immigrant. *Psychotherapy, 55*(1), 1–7. https://psycnet.apa.org/doi/10.1037/pst0000152
Alvarez, A. N., Liang, C. T. H., & Neville, H. A. (Eds.). (2016). *Cultural, racial, and ethnic psychology book series. The cost of racism for people of color: Contextualizing experiences of discrimination*. American Psychological Association. doi: https://doi.org/10.1037/14852-000.
American Psychological Association. (2008). *Report of the APA Task Force on gender identity and gender variance*. Retrieved from http://www.apa.org/pi/lgbt/resources/policy/gender-identity-report.pdf.
American Psychological Association. (2012). Guidelines for psychological practice with lesbian, gay, and bisexual clients. *American Psychologist, 67*(1), 10–42. https://doi.org/10.1037/a0024659.
American Psychological Association. (2015). Guidelines for psychological practice with transgender and gender nonconforming people. *American Psychologist, 70*(9), 832–864. https://doi.org/10.1037/a0039906.
Atkinson, D. R., Morten, G., & Sue, D. W. (1989). A minority identity development model. In D. R. Atkinson, G. Morten, & D. W. Sue (Eds.), *Counseling American minorities* (5th ed., pp. 35–52). New York: McGraw-Hill.
Badgett, M. V. L., Choi, S. K., & Wilson, B. D. M., (2019). LGBT poverty in the United States: A study of differences between sexual orientation and gender identity groups. The Williams Institute. Retrieved from https://williamsinstitute.law.ucla.edu/wp-content/uploads/National-LGBT-Poverty-Oct-2019.pdf.
Battle, J., & Harris, A. (2013). Connectedness and the sociopolitical involvement of same-gender-loving black men. *Men and Masculinities, 16*(2), 260–267. https://doi.org/10.1177/1097184X13487909.
Bos, H. M. W., Picavet, C., & Sandfort, T. G. M. (2012). Ethnicity, gender socialization, and children's attitudes toward gay men and lesbian women. *Journal of Cross-Cultural Psychology, 43*(7), 1082–1094. https://doi.org/10.1177/0022022111420146.
Bowles, D. (2019, January 5). *Nahuatl's lack of grammatical gender.* Medium. Retrieved from https://medium.com/@davidbowles/nahuatls-lack-of-grammatical-gender-5896ed54f2d7
Budge, S. L., Thai, J. L., Tebbe, E. A., & Howard, K. A. (2016). The intersection of race, sexual orientation, socioeconomic status, trans identity, and mental health outcomes. *The Counseling Psychologist, 44*(7), 1025–1049. https://doi.org/10.1177/0011000015609046.
Cass, V. C. (1979). Homosexual identity formation: A theoretical model. *Journal of Homosexuality, 4*(3), 219–235. https://doi.org/10.1300/J082v04n03_01.
Cerezo, A. (2016). The impact of discrimination on mental health symptomatology in sexual minority immigrant Latinas. *Psychology of Sexual Orientation and Gender Diversity, 3*(3), 283–292. https://doi.org/10.1037/sgd0000172.

Cerezo, A., Morales, A., Quintero, D., & Rothman, S. (2014). Trans migrations: Exploring life at the intersection of transgender identity and immigration. *Psychology of Sexual Orientation and Gender Diversity, 1*(2), 170–180. https://doi.org/10.1037/sgd0000031.

Chavez-Dueñas, N. Y., & Adames, H. Y. (2020). Intersectionality awakening model of Womanista: A transnational treatment approach for Latinx women. *Women & Therapy*. Advance online publication. https://doi.org/10.1080/02703149.2020.1775022.

Chavez-Dueñas, N. Y., Adames, H. Y., Perez-Chavez, J. G., & Salas, S. P. (2019). Healing ethno-racial trauma in Latinx immigrant communities: Cultivating hope, resistance, and action. *American Psychologist, 74*(1), 49–62. https://doi.org/10.1037/amp0000289.

Collins, P. H. (2009). *Black feminist thought: Knowledge, consciousness, and the politics of empowerment* (2nd ed.). New York: Routledge.

Combahee River Collective. (1995). Combahee river collective statement. In B. Guy-Sheftall (Ed.), *Words of fire: An anthology of African American feminist thought* (pp. 232–240). New York: New Press. (Original work published 1977).

Contreras, J. M., Banaji, M. R., & Mitchell, J. P. (2013). Multivoxel patterns in fusiform face area differentiate faces by sex and race. *PLoS One, 8*(7), e69684. https://doi.org/10.1371/journal.pone.0069684.

Crenshaw, K. (1989). Demarginalizing the intersection of race and sex: A black feminist critique of antidiscrimination doctrine, feminist theory and antiracist politics. *University of Chicago Legal Forum, 1989*(1), 139–167.

Crenshaw, K. W. (1991). Mapping the margins: Intersectionality, identity politics, and violence against women of color. *Stanford Law Review, 43*, 1241–1299. https://doi.org/10.2307/1229039.

Cross, W. E., Jr., & Vandiver, B. J. (2001). Nigrescence theory and measurement: Introducing the cross racial identity scale (CRIS). In J. G. Ponterotto, J. M. Casas, L. A. Suzuki, & C. M. Alexander (Eds.), *Handbook of multicultural counseling* (2nd ed., pp. 371–393). Thousand Oaks, CA: Sage Publications.

Cruikshank, M. (1992). *The gay and lesbian liberation movement*. New York: Psychology Press.

Diamond, L. (2007). A dynamical systems approach to the development and expression of female same-sex sexuality. *Perspectives on Psychological Science, 2*, 142–161.

Dill, B. T., & Kohlman, M. H. (2011). Intersectionality: A transformative paradigm in feminist theory and social justice. In S. N. Hesse-Biber (Ed.), *Handbook of feminist research: Theory and praxis* (2nd ed., pp. 154–174). Los Angeles, CA: Sage Publications.

Erikson, E. H. (1980). *Identity and the life cycle*. New York: W. W. Norton & Co..

Essed, P. (1991). *Sage series on race and ethnic relations, Vol. 2. Understanding everyday racism: An interdisciplinary theory*. Newbury Park: Sage Publications.

Fassinger, R. E., & Miller, B. A. (1997). Validation of an inclusive model of sexual minority identity formation on a sample of gay men. *Journal of Homosexuality, 32*(2), 53–78. https://doi.org/10.1300/J082v32n02_04.

Gansen, H. M. (2017). Reproducing (and disrupting) heteronormativity: Gendered sexual socialization in preschool classrooms. *Sociology of Education, 90*(3), 255–272. https://doi.org/10.1177/0038040717720981.

Garnets, L. D., & Kimmel, D. C. (Eds.). (2003). *Psychological perspectives on lesbian, gay, and bisexual experiences* (2nd ed.). New York: Columbia University Press.

Grzanka, P. R. (2020). From buzzword to critical psychology: An invitation to take intersectionality seriously. *Women & Therapy, 43*(3–4), 244–261. https://doi.org/10.1080/02703149.2020.1729473.

Helms, J. E. (1990). *Black and white racial identity: Theory research, and practice*. New York: Greenwood Press.

Helms, J. E. (1994). The conceptualization of racial identity. In E. Trickett, R. Watts, & D. Birman (Eds.), *Human diversity: Perspectives on people in context* (pp. 285–311). San Francisco, CA: Jossey-Bass.

Helms, J. E. (1995). An update of Helm's White and people of color racial identity models. In J. G. Ponterotto, J. M. Casas, L. A. Suzuki, & C. M. Alexander (Eds.), *Handbook of multicultural counseling* (pp. 181–198). Thousand Oaks, CA: Sage Publications, Inc..

Helms, J. E., & Cook, D. A. (1999). *Using race and culture in counseling and psychotherapy: Theory and process*. Boston: Allyn & Bacon.

History. Editors (2020, June 2). *Gay marriage, History.* Retrieved from www.history.com/topics/gay-marriage

Hughes, D., Rodriguez, J., Smith, E. P., Johnson, D. J., Stevenson, H. C., & Spicer, P. (2006). Parents' ethnic-racial socialization practices: A review of research and directions for future study. *Developmental Psychology, 42*(5), 747–770. https://doi.org/10.1037/0012-1649.42.5.747.

James, S. (2019, June 20). *What was your stonewall? Pivotal L.G.B.T.Q. moments across the U.S.* The New York Times. Retrieved from https://www.nytimes.com/2019/06/20/us/stonewalls-across-us-lgbtq.html

Jones, J.M. (1997). Prejudice and racism (2nd ed.). McGraw-Hill.

Kaufman, D. (2011, March 4). *The root: The misguided black vote on gay marriage.* NPR. Retrieved from https://www.npr.org/2011/03/04/134257733/the-root-the-misjudged-black-vote-on-gay-marriage

Kiesling, E. (2017). The missing colors of the rainbow: Black queer resistance. *European Journal of American Studies, 11*(3), 26. https://doi.org/10.4000/ejas.11830.

Kinsey, A. C., Pomeroy, W. B., Martin, C. E., & Gebhard, P. H. (1953). *Sexual behavior in the human female*. Philadelphia: Saunders.

Kumar, S. (2019). *LGBT community in India: A study*. Chhattisgarh: Educreation Publishing.

Lerner, R. M. (2002). *Concepts and theories of human development* (3rd ed.). Mahwah, NJ: Lawrence Erlbaum Associates Publishers.

Lesane-Brown, C. L. (2006). A review of race socialization within black families. *Developmental Review, 26*(4), 400–426. https://doi.org/10.1016/j.dr.2006.02.001.

Lewis, J. A., & Neville, H. A. (2015). Construction and initial validation of the gendered racial microaggressions scale for black women. *Journal of Journal of Counseling Psychology, 62*(2), 289–302. https://doi.org/10.1037/cou0000062.

Maccoby, E. E. (1988). Gender as a social category. *Developmental Psychology, 24*(6), 755–765.

Marcos, S. (2001). *Our word is our weapon: Selected writings*. New York: Seven Stories Press.

McCarn, S. R., & Fassinger, R. E. (1996). Revisioning sexual minority identity formation: A new model of lesbian identity and its implications. *The Counseling Psychologist, 24*(3), 508–534. https://doi.org/10.1177/0011000096243011.

Milan, T., & Katrin Milan, K. (2016). *A queer vision of love and marriage.* Ted Talk. Retrieved from https://www.ted.com/talks/tiq_milan_and_kim_katrin_milan_a_queer_vision_of_love_and_marriage/transcript?language=en#t-496750

Mosley, D. V., Chen, G. A., Lewis, J. A., Neville, H. A., French, B. H., Adames, H. Y., & Chavez-Dueñas, N. Y. (2019a, July 12). *LGBTQ+ people of color healing from hatred: How gaining critical consciousness heals us all.* Psychology Today. Retrieved from https://www.psychology-today.com/us/blog/healing-through-social-justice/201906/lgbtq-people-color-healing-hatred

Mosley, D. V., Gonzalez, K. A., Abreu, R. L., & Kaivan, N. C. (2019b). Unseen and underserved: A content analysis of wellness support services for bi + people of color and indigenous people on U.S. campuses. *Journal of Bisexuality.* Advance online publication. https://doi.org/10.1080/15299716.2019.1617552.

Nadal, K. L. (2011). *Filipino American psychology: A handbook of theory, research, and clinical practice*. Hoboken, NJ: John Wiley & Sons.

Nakamura, N., & Logie, C. H. (Eds.). (2020). LGBTQ mental health: International perspectives and experiences. *American Psychological Association.* https://doi.org/10.1037/0000159-000.

National Coalition of Anti-Violence Programs. (2014). *Lesbian, gay, bisexual, transgender, queer and HIV-affected hate violence, 2013* National Coalition of Anti-Violence Programs. Retrieved from https://avp.org/wp-content/uploads/2017/04/2013_ncavp_hvreport_final.pdf

Neblett, E. W., Jr., White, R. L., Ford, K. R., Philip, C. L., Nguyên, H. X., & Sellers, R. M. (2008). Patterns of racial socialization and psychological adjustment: Can parental communications about race reduce the impact of racial discrimination? *Journal of Research on Adolescence, 18*(3), 477–515. https://doi.org/10.1111/j.1532-7795.2008.00568.x.

Newsweek Staff. (1991). What is queer nation? Newsweek. Retrieved from https://www.news-week.com/what-queer-nation-202866.

Parham, T. A., White, J. L., & Ajamu, A. (1999). *The psychology of Blacks: An African centered perspective* (3rd ed.). Upper Saddle River, NJ: Prentice Hall.

Parks, C. W. (2001). African-American same-gender-loving youths and families in urban schools. *Journal of Gay & Lesbian Social Services: Issues in Practice, Policy & Research, 13*(3), 41–56. https://doi.org/10.1300/J041v13n03_03.

Peplau, L. A., & Garnets, L. D. (2000). A new paradigm for understanding women's sexuality and sexual orientation. *Journal of Social Issues, 56*(2), 329–350. https://doi.org/10.1111/0022-4537.00169.

Pew Research Center. (2013, June 13). *A survey of LGBT Americans.* Pew Research Center. Retrieved from https://www.pewsocialtrends.org/2013/06/13/a-survey-of-lgbt-americans/

Phinney, J. S. (1992). The multigroup ethnic identity measure: A new scale for use with adolescents and young adults from diverse groups. *Journal of Adolescent Research, 7*, 156–176.

Schmidt, J. (2010). *Migrating genders: Westernisation, migration, and Samoan fa'afafine.* Burlington, VT: Ashgate.

Shively, M. G., & De Cecco, J. P. (1977). Component of sexual identity. *Journal of Homosexuality, 3*(1), 41–48. https://doi.org/10.1300/J082v03n01_04.

Stephen, L. (2002). Sexualities and genders in Zapotec Oaxaca. *Latin American Perspectives, 123*(29), 41–59.

Syed, M., & Fish, J. (2018). Revisiting Erik Erikson's legacy on culture, race, and ethnicity. *Identity: An International Journal of Theory and Research, 18*(4), 274–283.

Tate, C. C., Youssef, C. P., & Bettergarcia, J. N. (2014). Integrating the study of transgender spectrum and cisgender experiences of self-categorization from a personality perspective. *Review of General Psychology, 18*(4), 302–312. https://doi.org/10.1037/gpr0000019.

Tran, C. (2018, June 11). *When remembering Stonewall, we need to listen to those who were there. Them.* Retrieved from https://www.them.us/story/who-threw-the-first-brick-at-stonewall.

U.S. Department of Justice. (2019, March 7). *Hate crime laws.* U.S. Department of Justice. Retrieved from https://www.justice.gov/crt/hate-crime-laws

Unger, R. K. (1979). Toward a redefinition of sex and gender. *American Psychologist, 34*(11), 1085–1094.

Wienclaw, R. A. (2011). Gender roles. In The Editors of Salem Press (Ed.), *Sociology reference guide: Gender roles and equality* (pp. 33–40). Pasadena, CA: Salem Press.

Sexual and Gender Minority People's Physical Health and Health Risk Behaviors

Ethan H. Mereish and M. Son Taylor

1 Sexual and Gender Minority People's Physical Health and Health Risk Behaviors

Although the literature on physical and sexual health and health risk behaviors among sexual and gender minority (i.e., queer) people is burgeoning, it is limited in its methodology and nuanced understanding of subgroups and intersectional experiences. This chapter has three main goals. First, we provide a review of the literature on sexual orientation and gender identity disparities in physical health, sexual health, and health risk behaviors among queer people. Some of the physical health literature reviewed covers disparities in cancer, obesity, cardiovascular disease, and sleep disturbance. We review some of the literature on sexual health, including sexually transmitted infections and pregnancy rates. We also discuss the research on health risk behaviors, such as substance use, physical activity, dietary behaviors, sexual behavior, and health screenings. Second, we describe several etiological factors that explain these disparities. These factors are adverse life experiences, minority stress, structural stigma, and other systemic oppression and barriers. Lastly, we end with a case to help illustrate how these etiological factors shape physical health and health behaviors and to demonstrate some intervention approaches with a biracial, pansexual, non-binary youth.

Consistent with this book's theme, we take an intersectional lens in understanding the experience of queer people and their physical health and health risk behaviors, especially highlighting queer people at the margins of society. We note that there is a dearth of literature on gender minority people as well as queer people of color's physical health outcomes; thus, some of the concepts reviewed may apply to queer people more broadly but there are unique distinctions across sexual

E. H. Mereish (✉) · M. S. Taylor
Department of Health Studies, American University, Washington, DC, USA
e-mail: mereish@american.edu

© The Author(s), under exclusive license to Springer Nature
Switzerland AG 2021
K. L. Nadal and M. R. Scharrón-del Río (ed.), *Queer Psychology*,
https://doi.org/10.1007/978-3-030-74146-4_5

orientation, gender identity, race, and other marginalized identity experiences. Finally, despite disparities in these health outcomes, we underscore that queer people are resilient and attention to their strengths in engaging in health promoting behaviors is understudied.

1.1 Physical Health

Queer people have an elevated risk for experiencing a range of physical health concerns compared to their heterosexual and cisgender peers. These range from queer people reporting poorer overall rating of their physical health (Simoni et al, 2017), and greater reporting of physical pain and distressing somatic symptoms (e.g., headaches, migraines; Hammond & Stinchcombe, 2019), inflammatory conditions (e.g., arthritis, asthma; Fredriksen-Goldsen et al, 2012), and metabolic diseases (e.g., diabetes; Beach et al, 2018), to having greater risk for physical disabilities (Fredriksen-Goldsen et al, 2012). In this section, we review some of the literature on physical health concerns and focus on cancer, obesity, cardiovascular disease, and sleep disturbance.

1.1.1 Cancer

Several population and epidemiological studies, almost all conducted with sexual minorities, show that queer people are at greater risk for multiple types of cancers, including breast, cervical, colorectal, lung, and skin cancers (Boehmer et al, 2014; Machalek et al, 2012). Among queer communities, some groups are at particular risk. For example, sexual minority women (SMW) are at higher risk of developing breast cancer (Boehmer et al, 2014) and have greater risk of dying from breast cancer than did women who reported living with a male spouse or cohabiting relationship partner (Cochran & Mays, 2012). Transgender women on hormone treatment are 46 times more likely to develop breast cancer than cisgender men, and transgender men on hormone treatment are half as likely to develop breast cancer compared to cisgender women (Joint et al, 2018).

There are also sexual orientation disparities in cancer among cisgender men. Sexual minority men (SMM) are more likely to be at risk for lung and colorectal cancer compared to heterosexual men (Boehmer et al, 2012). Additionally, sexual minority men are twice as likely to develop skin cancer than their heterosexual peersand are more likely to tan indoors than heterosexual men (Mansh et al, 2015; Rosario et al, 2016). SMM are also at risk for developing anal cancer due to their elevated risk to becoming infected with anal human papillomavirus (Machalek et al, 2012).

1.1.2 Obesity

Obesity disproportionally affects SMW and transgender people (Simoni et al, 2017) and not queer cisgender men. Studies consistently show that SMW are more likely to be overweight or obese than heterosexual women, with these disparities starting in adolescence (Simoni et al, 2017). Latina and Black SMW are 20% more likely to be overweight than White heterosexual women (Mays et al, 2002). Moreover, gender minority youth (GMY) have higher prevalence of overweight or obesity compared to cisgender youth (Bishop et al, 2020).

1.1.3 Cardiovascular Disease

Emerging research on cardiovascular disease among queer communities shows mixed findings. Specifically, a recent systematic review of the literature shows that sexual minority adults have several and greater risk factors for cardiovascular disease (CVD) compared to heterosexual adults (e.g., tobacco use, poor mental health, obesity risk for women); however, there is limited research and mixed findings in terms of differences in diagnoses of CVD (Caceres et al, 2017). Similarly, gender minority individuals have greater risk factors for CVD than cisgender individuals (Alzahrani et al, 2019). Gender-affirming hormones may be potentially an additional risk factor for cardiovascular disease among transgender individuals (Kidd et al, 2018; Streed et al, 2017). Recent work shows that transgender women report higher rates of coronary heart disease, stroke, and myocardial infarction than cisgender women (Caceres et al, 2020).

1.1.4 Sleep

Sleep is a significant factor contributing to poor physical health conditions and chronic disease (Cappuccio et al, 2011; X. Chen et al, 2014). Queer youth and adults are more likely to experience poor sleep quality and sleep disturbances than their heterosexual peers (Chen & Shiu, 2017; Galinsky et al, 2018; Li et al, 2017). Moreover, a population based study found that queer people, including gender minorities, were more likely to experience sleep deprivation (i.e., very short sleep) than heterosexual cisgender adults; sleep deprivation was also associated with greater odds of chronic conditions, including greater risk for stroke, heart attacks, coronary heart disease, asthma, chronic obstructive pulmonary disease, arthritis, and cancer among sexual minority adults (Dai & Hao, 2019).

1.2 Sexual Health

Queer people historically experience significant sexual health disparities compared to their heterosexual and cisgender peers. These include disparities in sexually transmitted infections (STIs) such as HIV prevalence (Everett, 2013; Herbst et al, 2008) and reproductive health (Nicopoullos et al, 2011). Sexual health disparities disproportionally affect queer people of color and transgender communities.

1.2.1 HIV/AIDS

There have been great strides to improve the health of those affected by HIV/AIDS since the 1980s; however, disparities continue to affect the queer community, specifically queer people of color and transgender women. According to the Centers for Disease Control and Prevention (2018), 70% of new U.S. HIV diagnoses were gay and bisexual adolescent and adult men. Additionally, one in six gay and bisexual men are likely to develop HIV in their lifetime. This risk is significantly higher for racial minority men. Specifically, one in two Black SMM and one in four Latino SMM are at risk for contracting HIV in their lifetime (Centers for Disease Control and Prevention, 2018).

Transgender people are also at greater risk for becoming infected with HIV, especially transgender people of color (Becasen et al, 2018). Among transgender women in the U.S. who have HIV, 44% of them are Black and 26% are Hispanic (Becasen et al, 2018). Similarly, over half (58%) of new HIV cases among transgender men were among Black transgender men (Clark et al, 2017).

1.2.2 Sexually Transmitted Infections

Disparities in sexually transmitted infections (STIs) begin in adolescence and continue into adulthood. Sexual minority youth (SMY) are twice as likely to contract gonorrhea, chlamydia, and HIV compared to heterosexual youth (Benson & Hergenroeder, 2005). Some subgroups within the queer umbrella experience heightened risk. For example, bisexual and other plurisexual individuals are more likely to contract STIs than their monosexual counterparts, including heterosexual, lesbian, and gay individuals (Everett, 2013). Additionally, there is some evidence to demonstrate that STI disparities are elevated for queer people of color (Mojola & Everett, 2012). Transgender people also have high STI prevalence (Van Gerwen et al, 2020).

1.2.3 Pregnancy

Emerging literature has demonstrated sexual orientation disparities in teen pregnancy among young women. Compared to heterosexual youth, bisexual youth are almost five times more likely and lesbian youth are almost twice as likely to experience teenage pregnancy (Charlton et al, 2018). In contrast to youth, SMW have fewer pregnancies than heterosexual women (Howlader et al, 2015; Zaritsky & Dibble, 2010). Pregnancy in adulthood has long been considered a protective factor for breast cancer; therefore, reduced pregnancy rates in SMW might be related to their increased cancer risk (Russo et al, 2005). Pregnancy prevalence rates among transgender youth are not significantly different from rates in the general Canadian youth population (Veale et al, 2016).

1.3 Health Risk Behaviors Are One Factor Explaining Physical and Sexual Health Disparities

Due to stigma, systemic and individual-level forms of oppression, societal norms, and lack of access to appropriate healthcare and health education, some queer people engage in health risk behaviors. These health risk behaviors can partially explain the aforementioned disparities in physical and sexual health as they have significant, long-term, and deleterious effects on queer people's health. Examples of these health risk behaviors include alcohol, tobacco, and other types of substance use, less engagement in physical activity, poor dietary behaviors, greater likelihood to engage in risky sexual behaviors, and lower likelihood to obtain recommended health screenings. Many of these disparities begin in adolescence and persist into adulthood.

1.3.1 Alcohol Use

Several epidemiological studies show that queer people are at greater risk for alcohol use and misuse and experience greater negative consequences from drinking compared to their heterosexual and cisgender peers. This is further exacerbated for SMW and bisexual individuals. Queer youth initiate alcohol use at younger ages and engage in greater binge drinking than their heterosexual and cisgender peers (Day et al, 2017; Mereish, 2019). Moreover, despite general decline in alcohol and tobacco use in the U.S., queer youth continue to show higher rates than their heterosexual peers (Fish et al, 2017; Watson et al, 2018).

Although there is research demonstrating alcohol use disparities between SMM and heterosexual men (Gilbert et al, 2017), other work shows no differences or mixed findings (Hughes et al, 2016). In contrast, the research evidence has been consistent for women, wherein SMW are more likely to engage in hazardous drinking than heterosexual women (Hughes et al, 2016). Bisexual people are more likely to use alcohol, binge drink, and experience alcohol use disorder compared to their lesbian, gay, or heterosexual peers, and these disparities are documented across multiple racial groups (Schuler & Collins, 2020; Schuler et al, 2020).

1.3.2 Nicotine Use

Queer people are at greater risk for nicotine use, such as smoking cigarettes, e-cigarettes or vaping, than their heterosexual and cisgender peers. This is concerning as nicotine use has myriad negative physical health effects. Transgender people are twice as likely to report smoking than cisgender people (Shires & Jaffee, 2016). Similarly, SMY and adults are more likely to use nicotine than their heterosexual peers (Agaku et al, 2014), and begin to do so at younger ages and more frequently (Watson et al, 2018). Similar to alcohol use, these disparities are greater for bisexual individuals compared to their heterosexual, lesbian, and gay peers (Schuler & Collins, 2020). Additionally, there are racial differences in tobacco use (Schuler et al. 2020). Black SMY are 66% more likely to use tobacco products than their White queer counterparts, and 225% more likely than their Black heterosexual peers (Blosnich et al, 2011). Sexual minority Hispanic youth are twice as likely to smoke cigarettes than their heterosexual Hispanic peers (Blosnich et al, 2011).

1.3.3 Other Substance Use

Queer people are more likely to use marijuana and illicit substances, such as inhalants and hallucinogen, than heterosexual and cisgender peers. SMY are three times more likely to use marijuana, synesthetic marijuana, and prescription drugs than heterosexual youth (Goldbach et al, 2017). Compared to heterosexual adults, sexual minority adults are twice as likely to have used an illicit drug or marijuana, or misused prescription pain killers than their heterosexual peers in the past year (Medley et al, 2016). Sexual minorities are also more likely to experience substance use problems than heterosexual adults, and heightened risk is rendered by race and gender (Mereish & Bradford, 2014) as well as sexual identity (Schuler et al, 2019). For instance, bisexual women are six times more likely to use hallucinogens, five times more likely to use methamphetamines, four times more likely to use opiates or ecstasy than heterosexual women (Kerr et al, 2015).

A survey of over 1200 transgender adults found that one fourth used cannabis and about one tenth used illicit drugs in the past 3 months (Gonzalez et al, 2017), with transgender men reporting the higher rates than transgender women (Gonzalez et al, 2017). Transgender Australians with non-binaries gender identities (e.g., non-binary, agender) are twice as likely to report illicit drug use than transgender people with binary identities (i.e., transgender women, transgender man; Cheung et al, 2020).

1.3.4 Physical Activity

The literature on physical activity, such as regular exercise, has been emerging over the past decade and has revealed some inconsistent findings that vary by gender. Among SMY, some evidence shows that queer youth are less likely than their heterosexual and cisgender peers to participate in physical activity, specifically team sports and engage in recommended daily physical activity (Bishop et al, 2020; Mereish & Poteat, 2015a). Findings from the Centers for Disease Control and Prevention's Youth Risk Behavior Surveillance System survey of 25 states showed that about 15% of SMY were physically active compared to 29% of heterosexual youth (Kann et al. 2018). Similarly, GMY are less likely to participate in sports and obtain the recommended daily exercise compared to cisgender youth (Bishop et al, 2020).

Among sexual minority adults, these findings are less consistent. Some work shows no sexual orientation differences in physical activity (Blosnich et al, 2014; Dilley et al, 2010), whereas one study shows that SMW are more physically active than heterosexual women (Everett & Mollborn, 2013), and and another study shows that they are less likely to be physically active (Zaritsky & Dibble, 2010). For instance, one study found that SMW obtain more hours of metabolic equivalent task exercise than heterosexual women, but SMW report sitting 4–5 hours more a week compared to heterosexual women (VanKim et al, 2017). Additionally, young sexual minorities are more likely to be physically inactive than heterosexuals (Rosario et al, 2016).

1.3.5   Dietary Behaviors

Some evidence shows that queer youth's diets are significantly lacking in nutrition compared to heterosexual and cisgender youth. SMY are less likely to eat breakfast, fruits, and vegetables and drink milk and water than heterosexual youth (Kann et al, 2018). SMY are significantly more likely to drink soda three times or more a day compared to heterosexual youth (Kann et al, 2018). Similarly, GMY are more likely to skip meals and consume fast food and soft drinks, and less likely to eat fruit or drink milk than cisgender youth (Bishop et al, 2020).

Lesbian women consume less daily vegetables compared to heterosexual women (Minnis et al, 2016). Gay men tend to eat one additional meal that is prepared outside of their home over a week than heterosexual men (Minnis et al, 2016). Gay men and SMW are more likely to consume sugar-sweetened beverages (e.g., soda or juice), than their heterosexual peers (Minnis et al, 2016). Black SMW are less likely to eat fruits and vegetables than White SMW (Molina et al, 2013). Lesbian women living in rural communities are more likely to have a high protein diet compared to lesbian women in urban areas (Barefoot et al, 2015). Moreover, young gay men are three times more likely to engage in vomiting for weight control than heterosexual men (Rosario et al, 2016).

1.3.6   Sexual Behavior

Studies show that some queer people engage in sexual behaviors that put them at greater risk for contracting STIs or becoming pregnant. For example, lesbian youth start engaging in sexual behaviors about 1 year younger than heterosexual young women (Ybarra et al, 2016); however, they are less likely use hormonal contraception compared to their bisexual and heterosexual youth counterparts (Charlton et al, 2013). Condom usage is significantly lower among SMY males compared to their heterosexual peers (Kann et al, 2018). Some gay and bisexual transgender men engage in high-risk sexual activity and 16% of them engaged in sex work during their lifetime (Bauer et al, 2013). Transgender women also have high rates of condom-less sex and sex work (Operario et al, 2011; Reback & Fletcher, 2014).

1.3.7   Health Screenings and Preventive Interventions

Routine health check-ups or screenings, such as vaginal or anal Pap smears, mammograms or regular STI testing, are essential for preventing and treating physical health conditions and ensuring optimal sexual health. However, the literature shows that queer people are less likely to engage or obtain these routine health check-ups (Charlton et al, 2011; Reiter & McRee, 2015). SMW are less likely to receive Pap tests and mammograms than women with only male sexual partners (Agenor et al, 2014; Buchmueller & Carpenter, 2010). A study of SMM living in NYC found that more Black (62%), Latino/Hispanic (54%), and Multiracial (54%) SMM sought out sexual health screenings compared to White (29%) and Asian (21%) SMM (Siconolfi et al, 2013). Gender minority adults also have low rates of obtaining a routine annual health checkup (Gonzales & Henning-Smith, 2017). Transgender men are also less likely to have an up-to-date pap test compared to cisgender women (Peitzmeier et al, 2014).

STI testing, such as HIV testing, is a critical part of preventing HIV infections and initiating treatment. SMM men are more likely to be tested for HIV than heterosexual men; however, bisexual men are less likely to do so than gay men (Lunn et al, 2017). Additionally, gay and bisexual transgender men have low rates of HIV testing (Bauer et al, 2013). A national study found that gay men and bisexual women had greater odds of obtaining an HIV test in their lifetime compared to their heterosexual peers within their same racial/ethnic group (Agénor et al, 2019). Moreover, the same study found that queer people across racial and ethnic groups were more likely to receive an HIV test in their lifetime compared to White heterosexual people, except for some Asian subgroups (e.g., Asian heterosexual, bisexual, and lesbian women and Asian bisexual and heterosexual men; Agénor et al, 2019). Lower rates of testing among Asian subgroups is attributed to HIV stigma and lack of access to sexual health information (Kang et al, 2003).

Pre-exposure prophlyaxis (PrEP) is a preventative medication that prevents contracting HIV (Grant et al, 2010). The use of PrEP among SMM and transgender individuals has been increasing (Wu et al, 2016). However, there are racial disparities in the uptake of PrEP, with Black and Latinx SMM are less likely to do so than White SMM (Kanny et al, 2019).

1.4   Etiological Factors

Multiple etiological influences explain the etiology of the aforementioned disparities in physical and sexual health outcomes and health risk behaviors. In addition to general factors that are known to influence these outcomes across populations (e.g., general stressors, mental health, societal norms), there are unique processes specific to queer people that contribute to their health.

1.4.1   Adverse Lifetime Experiences

Adverse and traumatic stressors over one's lifetime have long-term effects on physical health. These stressors have a toxic toll on physiological resources and stress response systems (McEwen, 2005). Adverse experiences make individuals more vulnerable to developing diseases as they weaken the immune system, exacerbate metabolic functions, and create physiological inflammation (Bennett et al, 2018).

Queer people experience heightened risk of a range of adverse stressors across their lifetime compared to heterosexual and cisgender people. For instance, queer people report higher prevalence of traumatic and adverse stressors, including childhood physical and sexual abuse, verbal, emotional, and physical victimization, and interpersonal violence than heterosexual and cisgender people (Dank et al, 2014; Friedman et al, 2011; Katz-Wise & Hyde, 2012; Reisner et al, 2015). These disparities are further exacerbated for transgender people, especially transgender women of color. Queer people are also more likely to experience homelessness in adolescence and adulthood (Corliss et al, 2011; Durso & Gates, 2012; Keuroghlian et al, 2014).

1.4.2   Interpersonal and Intrapersonal Stigma

In addition to general adverse life stressors, queer people experience unique and chronic stressors (i.e., minority stressors) related to their stigmatized and marginalized sexual orientation and gender identities, which also have negative effects on their health (Brooks, 1981; Meyer, 2003). These types of stressors are called minority stressors and range from distal minority stressors, which are external experiences of stigma (e.g., transphobic, biphobic, or heterosexist discrimination), to proximal minority stressors, which include internalized stigma (i.e., internalization of stigma into one's self-concept), identity concealment, and anticipation of stigmatizing experiences (Meyer, 2003; Testa et al, 2015). Research shows that minority stressors are associated with poor physical health outcomes for sexual minorities (Frost et al, 2015; Lick et al, 2013; Mereish & Poteat, 2015b). For example, experiences with discrimination and sexual identity concealment are negatively associated with physical and mental health-related quality of life among older queer adults (Fredriksen-Goldsen et al, 2014). Similarly, heterosexist discrimination and harassment and internalized heterosexism are associated with greater cardiovascular disease risk factors through their determinantal effects on sense of agency among sexual minorities (Mereish & Goldstein, 2020).

Several processes have been theorized to explain how minority stressors instigate poor physical health outcomes and greater health risk behaviors. Both distal and proximal minority stressors are posited to lead to poor mental health and a dysregulated physiological stress response; consequently, these have negative consequences to physiological functioning functioning (e.g., inflammation, gene expression alterations) and lead to poor physical health outcomes (e.g., cardiovascular disease, diabetes, cancer; Flentje et al, 2019; Li et al, 2020). Additionally, it is posited that minority stressors may lead to health risk behaviors (Lick et al, 2013). Queer people may engage in substance use, over eating, or risky sexual behaviors to manage or escape negative emotions related to stigma experiences, and some may avoid engaging in health promoting behaviors to protect themselves in stigmatizing contexts (e.g., transphobia related to bathroom use); and, in turn, these behaviors lead to long-term poor health (Lick et al, 2013). For instance, a large study of over 27,000 transgender people in the U.S. and its territories found that 59% of the sample avoided using public restrooms due to transphobia they might encounter, 32% restricted their food and liquids intake to avoid using restrooms, and 8% had a urinary tract infection or kidney-related problems due to avoiding restroom usage (James et al, 2016). Furthermore, minority stress may lead to compromised relational processes, such as feelings of shame and social isolation, which lead to poor mental and physical health (Mereish & Poteat, 2015b). Given that poor mental health has harmful effects on physical health, somatization of the mental distress of minority stress may also lead to poor physical health (Mereish & Poteat, 2015b).

Minority stressors are pervasive for queer people in every context in their lives (e.g., family, schools, workplace, communities, religious organizations), and they are also common in healthcare settings. Transgender people report significant transphobic experiences from their health providers. Over a third of transgender people report having negative experience from their health provider specifically related to them being transgender, including being refused treatement, and verbal, physical, or sexual harrassment by a health care provider (James et al, 2016). These negative experiences are also more common among transgender people of color and transgender people with disabilities. Health providers' negative attitudes toward and lack of cultural competence with queer people has significant effects on their health. For example, a fourth of transgender adults in a large study of transgender health reported avoiding seeing a doctor when needed because they were afraid of experiencing transphobia from their provider (James et al, 2016). Sexual minorities also report experiencing discrimination and heterosexism from their health providers (Baptiste-Roberts et al, 2017; Tabaac et al, 2019). Evidence shows that heterosexual health care providers have pervasive implicit homophobic attitudes toward sexual minorities (Sabin et al, 2015) (Fig. 1).

1.4.3 Structural Stigma

In addition to intrapersonal (e.g., internalized heterosexism) and interpersonal (e.g., transphobic discrimination) experiences with minority stress and stigma, queer people experience structural stigma (Hatzenbuehler, 2016). Structural stigma is evidenced at institutional and structural levels and includes policies, practices, and cultural norms that limit opportunities, constrain resources, and have negative implications for queer people's lives (Hatzenbuehler, 2016). Similar to minority stressors, structural stigma has toxic effects on physical health through dysregulated physiological stress response mechanisms as well as health behaviors. Compared to sexual minorities living in communities with low structural stigma, sexual minorities living in communities with high structural stigma have greater cardiometabolic risk over time (Hatzenbuehler et al, 2014b) and a 12-year lower life expectancy (Hatzenbuehler et al, 2014a). Moreover, a study of 38 European countries' levels of structural stigma (i.e., country laws and policies affecting sexual minorities, such as same-sex marriage or employment nondiscrimination laws, heterosexist attitudes held by the citizens of each country) found that SMM living in countries with high structural stigma were more likely to engage in risky sexual behavior and less likely to have access to HIV-preventive services (Pachankis et al, 2015).

There are other forms of institutional and structural oppression that queer people experience that have significant effects on their health. Sexual minorities in same-sex relationships are less likely to have health insurance coverage than individuals in other-sex relationships (Buchmueller & Carpenter, 2010). Transgender people report major structural barriers in accessing gender affirming health care. More than half of transgender people seeking gender affirming surgery and a quarter seeking gender affirming hormones are denied by their health insurance (James et al, 2016). Additionally, transgender people are three times more likely to be unemployed and twice more likely to live in poverty and be homeless than general U.S. adult population (James et al, 2016). Same-sex couples, and especially lesbian couples, Black

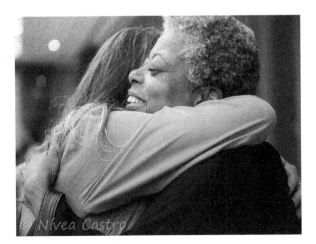

Fig. 1 Two friends hug at an event hosted by the Center for LGBTQ Studies. Photo by Nivea Castro

couples, and couples living in rural areas, are more likely to live in poverty than other-sex couples (Albelda et al, 2009). Furthermore, queer people have less access to inclusive and affirming education in school, such as sexual education (Guttmacher Institute, 2017).

1.5 Case Study

Sam is a 17-year-old biracial American Indian and Haitian American non-binary pansexual teenager who uses they/them pronouns. They perform well academically and excel in their reading and creative writing classes. Sam attends a high school that does not have gender neutral bathrooms, and their school does not have any LGBTQ-enumerated anti-bullying or anti-harassment policies. Sam is frequently bullied at school, including in bathrooms and locker rooms when they used to attend physical education (PE) class. Given the school's lack of gender-neutral bathrooms and locker rooms, Sam does not have access to a safe place to change and is required by the PE teacher to go the locker room that corresponds with their sex assigned at birth. Sam was often called homophobic, transphobic, and racist epithets and occasionally receives physical threats from their peers in these contexts. To avoid harassment and to feel safe, Sam no longer attends PE class, their primary source of physical exercise. Moreover, they limit drinking water and other liquids to avoid using the bathrooms at school. These experiences also contribute to Sam feeling alone, isolated, and ashamed, and in turn instigate feelings of depression and anxiety.

Sam's father is a truck driver who is often not home and their mother works as a babysitter and housekeeper. Due to their family's financial burdens, Sam cannot afford to pack lunch or buy a school lunch. Although Sam qualifies for free lunch at school, they typically consume soda and candy from the school's cafeteria vending machines as they attend an under resourced school that has poor quality food for students. Sam and their family also live in an area that is considered a "food desert", which limits their family's access to nutritious meals. Sam's parents do not allow Sam to participate in after school activities (e.g., sports) due to costs and time associated with these activities that conflicts with their parents' work schedules.

After Sam went through puberty, they experienced significant weight gain. This weight gain was exacerbated by their lack of access to a healthy and balanced diet as well as lack of regular physical activity. Therefore, Sam presents as obese and they are noticeably larger than their peers at school. Sam's chest and body size result in them experiencing significant gender dysphoria and psychological distress.

The school nurse likes Sam and has treated them for multiple urinary tract infections (UTIs). When the nurse discovered the cause of Sam's UTIs is related to their restricted liquid intake during school to avoid using school bathrooms and related harassment, he began to let Sam use the nurse's bathroom. Although the school nurse wants to help Sam, he often misgenders them as he often says to Sam that they/them pronouns are difficult to use.

Sam often spends their free time playing games on their phone and exploring queer and POC online groups, YouTube channels, and social media accounts. In a social media outlet, Sam discovered chest binding. They began binding their chest with duct tape they stole from school to compress their chest, so it appeared flat and more masculine and to affirm their non-binary gender identity. Experiencing their chest in a way that is aligned with their gender identity helped alleviate their symptoms of body dysmorphia and psychological distress. However, chest binding quickly began to cause frequent skin irritation, loss of breath, and back pain due to the use of duct tape, an unsafe method to bind. These complications also exacerbated Sam's asthma.

During a school day, Sam experienced shortness of breath and fell to the ground as they were unable to breath. A teacher called the school nurse to help, and the nurse assumed Sam was having an asthma attack and provided them with their inhaler. However, Sam's symptoms did not improve and the nurse called them an ambulance and alerted their parents that they are being sent to the hospital. Once Sam was carried away into the ambulance, the emergency medical technicians (EMTs) misgendered Sam and called them by their deadname (i.e., legal/given name). In an attempt to assess Sam's breathing difficulties, the EMTs cut open Sam's shirt and saw their chest compressed in duct tape and cut off the tape. When Sam was evaluated at the emergency room, Sam's doctor revealed that Sam experienced a small pneumothorax (i.e., collapsed lung) due to a compressed rib as a result of binding their chest tightly with duct tape over the past few months. In addition to their physical symptoms, Sam was anxious and distressed and their gender dysphoria was exacerbated as medical providers had to touch their chest to provide medical care. Sam also overheard two nurses whispering transphobic comments about them, making Sam feel distrustful of the medical providers and unsafe. Moreover, Sam's gender identity was outed to their parents and they discovered they were binding their chest, creating even more difficulties and distress for Sam.

Despite the lack of culturally competent medical care provided by the health providers, the hospital had an integrated care model, which included behavioral health providers. A psychologist, Dr. Gedeon reviewed Sam's chart and noticed the doctor's notes about Sam being transgender. Upon meeting Sam, Dr. Gedeon asked them for their name and pronouns and noticed that her name tag had her pronouns listed. The psychologist assessed Sam's mental and physical health concerns, helped them practice some coping skills to manage their immediate distress, and they set some goals to address their anxiety and bodyweight. She also referred Sam to a mental health provider at a local LGBTQ youth community center and provided Sam's parents with psycho-education to ensure they followed up on this referral.

Sam's parents reluctantly took them to the LGBTQ youth community center, Youth PRIDE, where they connected with the center's psychologist, Dr. Gomez. During their weekly sessions, Dr. Gomez took the time to build an affirming therapeutic relationship and learned more about Sam's strengths and resilience. Knowing that Sam enjoyed creative writing, Dr. Gomez asked Sam to share some of their writing with her and used therapeutic journaling interventions to help Sam feel more affirmed with their intersecting identities as well as better express and manage their thoughts and feelings. As a result, Sam was able to talk more freely about their experiences and identify skills to cope with racism, transphobia, and heterosexism, body dysmorphia, and related mental health concerns. Sam also developed tools they needed to talk to their family about being pansexual and non-binary and Dr. Gomez worked with Sam's parents to help them better understand ways to support them. She also connected their parents with other parents of transgender youth to help them become better parents and allies to Sam, which helped Sam's parents to allow them to bind their chest again. Sam received their first chest binder that is in a color that is similar to Sam's skin tone, which helped affirm their gender and racial identities. Sam also connected with other queer youth of color at Youth Pride and began to experience a sense of community that they longed for and that they were initially only able to access through social media.

Following up on the initial goals Sam set with Dr. Gedeon, Dr. Gomez worked with Sam to create a physical wellness plan, which included weekly physical activity in ways that were safe, enjoyable, and accessible to Sam (e.g., weekly free dancing and yoga classes at the Youth Pride, daily walks). She also worked with Sam to identify healthy foods in the cafeteria instead of consuming unhealthy snacks. In addition, Dr. Gomez helped Sam feel welcomed at Youth Pride's free nutritious community dinners. She also helped their parents connect with a city program tailored to providing low-income families with better access to healthy foods. Lastly, Dr. Gomez helped empower Sam and their parents to work with the school social worker and to advocate for a gender-neutral bathroom in their school (Fig. 2).

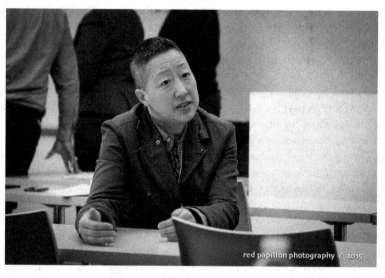

Fig. 2 Professor Sel Hwang, an expert on LGBTQ+ health issues, discusses their work at a conference. Photo by Riya Ortiz/Red Papillon Photography

References

Agaku, I. T., King, B. A., Husten, C. G., Bunnell, R., Ambrose, B. K., Hu, S. S., Holder-Hayes, E., Day, H. R., & Centers for Disease Control and Prevention (CDC). (2014). Tobacco product use among adults—United States, 2012-2013. *MMWR. Morbidity and Mortality Weekly Report, 63*(25), 542–547.

Agenor, M., Krieger, N., Austin, S. B., Haneuse, S., & Gottlieb, B. R. (2014). At the intersection of sexual orientation, race/ethnicity, and cervical cancer screening: Assessing pap test use disparities by sex of sexual partners among black, Latina, and white U.S. women. *Social Science & Medicine, 116*, 110–118. https://doi.org/10.1016/j.socscimed.2014.06.039.

Agénor, M., Pérez, A. E., Koma, J. W., Abrams, J. A., McGregor, A. J., & Ojikutu, B. O. (2019). Sexual orientation identity, race/ethnicity, and lifetime HIV testing in a National Probability Sample of U.S. women and men: An intersectional approach. *LGBT Health, 6*(6), 306–318. https://doi.org/10.1089/lgbt.2019.0001.

Albelda, R., Badgett, M. V. L., Gates, G., & Schneebaum, A. (2009). Poverty in the lesbian, gay, and bisexual community. Los Angeles: Williams Institute, UCLA.

Alzahrani, T., Nguyen, T., Ryan, A., Dwairy, A., McCaffrey, J., Yunus, R., Forgione, J., Krepp, J., Nagy, C., Mazhari, R., & Reiner, J. (2019). Cardiovascular disease risk factors and myocardial infarction in the transgender population. *Circulation: Cardiovascular Quality and Outcomes, 12*(4), e005597. https://doi.org/10.1161/CIRCOUTCOMES.119.005597.

Baptiste-Roberts, K., Oranuba, E., Werts, N., & Edwards, L. V. (2017). Addressing health care disparities among sexual minorities. *Obstetrics and Gynecology Clinics of North America, 44*(1), 71–80. https://doi.org/10.1016/j.ogc.2016.11.003.

Barefoot, K. N., Warren, J. C., & Smalley, K. B. (2015). An examination of past and current influences of rurality on lesbians' overweight/obesity risks. *LGBT Health, 2*(2), 154–161. https://doi.org/10.1089/lgbt.2014.0112.

Bauer, G. R., Redman, N., Bradley, K., & Scheim, A. I. (2013). Sexual health of trans men who are gay, bisexual, or who have sex with men: Results from Ontario, Canada. *International Journal of Transgenderism, 14*(2), 66–74. https://doi.org/10.1080/15532739.2013.791650.

Beach, L. B., Elasy, T. A., & Gonzales, G. (2018). Prevalence of self-reported diabetes by sexual orientation: Results from the 2014 behavioral risk factor surveillance system. *LGBT Health, 5*(2), 121–130. https://doi.org/10.1089/lgbt.2017.0091.

Becasen, J. S., Denard, C. L., Mullins, M. M., Higa, D. H., & Sipe, T. A. (2018). Estimating the prevalence of HIV and sexual behaviors among the US transgender population: A systematic review and meta-analysis, 2006–2017. *American Journal of Public Health, 109*(1), e1–e8. https://doi.org/10.2105/AJPH.2018.304727.

Bennett, J. M., Reeves, G., Billman, G. E., & Sturmberg, J. P. (2018). Inflammation-nature's way to efficiently respond to all types of challenges: Implications for understanding and managing "the epidemic" of chronic diseases. *Frontiers in Medicine, 5*, 316–316. https://doi.org/10.3389/fmed.2018.00316.

Benson, P. A., & Hergenroeder, A. C. (2005). Bacterial sexually transmitted infections in gay, lesbian, and bisexual adolescents: Medical and public health perspectives. *Seminars in Pediatric Infectious Diseases, 16*(3), 181–191. https://doi.org/10.1053/j.spid.2005.04.007.

Bishop, A., Overcash, F., McGuire, J., & Reicks, M. (2020). Diet and physical activity behaviors among adolescent transgender students: School survey results. *Journal of Adolescent Health, 66*(4), 484–490. https://doi.org/10.1016/j.jadohealth.2019.10.026.

Blosnich, J. R., Farmer, G. W., Lee, J. G. L., Silenzio, V. M. B., & Bowen, D. J. (2014). Health inequalities among sexual minority adults: Evidence from ten U.S. states, 2010. *American Journal of Preventive Medicine, 46*(4), 337–349. https://doi.org/10.1016/j.amepre.2013.11.010.

Blosnich, J. R., Jarrett, T., & Horn, K. (2011). Racial and ethnic differences in current use of cigarettes, cigars, and hookahs among lesbian, gay, and bisexual young adults. *Nicotine & Tobacco Research, 13*(6), 487–491. https://doi.org/10.1093/ntr/ntq261.

Boehmer, U., Miao, X., Maxwell, N., & Ozonoff, A. (2014). Sexual minority population density and incidence of lung, colorectal and female breast cancer in California. *BMJ Open, 4*(3), e004461. https://doi.org/10.1136/bmjopen-2013-004461.

Boehmer, U., Ozonoff, A., & Miao, X. (2012). An ecological approach to examine lung cancer disparities due to sexual orientation. *Public Health, 126*(7), 605–612. https://doi.org/10.1016/j.puhe.2012.04.004.

Brooks, V. R. (1981). *Minority stress and lesbian women*. New York: Free Press.

Buchmueller, T., & Carpenter, C. S. (2010). Disparities in health insurance coverage, access, and outcomes for individuals in same-sex versus different-sex relationships, 2000–2007. *American Journal of Public Health, 100*(3), 489–495. https://doi.org/10.2105/AJPH.2009.160804.

Caceres, B. A., Brody, A., Luscombe, R. E., Primiano, J. E., Marusca, P., Sitts, E. M., & Chyun, D. (2017). A systematic review of cardiovascular disease in sexual minorities. *American Journal of Public Health, 107*(4), e13–e21. https://doi.org/10.2105/ajph.2016.303630.

Caceres, B. A., Jackman, K. B., Edmondson, D., & Bockting, W. O. (2020). Assessing gender identity differences in cardiovascular disease in US adults: An analysis of data from the 2014–2017 BRFSS. *Journal of Behavioral Medicine, 43*(2), 329–338. https://doi.org/10.1007/s10865-019-00102-8.

Cappuccio, F. P., Cooper, D., D'Elia, L., Strazzullo, P., & Miller, M. A. (2011). Sleep duration predicts cardiovascular outcomes: A systematic review and meta-analysis of prospective studies. *European Heart Journal, 32*(12), 1484–1492. https://doi.org/10.1093/eurheartj/ehr007.

Centers for Disease Control and Prevention. (2018). *Diagnoses of HIV infection in the United States and dependent areas, 2017*. Retrieved from Atlanta, Georgia: https://www.cdc.gov/hiv/pdf/library/reports/surveillance/cdc-hiv-surveillance-report-2017-vol-29.pdf

Charlton, B. M., Corliss, H. L., Missmer, S. A., Frazier, A. L., Rosario, M., Kahn, J. A., & Austin, S. B. (2011). Reproductive health screening disparities and sexual orientation in a cohort study of U.S. adolescent and young adult females. *Journal of Adolescent Health, 49*(5), 505–510. https://doi.org/10.1016/j.jadohealth.2011.03.013.

Charlton, B. M., Corliss, H. L., Missmer, S. A., Rosario, M., Spiegelman, D., & Austin, S. B. (2013). Sexual orientation differences in teen pregnancy and hormonal contraceptive use: An examination across 2 generations. *American Journal of Obstetrics and Gynecology, 209*(3), 204. e201–204.e208. https://doi.org/10.1016/j.ajog.2013.06.036.

Charlton, B. M., Roberts, A. L., Rosario, M., Katz-Wise, S. L., Calzo, J. P., Spiegelman, D., & Austin, S. B. (2018). Teen pregnancy risk factors among young women of diverse sexual orientations. Pediatrics, 141(4).

Chen, J., & Shiu, C.-S. (2017). Sexual orientation and sleep in the US: A national profile. *American Journal of Preventive Medicine, 52*(4), 433–442.

Chen, X., Gelaye, B., & Williams, M. A. (2014). Sleep characteristics and health-related quality of life among a national sample of American young adults: Assessment of possible health disparities. *Quality of Life Research, 23*(2), 613–625. https://doi.org/10.1007/s11136-013-0475-9.

Cheung, A. S., Leemaqz, S. Y., Wong, J. W., Chew, D., Ooi, O., Cundill, P., Silberstein, N., Locke, P., Zwickl, S., Grayson, R., Zajac, J. D., & Pang, K. C. (2020). Non-binary and binary gender identity in Australian trans and gender diverse individuals. *Archives of Sexual Behavior, 49*, 2673–2681.

Clark, H., Babu, A. S., Wiewel, E. W., Opoku, J., & Crepaz, N. (2017). Diagnosed HIV infection in transgender adults and adolescents: Results from the national HIV surveillance system, 2009–2014. *AIDS and Behavior, 21*(9), 2774–2783. https://doi.org/10.1007/s10461-016-1656-7.

Cochran, S. D., & Mays, V. M. (2012). Risk of breast cancer mortality among women cohabiting with same sex partners: Findings from the National Health Interview Survey, 1997–2003. *Journal of Women's Health, 21*(5), 528–533. https://doi.org/10.1089/jwh.2011.3134.

Corliss, H. L., Goodenow, C. S., Nichols, L., & Austin, S. B. (2011). High burden of homelessness among sexual-minority adolescents: Findings from a representative Massachusetts high school sample. *American Journal of Public Health, 101*(9), 1683–1689. https://doi.org/10.2105/AJPH.2011.300155.

Dai, H., & Hao, J. (2019). Sleep deprivation and chronic health conditions among sexual minority adults. *Behavioral Sleep Medicine, 17*(3), 254–268. https://doi.org/10.1080/15402002.2017.1342166.

Dank, M., Lachman, P., Zweig, J., & Yahner, J. (2014). Dating violence experiences of lesbian, gay, bisexual, and transgender youth. *Journal of Youth and Adolescence, 43*(5), 846–857. https://doi.org/10.1007/s10964-013-9975-8.

Day, J. K., Fish, J. N., Perez-Brumer, A., Hatzenbuehler, M. L., & Russell, S. T. (2017). Transgender youth substance use disparities: Results from a population-based sample. *Journal of Adolescent Health, 61*(6), 729–735. https://doi.org/10.1016/j.jadohealth.2017.06.024.

Dilley, J. A., Simmons, K. W., Boysun, M. J., Pizacani, B. A., & Stark, M. J. (2010). Demonstrating the importance and feasibility of including sexual orientation in public health surveys: Health disparities in the Pacific northwest. *American Journal of Public Health, 100*(3), 460–467. https://doi.org/10.2105/AJPH.2007.130336.

Durso, L.E., & Gates, G.J. (2012). Serving Our Youth: Findings from a National Survey of Service Providers Working with Lesbian, Gay, Bisexual, and Transgender Youth who are Homeless or At Risk of Becoming Homeless. Los Angeles: The Williams Institute with True Colors Fund and The Palette Fund.

Everett, B. G. (2013). Sexual orientation disparities in sexually transmitted infections: Examining the intersection between sexual identity and sexual behavior. *Archives of Sexual Behavior, 42*(2), 225–236. https://doi.org/10.1007/s10508-012-9902-1.

Everett, B. G., & Mollborn, S. (2013). Differences in hypertension by sexual orientation among U.S. young adults. *Journal of Community Health, 38*(3), 588–596. https://doi.org/10.1007/s10900-013-9655-3.

Fish, J. N., Watson, R. J., Porta, C. M., Russell, S. T., & Saewyc, E. M. (2017). Are alcohol-related disparities between sexual minority and heterosexual youth decreasing? *Addiction, 112*(11), 1931–1941. https://doi.org/10.1111/add.13896.

Flentje, A., Heck, N. C., Brennan, J. M., & Meyer, I. H. (2019). The relationship between minority stress and biological outcomes: A systematic review. *Journal of Behavioral Medicine.* https://doi.org/10.1007/s10865-019-00120-6.

Fredriksen-Goldsen, K. I., Kim, H.-J., & Barkan, S. E. (2012). Disability among lesbian, gay, and bisexual adults: Disparities in prevalence and risk. *American Journal of Public Health, 102*(1), e16–e21. https://doi.org/10.2105/AJPH.2011.300379.

Fredriksen-Goldsen, K. I., Kim, H.-J., Shiu, C., Goldsen, J., & Emlet, C. A. (2014). Successful aging among LGBT older adults: Physical and mental health-related quality of life by age group. *The Gerontologist, 55*(1), 154–168. https://doi.org/10.1093/geront/gnu081.

Friedman, M. S., Marshal, M. P., Guadamuz, T. E., Wei, C., Wong, C. F., Saewyc, E. M., & Stall, R. (2011). A meta-analysis of disparities in childhood sexual abuse, parental physical abuse, and peer victimization among sexual minority and sexual nonminority individuals. *American Journal of Public Health, 101*(8), 1481–1494. https://doi.org/10.2105/AJPH.2009.190009.

Frost, D. M., Lehavot, K., & Meyer, I. H. (2015). Minority stress and physical health among sexual minority individuals. *Journal of Behavioral Medicine, 38*(1), 1–8. https://doi.org/10.1007/s10865-013-9523-8.

Galinsky, A. M., Ward, B. W., Joestl, S. S., & Dahlhamer, J. M. (2018). Sleep duration, sleep quality, and sexual orientation: Findings from the 2013-2015 National Health Interview Survey. *Sleep Health, 4*(1), 56–62. https://doi.org/10.1016/j.sleh.2017.10.004.

Gilbert, P. A., Drabble, L., Daniel-Ulloa, J., & Trocki, K. F. (2017). Alcohol outcomes by sexual orientation and race/ethnicity: Few findings of higher risk. *Journal of Studies on Alcohol and Drugs, 78*(3), 406–414. https://doi.org/10.15288/jsad.2017.78.406.

Goldbach, J. T., Mereish, E. H., & Burgess, C. (2017). Sexual orientation disparities in the use of emerging drugs. *Substance Use & Misuse, 52*(2), 265–271.

Gonzales, G., & Henning-Smith, C. (2017). Barriers to care among transgender and gender nonconforming adults. *The Milbank Quarterly, 95*(4), 726–748. https://doi.org/10.1111/1468-0009.12297.

Gonzalez, C. A., Gallego, J. D., & Bockting, W. O. (2017). Demographic characteristics, components of sexuality and gender, and minority stress and their associations to excessive alcohol, Cannabis, and illicit (noncannabis) drug use among a large sample of transgender people in the United States. *The Journal of Primary Prevention, 38*(4), 419–445. https://doi.org/10.1007/s10935-017-0469-4.

Grant, R. M., Lama, J. R., Anderson, P. L., McMahan, V., Liu, A. Y., Vargas, L., Goicochea, P., Casapía, M., Guanira-Carranza, J. V., Ramirez-Cardich, M. E., Montoya-Herrera, O., Fernández, T., Veloso, V. G., Buchbinder, S. P., Chariyalertsak, S., Schechter, M., Bekker, L. G., Mayer, K. H., Kallás, E. G., Amico, K. R., Mulligan, K., Bushman, L. R., Hance, R. J., Ganoza, C., Defechereux, P., Postle, B., Wang, F., JJ, M. C., Zheng, J. H., Lee, J., Rooney, J. F., Jaffe, H. S., Martinez, A. I., Burns, D. N., Glidden, D. V., & iPrEx Study Team. (2010). Preexposure chemoprophylaxis for HIV prevention in men who have sex with men. *New England Journal of Medicine, 363*(27), 2587–2599. https://doi.org/10.1056/NEJMoa1011205.

Guttmacher Institute. (2017). *State Laws and Policies: Sex and HIV education*. Retrieved from https://www.guttmacher.org/state-policy/explore/sex-and-hiv-education#

Hammond, N. G., & Stinchcombe, A. (2019). Health behaviors and social determinants of migraine in a Canadian population-based sample of adults aged 45-85 years: Findings from the CLSA. *Headache, 59*(9), 1547–1564. https://doi.org/10.1111/head.13610.

Hatzenbuehler, M. L. (2016). Structural stigma: Research evidence and implications for psychological science. *The American Psychologist, 71*(8), 742–751. https://doi.org/10.1037/amp0000068.

Hatzenbuehler, M. L., Bellatorre, A., Lee, Y., Finch, B. K., Muennig, P., & Fiscella, K. (2014a). Structural stigma and all-cause mortality in sexual minority populations. *Social Science & Medicine, 103*, 33–41. https://doi.org/10.1016/j.socscimed.2013.06.005.

Hatzenbuehler, M. L., Slopen, N., & McLaughlin, K. A. (2014b). Stressful life events, sexual orientation, and cardiometabolic risk among young adults in the United States. *Health Psychology, 33*(10), 1185.

Herbst, J. H., Jacobs, E. D., Finlayson, T. J., McKleroy, V. S., Neumann, M. S., Crepaz, N., & HIV/AIDS Prevention Research Synthesis Team. (2008). Estimating HIV prevalence and risk behaviors of transgender persons in the United States: A systematic review. *AIDS and Behavior, 12*(1), 1–17. https://doi.org/10.1007/s10461-007-9299-3.

Howlader, N., Noone, A., Krapcho, M., Garshell, J., Miller, D., Altekruse, S., Kosary, C. L., Yu, M., Ruhl, J., & Tatalovich, Z. (2015). *SEER cancer statistics review, 1975–2012*. Bethesda, MD: National Cancer Institute.

Hughes, T. L., Wilsnack, S. C., & Kantor, L. W. (2016). The influence of gender and sexual orientation on alcohol use and alcohol-related problems: Toward a global perspective. *Alcohol Research: Current Reviews, 38*(1), 121–132.

James, S. E., Herman, J. L., Rankin, S., Keisling, M., Mottet, L., & Anafi, M. (2016). The Report of the 2015 U.S. Transgender Survey. Washington, DC: National Center for Transgender Equality.

Joint, R., Chen, Z. E., & Cameron, S. (2018). Breast and reproductive cancers in the transgender population: A systematic review. *BJOG: An International Journal of Obstetrics & Gynaecology, 125*(12), 1505–1512. https://doi.org/10.1111/1471-0528.15258.

Kang, E., Rapkin, B. D., Springer, C., & Kim, J. H. (2003). The "demon plague" and access to care among Asian undocumented immigrants living with HIV disease in new York City. *Journal of Immigrant Health, 5*(2), 49–58. https://doi.org/10.1023/A:1022999507903.

Kann, L., McManus, T., Harris, W. A., Shanklin, S. L., Flint, K. H., Queen, B., Lowry, R., Chyen, D., Whittle, L., Thornton, J., Lim, C., Bradford, D., Yamakawa, Y., Leon, M., Brener, N., & Ethier, K. A. (2018). Youth risk behavior surveillance—United States, 2017. *Morbidity and mortality weekly report. Surveillance summaries (Washington, D.C.:2002), 67*(8), 1–114. https://doi.org/10.15585/mmwr.ss6708a1.

Kanny, D., Jeffries, W. L., IV, Chapin-Bardales, J., Denning, P., Cha, S., Finlayson, T., Wejnert, C., & Anderson, B. (2019). Racial/ethnic disparities in HIV preexposure prophylaxis among men who have sex with men—23 urban areas, 2017. *Morbidity and Mortality Weekly Report, 68*(37), 801.

Kerr, D., Ding, K., Burke, A., & Ott-Walter, K. (2015). An alcohol, tobacco, and other drug use comparison of lesbian, bisexual, and heterosexual undergraduate women. *Substance Use & Misuse, 50*(3), 340–349.

Katz-Wise, S. L., & Hyde, J. S. (2012). Victimization experiences of lesbian, gay, and bisexual individuals: A meta-analysis. *The Journal of Sex Research, 49*(2–3), 142–167. https://doi.org/1 0.1080/00224499.2011.637247.

Keuroghlian, A. S., Shtasel, D., & Bassuk, E. L. (2014). Out on the street: A public health and policy agenda for lesbian, gay, bisexual, and transgender youth who are homeless. *The American Journal of Orthopsychiatry, 84*(1), 66–72. https://doi.org/10.1037/h0098852.

Kidd, J. D., Dolezal, C., & Bockting, W. O. (2018). The relationship between tobacco use and legal document gender-marker change, hormone use, and gender-affirming surgery in a United States sample of trans-feminine and trans-masculine individuals: Implications for cardiovascular health. *LGBT Health, 5*(7), 401–411. https://doi.org/10.1089/lgbt.2018.0103.

Li, M. J., Takada, S., Okafor, C. N., Gorbach, P. M., Shoptaw, S. J., & Cole, S. W. (2020). Experienced homophobia and gene expression alterations in black and Latino men who have sex with men in Los Angeles County. *Brain, Behavior, and Immunity, 83*, 120–125. https://doi.org/10.1016/j.bbi.2019.09.021.

Li, P., Huang, Y., Guo, L., Wang, W., Xi, C., Lei, Y., Luo, M., Pan, S., Deng, X., Zhang, W.-H., & Lu, C. (2017). Is sexual minority status associated with poor sleep quality among adolescents? Analysis of a national cross-sectional survey in Chinese adolescents. *BMJ Open, 7*(12), e017067. https://doi.org/10.1136/bmjopen-2017-017067.

Lick, D. J., Durso, L. E., & Johnson, K. L. (2013). Minority stress and physical health among sexual minorities. *Perspectives on Psychological Science, 8*(5), 521–548. https://doi.org/10.1177/1745691613497965.

Lunn, M. R., Cui, W., Zack, M. M., Thompson, W. W., Blank, M. B., & Yehia, B. R. (2017). Sociodemographic characteristics and health outcomes among lesbian, gay, and bisexual U.S. adults using healthy people 2020 leading health indicators. *LGBT Health, 4*(4), 283–294. https://doi.org/10.1089/lgbt.2016.0087.

Machalek, D. A., Poynten, M., Jin, F., Fairley, C. K., Farnsworth, A., Garland, S. M., Hillman, R. J., Petoumenos, K., Roberts, J., Tabrizi, S. N., Templeton, D. J., & Grulich, A. E. (2012). Anal human papillomavirus infection and associated neoplastic lesions in men who have sex with men: A systematic review and meta-analysis. *The Lancet Oncology, 13*(5), 487–500. https://doi.org/10.1016/S1470-2045(12)70080-3.

Mansh, M., Katz, K. A., Linos, E., Chren, M.-M., & Arron, S. (2015). Association of skin cancer and indoor tanning in sexual minority men and women. *JAMA Dermatology, 151*(12), 1308–1316. https://doi.org/10.1001/jamadermatol.2015.3126.

Mays, V. M., Yancey, A. K., Cochran, S. D., Weber, M., & Fielding, J. E. (2002). Heterogeneity of health disparities among African American, Hispanic, and Asian American women: Unrecognized influences of sexual orientation. *American Journal of Public Health, 92*(4), 632–639. https://doi.org/10.2105/AJPH.92.4.632.

McEwen, B. S. (2005). Stressed or stressed out: What is the difference? *Journal of psychiatry & neuroscience: JPN, 30*(5), 315–318.

Medley, G., Lipari, R., Bose, J., Cribb, D., Kroutil, L., & McHenry, G. (2016). Sexual orientation and estimates of adult substance use and mental health: Results from the 2015 National Survey on drug use and health. *NSDUH Data Review*, 1–54.

Mereish, E. H. (2019). Substance use and misuse among sexual and gender minority youth. *Current Opinion in Psychology, 30*, 123–127.

Mereish, E. H., & Bradford, J. B. (2014). Intersecting identities and substance use problems: Sexual orientation, gender, race, and lifetime substance use problems. *Journal of Studies on Alcohol and Drugs, 75*(1), 179–188. https://doi.org/10.15288/jsad.2014.75.179.

Mereish, E. H., & Goldstein, C. (2020). Minority stress and cardiovascular disease risk among sexual minorities: Mediating effects of diminished sense of mastery. *International Journal of Behavioral Medicine, 27*, 726–736.

Mereish, E. H., & Poteat, V. P. (2015a). Let's get physical: Sexual orientation disparities in physical activity, sports involvement, and obesity among a population-based sample of adolescents. *American Journal of Public Health, 105*(9), 1842–1848. https://doi.org/10.2105/AJPH.2015.302682.

Mereish, E. H., & Poteat, V. P. (2015b). A relational model of sexual minority mental and physical health: The negative effects of shame on relationships, loneliness, and health. *Journal of Counseling Psychology, 62*(3), 425–437. https://doi.org/10.1037/cou0000088.

Meyer, I. H. (2003). Prejudice, social stress, and mental health in lesbian, gay, and bisexual populations: Conceptual issues and research evidence. *Psychological Bulletin, 129*(5), 674.

Minnis, A. M., Catellier, D., Kent, C., Ethier, K. A., Soler, R. E., Heirendt, W., Halpern, M. T., & Rogers, T. (2016). Differences in chronic disease behavioral indicators by sexual orientation and sex. *Journal of Public Health Management and Practice: JPHMP, 22*(Suppl 1), S25–S32. https://doi.org/10.1097/PHH.0000000000000350.

Mojola, S. A., & Everett, B. (2012). STD and HIV risk factors among U.S. young adults: Variations by gender, race, ethnicity and sexual orientation. *Perspectives on Sexual and Reproductive Health, 44*(2), 125–133. https://doi.org/10.1363/4412512.

Molina, Y., Lehavot, K., Beadnell, B., & Simoni, J. (2013). Racial disparities in health behaviors and conditions among lesbian and bisexual women: The role of internalized stigma. *LGBT Health, 1*(2), 131–139. https://doi.org/10.1089/lgbt.2013.0007.

Nicopoullos, J. D. M., Almeida, P., Vourliotis, M., & Gilling-Smith, C. (2011). A decade of the sperm-washing programme: Correlation between markers of HIV and seminal parameters. *HIV Medicine, 12*(4), 195–201. https://doi.org/10.1111/j.1468-1293.2010.00868.x.

Operario, D., Nemoto, T., Iwamoto, M., & Moore, T. (2011). Unprotected sexual behavior and HIV risk in the context of primary partnerships for transgender women. *AIDS and Behavior, 15*(3), 674–682. https://doi.org/10.1007/s10461-010-9795-8.

Pachankis, J. E., Hatzenbuehler, M. L., Hickson, F., Weatherburn, P., Berg, R. C., Marcus, U., & Schmidt, A. J. (2015). Hidden from health: Structural stigma, sexual orientation concealment, and HIV across 38 countries in the European MSM Internet Survey. *AIDS (London, England), 29*(10), 1239–1246. https://doi.org/10.1097/QAD.0000000000000724.

Peitzmeier, S. M., Khullar, K., Reisner, S. L., & Potter, J. (2014). Pap test use is lower among female-to-male patients than non-transgender women. *American Journal of Preventive Medicine, 47*(6), 808–812. https://doi.org/10.1016/j.amepre.2014.07.031.

Reback, C. J., & Fletcher, J. B. (2014). HIV prevalence, substance use, and sexual risk behaviors among transgender women recruited through outreach. *AIDS and Behavior, 18*(7), 1359–1367. https://doi.org/10.1007/s10461-013-0657-z.

Reisner, S. L., Greytak, E. A., Parsons, J. T., & Ybarra, M. L. (2015). Gender minority social stress in adolescence: Disparities in adolescent bullying and substance use by gender identity. *Journal of Sex Research, 52*(3), 243–256. https://doi.org/10.1080/00224499.2014.886321.

Reiter, P. L., & McRee, A.-L. (2015). Cervical cancer screening (Pap testing) behaviours and acceptability of human papillomavirus self-testing among lesbian and bisexual women aged 21–26 years in the USA. *Journal of Family Planning and Reproductive Health Care, 41*(4), 259. https://doi.org/10.1136/jfprhc-2014-101004.

Rosario, M., Li, F., Wypij, D., Roberts, A. L., Corliss, H. L., Charlton, B. M., Frazier, A. L., & Austin, S. B. (2016). Disparities by sexual orientation in frequent engagement in cancer-related risk behaviors: A 12-year follow-up. *American Journal of Public Health, 106*(4), 698–706. https://doi.org/10.2105/AJPH.2015.302977.

Russo, J., Moral, R., Balogh, G. A., Mailo, D., & Russo, I. H. (2005). The protective role of pregnancy in breast cancer. *Breast Cancer Research, 7*(3), 131. https://doi.org/10.1186/bcr1029.

Sabin, J. A., Riskind, R. G., & Nosek, B. A. (2015). Health care providers' implicit and explicit attitudes toward lesbian women and gay men. *American Journal of Public Health, 105*(9), 1831–1841. https://doi.org/10.2105/AJPH.2015.302631.

Schuler, M. S., & Collins, R. L. (2020). Sexual minority substance use disparities: Bisexual women at elevated risk relative to other sexual minority groups. *Drug and Alcohol Dependence, 206*, 107755. https://doi.org/10.1016/j.drugalcdep.2019.107755.

Schuler, M. S., Prince, D. M., Breslau, J., & Collins, R. L. (2020). Substance use disparities at the intersection of sexual identity and race/ethnicity: Results from the 2015–2018 National Survey on Drug Use and Health. *LGBT Health.* https://doi.org/10.1089/lgbt.2019.0352.

Schuler, M. S., Stein, B. D., & Collins, R. L. (2019). Differences in substance use disparities across age groups in a national cross-sectional survey of lesbian, gay, and bisexual adults. *LGBT Health, 6*(2), 68–76. https://doi.org/10.1089/lgbt.2018.0125.

Shires, D. A., & Jaffee, K. D. (2016). Structural discrimination is associated with smoking status among a national sample of transgender individuals. *Nicotine & Tobacco Research, 18*(6), 1502–1508. https://doi.org/10.1093/ntr/ntv221.

Siconolfi, D. E., Kapadia, F., Halkitis, P. N., Moeller, R. W., Storholm, E. D., Barton, S. C., Solomon, T. M., & Jones, D. (2013). Sexual health screening among racially/ethnically diverse young gay, bisexual, and other men who have sex with men. *Journal of Adolescent Health, 52*(5), 620–626. https://doi.org/10.1016/j.jadohealth.2012.10.002.

Simoni, J. M., Smith, L., Oost, K. M., Lehavot, K., & Fredriksen-Goldsen, K. (2017). Disparities in physical health conditions among lesbian and bisexual women: A systematic review of population-based studies. *Journal of Homosexuality, 64*(1), 32–44. https://doi.org/10.108 0/00918369.2016.1174021.

Streed, C. G., Harfouch, O., Marvel, F., Blumenthal, R. S., Martin, S. S., & Mukherjee, M. (2017). Cardiovascular disease among transgender adults receiving hormone therapy. *Annals of Internal Medicine, 167*(4), 256–267. https://doi.org/10.7326/M17-0577.

Tabaac, A. R., Benotsch, E. G., & Barnes, A. J. (2019). Mediation models of perceived medical heterosexism, provider–patient relationship quality, and cervical Cancer screening in a community sample of sexual minority women and gender nonbinary adults. *LGBT Health, 6*(2), 77–86. https://doi.org/10.1089/lgbt.2018.0203.

Testa, R. J., Habarth, J., Peta, J., Balsam, K., & Bockting, W. (2015). Development of the gender minority stress and resilience measure. *Psychology of Sexual Orientation and Gender Diversity, 2*(1), 65.

Van Gerwen, O. T., Jani, A., Long, D. M., Austin, E. L., Musgrove, K., & Muzny, C. A. (2020). Prevalence of sexually transmitted infections and human immunodeficiency virus in transgender persons: A systematic review. *Transgender Health, 5*(2), 90–103. https://doi.org/10.1089/trgh.2019.0053.

VanKim, N. A., Austin, S. B., Jun, H.-J., & Corliss, H. L. (2017). Physical activity and sedentary behaviors among lesbian, bisexual, and heterosexual women: Findings from the Nurses' health study II. *Journal of Women's Health, 26*(10), 1077–1085. https://doi.org/10.1089/jwh.2017.6389.

Veale, J., Watson, R. J., Adjei, J., & Saewyc, E. (2016). Prevalence of pregnancy involvement among Canadian transgender youth and its relation to mental health, sexual health, and gender identity. *The international Journal of Transgenderism, 17*(3–4), 107–113. https://doi.org/1 0.1080/15532739.2016.1216345.

Watson, R. J., Lewis, N. M., Fish, J. N., & Goodenow, C. (2018). Sexual minority youth continue to smoke cigarettes earlier and more often than heterosexuals: Findings from population-based data. *Drug and Alcohol Dependence, 184*, 64–70. https://doi.org/10.1016/j.drugalcdep.2017.11.025.

Wu, H., Mendoza, M. C. B., Huang, Y.-L. A., Hayes, T., Smith, D. K., & Hoover, K. W. (2016). Uptake of HIV preexposure prophylaxis among commercially insured persons—United States, 2010–2014. *Clinical Infectious Diseases, 64*(2), 144–149. https://doi.org/10.1093/cid/ciw701.

Ybarra, M. L., Rosario, M., Saewyc, E., & Goodenow, C. (2016). Sexual behaviors and partner characteristics by sexual identity among adolescent girls. *Journal of Adolescent Health, 58*(3), 310–316. https://doi.org/10.1016/j.jadohealth.2015.11.001.

Zaritsky, E., & Dibble, S. L. (2010). Risk factors for reproductive and breast cancers among older lesbians. *Journal of Women's Health, 19*(1), 125–131. https://doi.org/10.1089/jwh.2008.1094.

Context Matters: Minority Stress and Mental Health Experiences of Diverse LGBTQ People

Brandon L. Velez, David Zelaya, and Jillian Scheer

1 Mental Health Disparities

In 2016, the National Institute for Health (NIH) officially designated sexual and gender minority people as health disparities populations and declared that more research is needed to understand their mental and physical health. Researchers have documented that the prevalence of psychiatric diagnoses—such as mood disorders (e.g., major depressive disorder), anxiety disorders, and substance use disorders— and mental health service utilization are higher among lesbian, gay, bisexual, trans- gender, and queer (LGBTQ) individuals compared to their heterosexual and/or cisgender counterparts (e.g., Cochran et al., 2003; Mongelli et al., 2019; Lefevor et al., 2019). For example, LGBQ people are 1.5 times more likely to receive mental health or substance use diagnoses than heterosexual people (King et al., 2008) and transgender individuals are 1.7 times more likely to receive such diagnoses than cisgender individuals (Meyer et al., 2017). Furthermore, suicidal ideation and attempts are greater among LGBQ people—and bisexual people in particular—than heterosexual people (Salway et al., 2019). Similarly, a large sample (N = 27,715) of transgender adults in the United States (U.S.) found that 40% had ever attempted suicide (James et al., 2016)—which is much higher than the 4.6% observed in the

B. L. Velez (✉)
Department of Counseling and Clinical Psychology,
Teachers College—Columbia University, New York, NY, USA
e-mail: blv2106@tc.columbia.edu

D. Zelaya
Department of Behavioral & Social Sciences, Brown University School of Public Health,
Providence, RI, USA

J. Scheer
Syracuse University, College of Arts and Sciences, Syracuse, NY, USA
e-mail: jrscheer@syr.edu

© The Author(s), under exclusive license to Springer Nature
Switzerland AG 2021
K. L. Nadal and M. R. Scharrón-del Río (ed.), *Queer Psychology*,
https://doi.org/10.1007/978-3-030-74146-4_6

103

general population (Kessler et al., 1999). Highlighting heterogeneity within the LGBQ community, research also suggests that sexual orientation-based mental health disparities may be larger for people who identify as bisexual, questioning, queer, pansexual, demisexual, or asexual than for gay/lesbian people and that gender identity-based disparities may be larger among gender nonconforming people than among transgender women or men (Borgogna et al., 2019; Bostwick et al., 2010; Lefevor et al., 2019) (Fig. 1).

Importantly, the clear existence of these disparities does not—in-and-of itself—shed light on their cause. Scholars working in psychology, public health, and allied disciplines have taken up this question and generated a robust body of literature in the last several decades. To better understand the factors influencing diverse LGBTQ people's mental health, this chapter will discuss three frameworks that scholars concerned with LGBTQ often employ in their work: minority stress theory, syndemic theory, and intersectionality. The chapter also briefly touches upon mental health interventions and the strengths and resilience of LGBTQ people. The chapter closes with a clinical vignette that illustrates some of the processes described throughout the chapter.

2   Minority Stress Theory

Minority stress theory (Brooks, 1981; DiPlacido, 1998; Meyer, 2003) is a conceptual framework that was designed to help explain the mental health disparities observed between LGBQ people and heterosexual people and has been extended to

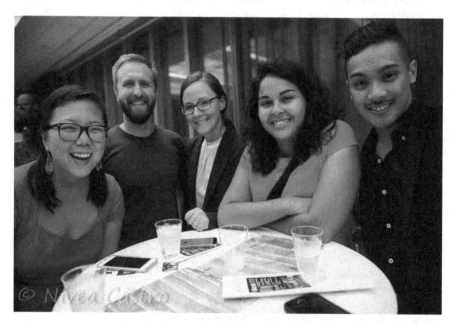

Fig. 1 A group of friends at an LGBTQ community event. Photo Courtesy of Nivea Castro

also consider disparities between transgender and cisgender people (Breslow et al., 2015; Testa et al., 2015). Minority stress theory draws from the broader psychological literature on stress, which could be conceptualized as any event or situation that requires individuals to adapt to new circumstances (Dohrenwend, 1998). Historically, psychological research focused on stressors such as severe trauma (e.g., surviving a natural disaster), major developmental milestones (e.g., marriage), chronic stressors (e.g., coping with a long-term illness), everyday hassles (e.g., morning traffic), or role strains (e.g., work-family conflict). Each of these stressors may tax or even exceed an individual's ability to cope, which sometimes precipitates the development of mental health concerns regardless of individuals' sexual or gender identities.

Importantly, LGBTQ people also encounter social stressors that stem from heterosexism and cissexism—that is, systems of oppression experienced by sexual and gender minority people. According to minority stress theory (Meyer, 2003; Testa et al., 2015), it is the addition of these *minority stressors* on top of other stressors that accounts for the higher prevalence of mental health concerns among LGBTQ people relative to their heterosexual and cisgender peers.

Meyer (2003) described four minority stress processes. Though these processes were originally described in reference to LGBQ people's experiences of heterosexism, scholars have subsequently articulated analogous processes stemming from cissexism that impact transgender people (e.g., Testa et al., 2015). First, there is discrimination, or differential treatment, derogation, harassment, or victimization of people because of one's sexual minority and/or gender minority identity (see Chap. 7, this volume). Discrimination may be perpetrated by individuals (i.e., manifests interpersonally) or it may be enshrined in policy or law (i.e., manifests structurally). Research with bisexual individuals indicates that they may experience discrimination from both heterosexual and gay/lesbian communities (e.g., Brewster & Moradi, 2010). The second minority stressor is expectations of rejection, which refers to the anticipation that one will encounter discrimination in the future—and the anxious vigilance this anticipation promotes. Expectations of rejection overlaps conceptually with sexual orientation-based stigma consciousness and rejection sensitivity (Feinstein et al., 2014; Pinel, 1999). Expectations of rejection may occur, for example, when partners in a male same-sex couple hesitate to hold each other's hands in public for fear of drawing attention to their sexual minority identities and thus becoming potential targets of heterosexist violence. The next stressor, internalized heterosexism (or internalized biphobia or transphobia for bisexual or transgender people), refers to LGBTQ people's endorsement of negative attitudes or beliefs about LGBTQ people, identities, and communities. Reducing such internalized prejudice and developing affirmative attitudes and beliefs are conceptualized as important processes in models of LGBTQ identity development (see Chaps. 3 and 4, this volume). The fourth stressor, identity concealment, refers to the stress that occurs when LGBTQ people must choose whether to conceal or disclose their sexual and/or gender minority identities to other people in their lives. Though sexual minority identity may be more easily concealed than other minority statuses, such as race or ethnicity, LGBQ people whose appearance, attire, or mannerisms are perceived to be gender nonconforming may be more likely to be assumed by others to be sexual minorities (Puckett et al., 2016). Similarly, transgender people who change their appearance—via clothing, hairstyle, or gender affirming medical procedures—may find it more difficult to conceal their transgender identity at the beginning of their physical transition.

A robust body of literature supports the major tenets of minority stress theory. For example, taking into account the frequency of experiences of discrimination attenuates the association of sexual minority status with psychiatric morbidity (e.g., Mays & Cochran, 2001; Rodriguez-Seijas et al., 2019). Furthermore, discrimination, expectations of rejection, and internalized heterosexism (or biphobia or transphobia) are consistently associated with poorer mental health among LGBTQ people (e.g., Breslow et al., 2015; Feinstein et al., 2012; Newcomb & Mustanski, 2010; Sarno et al., 2020). Findings regarding identity concealment are more complex. In some studies, greater concealment is associated with poorer mental health (e.g., Jackson & Mohr, 2016); in others, greater concealment is associated with better mental health (Pachankis & Bränström, 2018; van der Star et al., 2019). These discrepant findings may indicate that the mental health impact of concealment or disclosure depends on social context—that is, lower concealment and greater disclosure may be more beneficial to mental health in situations in which one will be supported rather than rejected for having a sexual and/or a gender minority identity (Chaudoir & Fisher, 2010).

Once it has been established that minority stressors are associated with poorer mental health among LGBTQ populations, the next line of questioning focuses on how or why. Meyer (2003) distinguished between distal and proximal stressors. Because discrimination occurs in the social environment and is thus external to the individual, discrimination is a distal stressor. In contrast, because expectations of rejection, internalized heterosexism, and concealment decisions occur within the individual, they are framed as proximal stressors. Importantly, LGBTQ people cognitively appraise or evaluate their experiences of discrimination, whereupon they "become proximal concepts with psychological importance to the individual (p. 676). That is, LGBTQ people's experiences of discrimination are postulated to strengthen expectations that one will be rejected in the future, enhance one's own negative attitudes toward LGBTQ people, and lead to more concealment of one's LGBTQ identity in the future to avoid experiencing more discrimination. Hatzenbuehler (2009) built upon the minority stress model by explicitly hypothesizing that the association of discrimination with mental health outcomes was partially mediated or accounted for by discrimination's influence on the three proximal stressors. In addition, he hypothesized that another way discrimination negatively impacted mental health was through its influence on general psychological processes—that is, affective, cognitive, and interpersonal variables that serve as antecedents of mental health concerns among people regardless of their sexual or gender identities. Such general psychological variables include emotion (dys)regulation processes like rumination; negative cognitive schemas like hopelessness or poor self-esteem; and social isolation or poor social support.

A growing number of studies provide some support for Hatzenbuehler's (2009) mediation model of minority stress. For example, expectations of rejection and internalized heterosexism (or biphobia or transphobia)—but not concealment—have been found to mediate the association of discrimination with poor mental health outcomes—like depression, social anxiety, psychological distress, and low psychological well-being—among samples of LGBTQ people (e.g., Breslow et al., 2015; Feinstein et al., 2012; Velez & Moradi, 2016). Studies have also found that maladaptive coping (e.g., rumination, detachment, self-blame) and social support also mediate the association of discrimination with poor mental health outcomes (e.g., Bandermann & Szymanski, 2014; Sarno et al., 2020; Schwartz et al., 2016). However, relatively less research has examined both proximal stressors and the general psychological processes as mediators of the discrimination-mental health association in the same study.

3 Syndemics

LGBTQ people might engage in health-risk behaviors, such as alcohol and substance use and suicidality, to manage the health-corrosive impact of minority stress (Baams et al., 2015; Hatzenbuehler & Pachankis, 2016; McCabe et al., 2010). For example, consistent evidence demonstrates the co-occurrence of distal stressors (e.g., racism), proximal stressors (e.g., internalized heterosexism), and health-risk behaviors (e.g., binge drinking) among gay and bisexual men of color (Dyer et al., 2012; Mizuno et al., 2012). Indeed, such psychosocial health conditions affecting LGBTQ people often cluster together, exacerbating serious health burdens facing this population (Stall et al., 2008; Stall et al., 2001; Tsai & Burns, 2015). Prior research has also documented a biological, social, and psychological interaction of these psychosocial health conditions, including inflammation, stigma, and depression (Mendenhall & Singer, 2020). Syndemic theory (Singer, 1994, 2000) is one framework that can help to explain the concentration and interaction (i.e., synergies) of co-occurring epidemics facing socially disadvantaged populations, such as low-income transgender women of color.

According to syndemic theory, multiple co-occurring epidemics, such as substance abuse, violence, HIV, sexual abuse, and depression, synergistically enhance LGBTQ individuals' disproportionate risk of poor overall mental health compared to cisgender, heterosexual individuals (Singer, 1996; Singer & Claire, 2003; Stall et al., 2003). Over the past ten years, syndemic research has primarily examined the role of violence (e.g., sexual abuse and intimate partner violence), stressors associated with oppression (e.g., racism and heterosexism), and mental and behavioral health issues (e.g., posttraumatic stress, depression, substance use) in HIV acquisition and transmission among Black and Latinx sexual minority men (Stall et al., 2003; Wilson et al., 2014) and transgender women, (Baral et al., 2013; Chakrapani et al., 2017; Operario et al., 2014), and physical health issues among LGBTQ people of color and white LGBTQ people (Scheer & Pachankis, 2019). Despite recent applications of syndemic theory to understanding the concentrated clustering of co-occurring epidemics among LGBTQ people with multiple marginalized identities, additional research needs to examine multiple forms of oppression—including racism, classism, nationalism, sexism, cissexism, and ableism—as key drivers of syndemic conditions among LGBTQ people who hold intersecting identities (Frye et al., 2014; Jackson et al., 2020; Quinn, 2019).

4 Intersectionality

Intersectionality is a concept and critical analytic perspective that has its roots in the scholarship and activism of Black women and other Women of Color (e.g., Collins, 2000; Combahee River Collective, 2007, original work 1977/1983; Crenshaw, 1989). Discussing the full scope of the contributions of intersectionality to psychology and other academic disciplines is beyond the scope of this chapter (but see Chap. 2, this volume; Cole, 2009). However, it is vital to incorporate an intersectional perspective in any consideration of the mental health of LGBTQ people—or any population, for that matter.

Intersectionality draws our attention to the fact that no system of oppression (and privilege)—such as heterosexism or cissexism—occurs in an ahistorical, acontextual vacuum. Rather, systems of oppression intersect like the streets of a busy traffic intersection (Crenshaw, 1989). Individuals—who can be understood in this metaphor to be the cars actively traversing the intersection—may experience an accident (i.e., discrimination) because of the flow of traffic in one direction (e.g., heterosexism), a second direction (e.g., cissexism), a third direction (e.g., racism)—or any combination of "directions" or systems of oppression. Another important insight offered by intersectionality is that systems of oppression are co-constituted—that is, beyond just co-occurring, systems of oppression mutually influence each other (Collins, 2000). Take for example the case of an undocumented Latina transgender woman who must engage in survival sex because she is not able to attain legal employment. If she encounters harassment from the police, this may reflect not only cissexism but also classist notions of what is legitimate work, sexist or misogynistic disdain for women's sexuality, and exploitation of racist or nativist policies and laws that make undocumented people particularly vulnerable during interactions with the police.

Psychological scholarship focused on the mental health of LGBTQ people has employed an intersectionality perspective in a variety of ways. For example, studies have sought to determine if racist stressors like racist discrimination or internalized racism are associated with mental health concerns among LGBQ people additively or above and beyond the influence of heterosexist stressors (e.g., Thoma & Huebner, 2013; Velez et al., 2019). Other studies have explored if the co-occurrence of other forms of oppression—like sexism and racism—has multiplicative effects on mental health (e.g., Szymanski, 2005; Szymanski & Gupta, 2009). Still other research has explored the possibility that the intersection of heterosexism or cissexism with another form of oppression produces experiences that are truly unique to certain populations. For example, one study found that the sexual objectification experienced by gay or bisexual Men of Color was shaped by racialized stereotypes of their bodies and sexualities (Brennan et al., 2013). Similarly, Balsam and colleagues' (2011) LGBT People of Color Microaggressions scale assesses stressors that may be uniquely stressful to this population, like racism experienced in the LGBTQ community, heterosexism experienced in communities of Color, and racism in dating and relationships (Fig. 2).

5 Strengths and Mental Health Promoters Among LGBTQ People

Though this chapter has thus far emphasized the mental health concerns of and stressors experienced by LGBTQ people, it is also important to acknowledge that—despite the toxic influence of heterosexism, cissexism, and other forms of oppression—many LGBTQ people thrive and find joy in their identities. Riggle and Rostosky (2011) conducted a series of large-scale qualitative studies that allowed LGBTQ people to describe in their own words the positive aspects of their sexual and/or gender minority identities. Themes that emerged from participant responses included feeling authentic to oneself; developing self-awareness and personal insight; feeling free to challenge society's rules regarding gender, relationships, and sexuality; feeling strong emotional connections with others; belonging to a

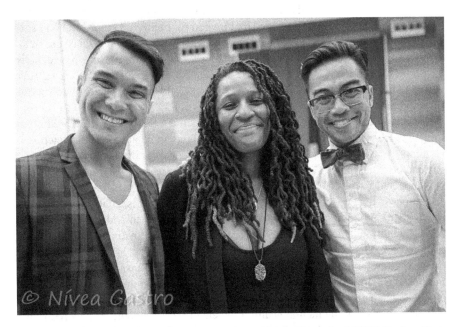

Fig. 2 QPOC Artists who performed at an event hosted by the Center for LGBTQ Studies. Photo Courtesy of Nivea Castro

community; feeling compassion and empathy for other people; and serving as posi- tive role models for other LGBTQ people. Among LGBTQ adolescents and adults, parental or family acceptance of one's LGBTQ identity is associated with better mental outcomes above and beyond the influence of parental rejection and general family acceptance (Kibrik et al., 2019; Ryan et al., 2009). Furthermore, one study found that LGBTQ-specific parental acceptance—but not general family support— buffered the associations of expectations of rejection and internalized heterosexism with depression in a sample of lesbian and gay adults (Feinstein et al., 2014). Thus, family acceptance may enhance mental health or serve as a source of resilience for LGBTQ people. Finally, research with transgender people and other gender minor- ity populations indicates that social (e.g., changing one's name or pronoun, dressing in ways that align with one's gender identity, disclosing one's gender minority iden- tity) and medical (e.g., hormone replacement therapy, gender affirming surgeries) gender affirmation experiences are associated with better mental health (Hughto et al., 2020).

6 Interventions

Evidence for the influence of heterosexist or cissexist stressors, stressors stemming from other systems of oppression, and syndemic conditions on the mental health of LGBTQ populations has important implications for treatment of LGBTQ people's transdiagnostic health needs. For example, LGBTQ people who report mental health symptoms should be screened and treated for comorbid behavioral and sex- ual health issues and referred to health care providers who offer substance use treat- ment, comprehensive sexual health evaluations, and routine testing for sexually transmitted infections (Centers for Disease Control and Prevention (CDC) 2015). Psychotherapeutic or counseling interventions should also explicitly address the roles of stressors stemming from societal oppression in precipitating LGBTQ peo- ple's mental health concerns. One such intervention is ESTEEM (Effective Skills to Empower Effective Men), a cognitive-behavioral therapy that targets the heterosex- ist minority stressors and general psychological processes that are associated with gay and bisexual men's syndemic conditions (Pachankis et al., 2015). ESTEEM has demonstrated preliminary efficacy in reducing depression, alcohol use problems, and co-occurring HIV-risk behaviors among young gay and bisexual men (Pachankis et al., 2015). In addition, ESTEEM was recently adapted to address co-occurring health conditions facing sexual minority women in a treatment called EQuIP (Empowering Queer Identities in Psychotherapy; Pachankis et al., 2020). Analogous psychotherapy treatments may be developed for transgender populations. Furthermore, similar interventions may be developed that more directly address the unique contributions of other systems of oppression—like racism, classism, able- ism, or ageism—on the mental health of diverse LGBTQ people. For more discus- sion of clinical work with LGBTQ populations, see Chap. 9 of this volume.

It is also important to underscore that though psychotherapy interventions are vital to addressing the mental health concerns of LGBTQ people, interventions are needed that work beyond the micro-level (individual or small group) and enact change at the meso-level (organizational, community) and macro-levels (societal) (Rostosky & Riggle, 2011). Psychologists and allied helping professionals must consider ways that they may draw from their knowledge of minority stress theory, syndemics, and intersectionality to develop and proliferate psychoeducational programming, organizational consultation practices, or policy initiatives and social justice activism that addresses the structural forces that shape the experiences and functioning of LGBTQ populations. Chapter 17 of this volume discusses the importance of LGBTQ activism (Fig. 3).

Vignette: Evan

Evan is a 23-year-old Dominican American trans man. He has described his sexual orientation as "questioning." Evan works a full-time minimum wage job at a local supermarket. Evan was referred by his primary care physician (PCP) to the hospitals' LGBTQ behavioral health clinic due to general life stressors, low mood, self-harm, and passive suicidal ideation. Evan also said that he would like to discuss the possibility of pursuing hormone-replacement therapy (HRT) and "top" surgery to more fully express his male gender identity. In addition, he would like to discuss family stress, perceived conflict between religion and his gender and sexual identities, and uncertainty regarding his sexual orientation.

Evan said that he grew up in a working-class family in upper Manhattan. Both of his parents were born in the Dominican Republic but moved to the U.S. before Evan was born. Evan has two younger siblings: Angie, a 15-year-old sister, and Juan, a 13-year-old brother. Evan said that while growing up, his family had limited resources, and for part of his life his family received welfare. However, his parents both worked multiple jobs to provide for the family and they instilled in their children the importance of working hard and persevering. Evan contributes half of his paycheck to his parents to supplement the family household income. His immediate family was also supported by a large extended family that lives throughout New York City.

Evan said that he realized he was transgender approximately three years ago. He came out as trans to friends a year ago and to his family three years ago. Until that time, Evan identified as a cisgender lesbian woman. He came out as a lesbian to his

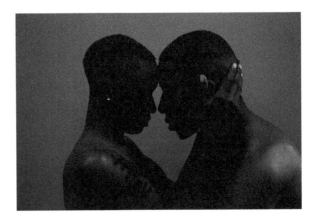

Fig. 3 An intimate moment shared between two Black men. Photo by Joshua McKnight

friends and family when he was 14 years old. His family was tolerant of his sexual orientation, which he attributed to the fact that he has a *tia* that is an out lesbian. However, his family—and his parents in particular—had a strong negative reaction to his disclosure of his transgender identity. They said that they did not understand why "she" needed to "pretend to be a man" and that it goes against the religious beliefs of the "*Iglesia Católica*." Evan's parents believe that he is too wrapped up in "American culture" and have said that if he lived in the Dominican Republic this would not be happening. To this day, they continue to call Evan by his birth name, Maria, and to refer to him with feminine pronouns despite Evan's explicit request that they use his chosen name and masculine pronouns. In contrast, Evan's siblings have been supportive and are using his chosen name and masculine pronouns.

Soon after coming out as transgender to his family and friends, Evan began dressing in more masculine attire and cutting his hair short. Recently, he has decided to begin pursuing more physical transitions. He asked his therapist if she would be capable of providing Evan with a letter of support to begin HRT, and his therapist said that this was a possibility but would require a psychological evaluation. Though Evan is excited about the prospect of pursuing medical interventions, he is unsure that his health insurance—which he receives from his parents—will cover the cost, which he anticipates will be high. Evan also worries that his parents will completely remove him from their insurance coverage if he broaches the subject of pursuing gender affirming medical procedures with them. Evan reports that his suicidal ideation and self-injurious behavior (nonlethal cutting of his arms) have become more frequent since he began worrying about barriers to transitioning. He wants to start HRT as soon as possible as he fears that his suicidal ideation and self-injurious behavior may worsen. Though Evan says he has never had a problem with drinking, he does admit that the frequency and severity of his drinking has increased within the last few months because he believes it is the quickest way to relax and forget about the stress in his life.

After coming out as a transgender man, Evan initially identified as heterosexual. Recently, however, he has found himself aware of a growing attraction to men. Despite these attractions, Evan is reluctant to act on them because he expects that gay or bisexual men will not be attracted to him and will reject him because he is transgender. Indeed, he stated that he feels uncomfortable and anxious in exclusively gay or bisexual male spaces—particularly if the men are predominantly White. Although he feels very supported by his group of close friends —which includes lesbian women and other transgender men—he is unsure of how they may react if he tells them about his attraction to men. Moreover, Evan feels guilty that he may need to come out to his family yet again—this time as a bisexual man.

7 Discussion of Vignette

The clinical case vignette of Evan underscores many of topics highlighted in this chapter. Evan has experienced cissexist discrimination in the form of rejection and mistreatment (e.g., misgendering) from his parents. His experiences disclosing a stigmatized identity have been mixed: though his parents rejected him, thus contributing to his distress, his siblings have supported him, which has been positive for their relationships. His reluctance to disclose his bisexual identity to his family may be conceptualized as stemming from expectations of (biphobic) rejection. The financial barriers Evan anticipates encountering in order to access gender affirming healthcare illustrate how the classism baked into the healthcare systems of the U.S. uniquely disadvantages poor or working class transgender people. Evan's reluctance to enter predominantly White (and presumably cisgender) gay or bisexual male spaces may reflect his awareness of racism stemming from his identity as a Dominican American and his experiences of sexism that he may have encountered earlier in life as a person assigned-female at birth. Evan's gender dysphoria, emotional distress (which may be signs of a possible mood disorder), and recently increased alcohol use illustrate the patterns described in syndemics theory. For example, if Evan's alcohol continues to increase in frequency and severity, alcohol's disinhibitive effects may make him more susceptible to engage in polysubstance use and risky sexual behavior, which would in turn have implications for his physical and sexual well-being.

References

Baams, L., Grossman, A. H., & Russell, S. T. (2015). Minority stress and mechanisms of risk for depression and suicidal ideation among lesbian, gay, and bisexual youth. *Developmental Psychology, 51*(5), 680–696. https://doi.org/10.1037/a0038994.

Balsam, K. F., Molina, Y., Beadnell, B., Simoni, J., & Walters, K. (2011). Measuring multiple minority stress: The LGBT people of color microaggressions scale. *Cultural Diversity and Ethnic Minority Psychology, 17*(2), 163. https://doi.org/10.1037/a0023244.

Bandermann, K. M., & Szymanski, D. M. (2014). Exploring coping mediators between heterosexist oppression and posttraumatic stress symptoms among lesbian, gay, and bisexual persons. *Psychology of Sexual Orientation and Gender Diversity, 1*, 213–224. https://doi.org/10.1037/sgd0000044.

Baral, S. D., Poteat, T., Strömdahl, S., Wirtz, A. L., Guadamuz, T. E., & Beyrer, C. (2013). Worldwide burden of HIV in transgender women: A systematic review and meta-analysis. *The Lancet Infectious Diseases, 13*(3), 214–222. https://doi.org/10.1016/s1473-3099(12)70315-8.

Borgogna, N. C., McDermott, R. C., Aita, S. L., & Kridel, M. M. (2019). Anxiety and depression across gender and sexual minorities: Implications for transgender, gender nonconforming, pansexual, demisexual, asexual, queer, and questioning individuals. *Psychology of Sexual Orientation and Gender Diversity, 6*(1), 54–63. https://doi.org/10.1037/sgd0000306.

Bostwick, W. B., Boyd, C. J., Hughes, T. L., & McCabe, S. E. (2010). Dimensions of sexual orientation and the prevalence of mood and anxiety disorders in the United States. *American Journal of Public Health, 100*(3), 468–475. https://doi.org/10.2105/AJPH.2008.152942.

Brennan, D. J., Asakura, K., George, C., Newman, P. A., Giwa, S., Hart, T. A., Souleymanov, R., & Betancourt, G. (2013). "Never reflected anywhere": Body image among ethnoracialized gay and bisexual men. *Body Image, 10*, 389–398. https://doi.org/10.1016/j.bodyim.2013.03.006.

Breslow, A. S., Brewster, M. E., Velez, B. L., Wong, S., Geiger, E., & Soderstrom, B. (2015). Resilience and collective action: Exploring buffers against minority stress for transgender individuals. *Psychology of Sexual Orientation and Gender Diversity, 2*(3), 253–265. https://doi.org/10.1037/sgd0000117.

Brewster, M. E., & Moradi, B. (2010). Perceived experiences of anti-bisexual prejudice: Instrument development and evaluation. *Journal of Counseling Psychology, 57*, 451–468. https://doi.org/10.1037/a0021116.

Brooks, V. R. (1981). *Minority stress and lesbian women.* Lexington, MA: Lexington Books.

Centers for Disease Control and Prevention. (2015). Sexually transmitted diseases treatment guidelines, 2015. *Morbidity and Mortality Weekly Report, 64*(3), 1–134.

Chakrapani, V., Newman, P. A., Shunmugam, M., Logie, C. H., & Samuel, M. (2017). Syndemics of depression, alcohol use, and victimisation, and their association with HIV-related sexual risk among men who have sex with men and transgender women in India. *Global Public Health, 12*(2), 250–265. https://doi.org/10.1080/17441692.2015.1091024.

Chaudoir, S. R., & Fisher, J. D. (2010). The disclosure processes model: Understanding disclosure decision making and postdisclosure outcomes among people living with a concealable stigmatized identity. *Psychological Bulletin, 136*(2), 236–256. https://doi.org/10.1037/a0018193.

Cochran, S. D., Sullivan, J. G., & Mays, V. M. (2003). Prevalence of mental disorders, psychological distress, and mental health services use among lesbian, gay, and bisexual adults in the United States. *Journal of Consulting and Clinical Psychology, 71*(1), 53–61. https://doi.org/10.1037/0022-006X.71.1.53.

Cole, E. R. (2009). Intersectionality and research in psychology. *American Psychologist, 64*(3), 170–180. https://doi.org/10.1037/a0014564.

Collins, P. H. (2000). *Black feminist thought: Knowledge, consciousness, and the politics of empowerment.* New York, NY: Routledge.

Combahee River Collective. (2007). A black feminist statement. In E. B. Freedman (Ed.), *The essential feminist reader* (pp. 325–330). New York, NY: Modern Library. (Original work published 1977).

Crenshaw, K. (1989). Demarginalizing the intersection of race and sex: A black feminist critique of antidiscrimination doctrine, feminist theory and antiracist politics. *University of Chicago Legal Forum, 139*(1), 139–167. Retrieved from: https://chicagounbound.uchicago.edu/uclf/vol1989/iss1/8.

DiPlacido, J. (1998). Minority stress among lesbians, gay men, and bisexuals: A consequence of heterosexism, homophobia, and stigmatization. In G. M. Herek (Ed.), *Stigma and sexual orientation: Vol. 4. Understanding prejudice against lesbians, gay men, and bisexuals* (pp. 138–159). Thousand Oaks, CA: Sage.

Dohrenwend, B. P. (1998). *Adversity, stress, and psychopathology.* New York: Oxford University Press.

Dyer, T. P., Shoptaw, S., Guadamuz, T. E., Plankey, M., Kao, U., Ostrow, D., Chmiel, J. S., Herrick, A., & Stall, R. (2012). Application of syndemic theory to black men who have sex with men in the multicenter AIDS cohort study. *Journal of Urban Health, 89*(4), 697–708. https://doi.org/10.1007/s11524-012-9674-x.

Feinstein, B."A., Goldfried, M."R., & Davila, J. (2012). The relationship between experiences of discrimination and mental health among lesbians and gay men: An examination of internalized homonegativity and stigma sensitivity as potential mechanisms. *Journal of Consulting and Clinical Psychology, 80*, 917–927. https://doi.org/10.1037/a0029425.

Feinstein, B. A., Wadsworth, L. P., Davila, J., & Goldfried, M. R. (2014). Do parental acceptance and family support moderate associations between dimensions of minority stress and depressive symptoms among lesbians and gay men? *Professional Psychology: Research and Practice, 45*(4), 239–246. https://doi.org/10.1037/a0035393.

Frye, V., Egan, J. E., Van Tieu, H., Cerdá, M., Ompad, D., & Koblin, B. A. (2014). "I didn't think I could get out of the fucking park." Gay men's retrospective accounts of neighborhood space, emerging sexuality and migrations. *Social Science & Medicine, 104*, 6–14. https://doi.org/10.1016/j.socscimed.2013.12.002.

Hatzenbuehler, M. L. (2009). How does sexual minority stigma "get under the skin"? A psychological mediation framework. *Psychological Bulletin, 135*, 707–730. https://doi.org/10.1037/a0016441.

Hatzenbuehler, M. L., & Pachankis, J. E. (2016). Stigma and minority stress as social determinants of health among lesbian, gay, bisexual, and transgender youth: Research evidence and clinical implications. *Pediatric Clinics, 63*(6), 985–997. https://doi.org/10.1016/j.pcl.2016.07.003.

Hughto, J. M. W., Gunn, H. A., Rood, B. A., & Pantalone, D. W. (2020). Social and medical gender affirmation experiences are inversely associated with mental health problems in a US non-probability sample of transgender adults. *Archives of Sexual Behavior, 49*(7), 2635–2647. https://doi.org/10.1007/s10508-020-01655-5.

Jackson, S. D., & Mohr, J. J. (2016). Conceptualizing the closet: Differentiating stigma concealment and nondisclosure processes. *Psychology of Sexual Orientation and Gender Diversity, 3*(1), 80–92. https://doi.org/10.1037/sgd0000147.

Jackson, S. D., Mohr, J. J., Sarno, E. L., Kindahl, A. M., & Jones, I. L. (2020). Intersectional experiences, stigma-related stress, and psychological health among Black LGBQ individuals. *Journal of Consulting and Clinical Psychology, 88*(5), 416–428. https://doi.org/10.1037/ccp0000489.

James, S. E., Herman, J. L., Rankin, S., Keisling, M., Mottet, L., & Anafi, M. (2016). The Report of the 2015 U.S. Transgender Survey. Washington, DC: National Center for Transgender Equality. Retrieved from https://transequality.org/sites/default/files/docs/usts/USTS-Full-Report-Dec17.pdf.

Kessler, R. C., Borges, G., & Walters, E. E. (1999). Prevalence of and risk factors for lifetime suicide attempts in the National Comorbidity Survey. *Archives of General Psychiatry, 56*(7), 617–626. https://doi.org/10.1001archpsyc.56.7.617.

Kibrik, E. L., Cohen, N., Stolowicz-Melman, D., Levy, A., Boruchovitz-Zamir, R., & Diamond, G. M. (2019). Measuring adult children's perceptions of their parents' acceptance and rejection of their sexual orientation: Initial development of the Parental acceptance and Rejection of Sexual Orientation Scale (PARSOS). *Journal of Homosexuality, 66*(11), 1513–1534. https://doi.org/10.1080/00918369.2018.1503460.

King, M., Semlyen, J., Tai, S. S., Killaspy, H., Osborn, D., Popelyuk, D., & Nazareth, I. (2008). A systematic review of mental disorder, suicide, and deliberate self harm in lesbian, gay, and bisexual people. *BMC Psychiatry, 8.* https://doi.org/10.1186/1471-244X-8-70.

Lefevor, G. T., Boyd-Rogers, C. C., Sprague, B. M., & Janis, R. A. (2019). Health disparities between genderqueer, transgender, and cisgender individuals: An extension of minority stress theory. *Journal of Counseling Psychology, 66*(4), 385–395. https://doi.org/10.1037/cou0000339.

Mays, V. M., & Cochran, S. D. (2001). Mental health correlates of perceived discrimination among lesbian, gay, and bisexual adults in the United States. *American Journal of Public Health, 91*(11), 1869–1876.

McCabe, S. E., Bostwick, W. B., Hughes, T. L., West, B. T., & Boyd, C. J. (2010). The relationship between discrimination and substance use disorders among lesbian, gay, and bisexual adults in the United States. *American Journal of Public Health, 100*(10), 1946–1952. https://doi.org/10.2105/ajph.2009.163147.

Mendenhall, E., & Singer, M. (2020). What constitutes a syndemic? Methods, contexts, and framing from 2019. *Current Opinion in HIV and AIDS, 15*(4), 213–217. https://doi.org/10.1097/coh.0000000000000628.

Meyer, I. H. (2003). Prejudice, social stress, and mental health in lesbian, gay, and bisexual populations: Conceptual issues and research evidence. *Psychological Bulletin, 129*, 674. https://doi.org/10.1037/0033-2909.129.5.674.

Meyer, I. H., Brown, T. N., Herman, J. L., Reisner, S. L., & Bockting, W. O. (2017). Demographic characteristics and health status of transgender adults in select US regions: Behavioral risk factor surveillance system, 2014. *American Journal of Public Health, 107*(4), 582–589. https://doi.org/10.2105/ajph.2016.303648.

Mizuno, Y., Borkowf, C., Millett, G. A., Bingham, T., Ayala, G., & Stueve, A. (2012). Homophobia and racism experienced by Latino men who have sex with men in the United States: Correlates of exposure and associations with HIV risk behaviors. *AIDS and Behavior, 16*(3), 724–735. https://doi.org/10.1007/s10461-011-9967-1.

Mongelli, F., Perrone, D., Balducci, J., Sacchetti, A., Ferrari, S., Mattei, G., & Galeazzi, G. M. (2019). Minority stress and mental health among LGBT populations: An update on the evidence. *Minerva Psichiatrica, 60*(1), 27–50. https://doi.org/10.23736/S0391-1772.18.01995-7.

Newcomb, M. E., & Mustanski, B. (2010). Internalized homophobia and internalizing mental health problems: A meta-analytic review. *Clinical Psychology Review, 30*, 1019–1029. https://doi.org/10.1016/j.cpr.2010.07.003.

Operario, D., Yang, M. F., Reisner, S. L., Iwamoto, M., & Nemoto, T. (2014). Stigma and the syndemic of HIV-related health risk behaviors in a diverse sample of transgender women. *Journal of Community Psychology, 42*(5), 544–557. https://doi.org/10.1002/jcop.21636.

Pachankis, J. E., & Bränström, R. (2018). Hidden from happiness: Structural stigma, sexual orientation concealment, and life satisfaction across 28 countries. *Journal of Consulting and Clinical Psychology, 86*(5), 403–415. https://doi.org/10.1037/ccp0000299.

Pachankis, J. E., Hatzenbuehler, M. L., Rendina, H. J., Safren, S. A., & Parsons, J. T. (2015). LGB-affirmative cognitive-behavioral therapy for young adult gay and bisexual men: A randomized controlled trial of a transdiagnostic minority stress approach. *Journal of Consulting and Clinical Psychology, 83*, 875–889. https://doi.org/10.1037/ccp0000037875.

Pachankis, J. E., McConocha, E. M., Clark, K. A., Wang, K., Behari, K., Fetzner, B. K., Brisbin, C. D., Scheer, J. R., & Lehavot, K. (2020). A transdiagnostic minority stress intervention for gender diverse sexual minority women's depression, anxiety, and unhealthy alcohol use. *Journal of Consulting and Clinical Psychology, 88*(7), 613. https://doi.org/10.1037/ccp0000508.

Pinel, E. C. (1999). Stigma consciousness: The psychological legacy of social stereo-types. *Journal of Personality and Social Psychology, 76*, 114–128. https://doi.org/10.1037/0022-3514.76.1.114.

Puckett, J. A., Maroney, M. R., Levitt, H. M., & Horne, S. G. (2016). Relations between gender expression, minority stress, and mental health in cisgender sexual minority women and men. *Psychology of Sexual Orientation and Gender Diversity, 3*(4), 489–498. https://doi.org/10.1037/sgd0000201.

Quinn, K. G. (2019). Applying an intersectional framework to understand syndemic conditions among young black gay, bisexual, and other men who have sex with men. *Social Science & Medicine, 112779*. https://doi.org/10.1016/j.socscimed.2019.112779.

Riggle, E. D. B., & Rostosky, S. S. (2011). *A positive view of LGBTQ: Embracing identity and cultivating well-being.* Lanham: Rowman & Littlefield Publishers.

Rodriguez-Seijas, C., Eaton, N. R., & Pachankis, J. E. (2019). Prevalence of psychiatric disorders at the intersection of race and sexual orientation: Results from the National Epidemiologic Survey of alcohol and related conditions-III. *Journal of Consulting and Clinical Psychology, 87*, 321–331. https://doi.org/10.1037/ccp0000377.

Rostosky, S. S., & Riggle, E. D. B. (2011). Marriage equality for same-sex couples: Counseling psychologists as social change agents. *The Counseling Psychologist, 39*, 956–972. https://doi.org/10.1177/0011000011398398.

Ryan, C., Huebner, D., Diaz, R. M., & Sanchez, J. (2009). Family rejection as a predictor of negative health outcomes in white and Latino lesbian, gay, and bisexual young adults. *Pediatrics, 123*, 346–352. https://doi.org/10.1542/peds.2007-3524.

Salway, T., Ross, L. E., Fehr, C. P., Burley, J., Asadi, S., Hawkins, B., & Tarasoff, L. A. (2019). A systematic review and meta-analysis of disparities in the prevalence of suicide ideation and attempt among bisexual populations. *Archives of Sexual Behavior, 48*(1), 89–111. https://doi.org/10.1007/s10508-018-1150-6.

Sarno, E. L., Newcomb, M. E., & Mustanski, B. (2020). Rumination longitudinally mediates the association of minority stress and depression in sexual and gender minority individuals. *Journal of Abnormal Psychology, 129*(4), 355–363. https://doi.org/10.1037/abn0000508.

Scheer, J. R., & Pachankis, J. E. (2019). Psychosocial syndemic risks surrounding physical health conditions among sexual and gender minority individuals. *LGBT Health, 6*(8), 377–385. https://doi.org/10.1089/lgbt.2019.0025.

Schwartz, D. R., Stratton, N., & Hart, T. A. (2016). Minority stress and mental and sexual health: Examining the psychological mediation framework among gay and bisexual men. *Psychology of Sexual Orientation and Gender Diversity, 3*, 313–324. https://doi.org/10.1037/sgd0000180.

Singer, M. (1994). AIDS and the health crisis of the US urban poor; the perspective of critical medical anthropology. *Social Science & Medicine, 39*(7), 931–948. https://doi.org/10.1016/0277-9536(94)90205-4.

Singer, M. (1996). A dose of drugs, a touch of violence, a case of AIDS: Conceptualizing SAVA. *Free Inquiry in Creative Sociology, 24*, 99–110.

Singer, M. (2000). A dose of drugs, a touch of violence, a case of AIDS: Conceptualizing the SAVA syndemic. *Free Inquiry in Creative Sociology, 28*(1), 13–24.

Singer, M., & Claire, S. (2003). Syndemics and public health: Reconceptualizing disease in bio-social context. *Medical Anthropology Quarterly, 17*, 423–441. https://doi.org/10.1525/maq.2003.17.4.423.

Stall, R., Friedman, M., & Catania, J. A. (2008). Interacting epidemics and gay men's health: A theory of syndemic production among urban gay men. *Unequal opportunity: Health disparities affecting gay and bisexual men in the United States: Oxford University Press, USA., 1*, 251–274.

Stall, R., Mills, T. C., Williamson, J., Hart, T., Greenwood, G., Paul, J., Pollack, L., Binson, D., Osmond, D., & Catania, J. A. (2003). Association of co-occurring psychosocial health problems and increased vulnerability to HIV/AIDS among urban men who have sex with men. *American Journal of Public Health, 93*(6), 939–942. https://doi.org/10.2105/ajph.93.6.939.

Stall, R., Paul, J. P., Greenwood, G., Pollack, L. M., Bein, E., Crosby, G. M., Mills, T. C., Binson, D., Coates, T. J., & Catania, J. A. (2001). Alcohol use, drug use and alcohol-related problems among men who have sex with men: The Urban Men's Health Study. *Addiction, 96*(11), 1589–1601. https://doi.org/10.1046/j.1360-0443.2001.961115896.x.

Szymanski, D. M. (2005). Heterosexism and sexism as correlates of psychological distress in lesbians. *Journal of Counseling & Development, 83*, 355–360.

Szymanski, D. M., & Gupta, A. (2009). Examining the relationship between multiple internalized oppressions and African American lesbian, gay, bisexual, and questioning persons' self-esteem and psychological distress. *Journal of Counseling Psychology, 56*(1), 110–118. https://doi.org/10.1037/a0012981.

Testa, R. J., Habarth, J., Peta, J., Balsam, K., & Bockting, W. (2015). Development of the gender minority stress and resilience measure. *Psychology of Sexual Orientation and Gender Diversity, 2*(1), 65–77. https://doi.org/10.1037/sgd0000081.

Thoma, B. C., & Huebner, D. M. (2013). Health consequences of racist and antigay discrimination for multiple minority adolescents. *Cultural Diversity and Ethnic Minority Psychology, 19*, 404–413. https://doi.org/10.1037/a0031739.

Tsai, A. C., & Burns, B. F. (2015). Syndemics of psychosocial problems and HIV risk: A systematic review of empirical tests of the disease interaction concept. *Social Science & Medicine, 139*, 26–35. https://doi.org/10.1016/j.socscimed.2015.06.024.

van der Star, A., Pachankis, J. E., & Bränström, R. (2019). Sexual orientation openness and depression symptoms: A population-based study. *Psychology of Sexual Orientation and Gender Diversity, 6*(3), 369–381. https://doi.org/10.1037/sgd0000335.

Velez, B. L., & Moradi, B. (2016). A moderated mediation test of minority stress: The role of collective identity. *The Counseling Psychologist, 44*, 1132–1157. https://doi.org/10.1177/0011000016665467.

Velez, B. L., Polihronakis, C. J., Watson, L. B., & Cox, R. (2019). Heterosexism, racism, and the mental health of sexual minority people of color. *The Counseling Psychologist, 47*, 129–159. https://doi.org/10.1177/0011000019828309.

Wilson, P. A., Nanin, J., Amesty, S., Wallace, S., Cherenack, E. M., & Fullilove, R. (2014). Using syndemic theory to understand vulnerability to HIV infection among black and Latino men in new York City. *Journal of Urban Health, 91*(5), 983–998. https://doi.org/10.1007/s11524-014-9895-2.

LGBTQ+ People and Discrimination: What We Have and Continue to Face in the Fight for Our Lives

Anneliese Singh, Rebekah Ingram Estevez, and Natalia Truszczynski

Writing about the experiences of LGBTQ+ people and discrimination is both a solemn and daunting task, as there is much to cover. LGBTQ+ communities have faced pervasive and persistent generational trauma and discrimination due to colonization and indigenous erasure of LGBTQ+ identities over many centuries that has extended into our current sociopolitical times (Singh et al., 2020). This trauma and discrimination has become embedded in societal institutions, such as education, healthcare, law, and more—which then plays out across interpersonal relationships in multiple settings (e.g., family, dating, friendship, work) to create inequities on a grand scale for LGBTQ+ people (Fig. 1).

We note this solemn and daunting task at the outset of this chapter, as it will be impossible to cover LGTBQ+ discrimination exhaustively. We also note the overwhelming nature of this task, as we want to also push against this discrimination even as we write. Yes, LGBTQ+ people and communities have faced, and continue to face, extensive societal bias and prejudice. Yet, a key understanding of LGBTQ+ discrimination has also been that LGBTQ+ people have also fought for their lives in a multitude of ways through coping and resilience to discrimination that we must acknowledge in psychology and the helping professions. We must also note that because of intersecting advantages and disadvantages, some in the LGBTQ+ community have been able to buffer the effects of discrimination through their

A. Singh (✉)
Office of Chief Diversity Officer, Tulane University, New Orleans, LA, USA
e-mail: anneliese@tulane.edu

R. I.Estevez · N. Truszczynski
Department of Counseling Psychology, University of Georgia, Athens, GA, USA
e-mail: rebeste@uga.edu; nattrus@uga.edu

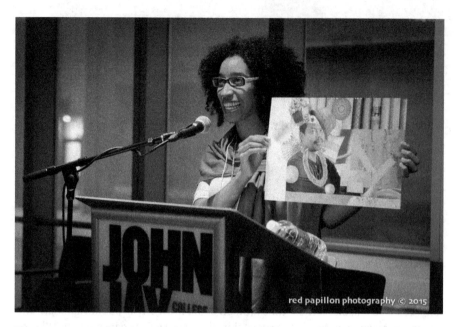

Fig. 1 Dr. Alexis Gumbs, author and poet, presents at the LGBTQ Scholars of Color Network Conference. Photo Courtesy of Riya Ortiz/Red Papillon Photography

privileged identities (e.g., white, able-bodied, middle and upper class, educational access, U.S. citizen, Christianity, etc.). So, as we write this chapter, we issue at the outset a debt of gratitude to the generations of Black feminist women, such as Sojourner Truth (1863), Kimberlé Crenshaw (1991), Brittany Cooper (2018), and many, many more who have gifted us the scholarship of intersectionality that demands we examine how interlocking oppressions influence well-being and access to the resources people need to survive and fight against societal inequity.

In this chapter, we cover essential constructs to know in order to understand LGBTQ+ discrimination, and the types of discrimination experiences LGBTQ+ communities face. We also review the LGBTQ+ resilience and coping literature, share a case study that highlights the impact of discrimination for LGBTQ+ people from an intersectionality theory perspective. We end with implications for practice, policy, and advocacy, so mental health professionals can seek to dismantle cis-het supremacy and other interlocking oppressions through reducing the harm our professions have and continue to inflict on LGBTQ+ communities.

1 Understanding LGBTQ+ Experiences of Discrimination: Essential Concepts

The LGBTQ+ community is heterogenous in nature, made of several microgroups encompassing varying sexual orientations (e.g. lesbian, queer) and gender identities (e.g. non-binary, trans man; Mink et al., 2014). Sexual orientation is a separate, though related, construct from gender identity. A person's sexual orientation reflects their sexual, emotional, and/or physical attraction to another person, while gender identity reflects a person's internally experienced sense of where they fall on the gender spectrum of identities such as woman, man, third gender, non-binary, and/or agender (American Psychological Association, 2015; Knutson et al., 2019).

In order to acknowledge the pervasive impact of LGBTQ+ discrimination, we must know terms related to the mechanisms of LGBTQ+ oppression. Society as a whole is steeped in heteronormativity—the social norm and policy-enforced belief that there are two genders (cisgender man and woman), two sexes (male and female), and that romantic and/or sexual relationships should consist of cisgender man/woman pairs and families should be headed by such gendered and sexually normative individuals (Oswald et al., 2005, as cited in Allen & Mendez, 2018). Heteronormativity is a powerful systemic force within the social, institutional, and political domains and confers privilege and power to groups whose identities align with these norms and values (Allen & Mendez, 2018; Mink et al., 2014). Thus, people whose sexual orientation and/or gender identity differ are subject to prejudice, discrimination, and rejection, the effects of which detrimentally impact health and wellbeing (Meyer, 2003; Meyer, 2015; Hendricks & Testa, 2012).

Importantly, expressions of heteronormativity intersect with other systems of power and oppression within which it is embedded—namely classism, ethnocentricity, racism, nationalism, and able-bodied bias, among others (Allen & Mendez, 2018; Crenshaw, 1989; Mink et al., 2014). Additionally, the classic model of heteronormativity has been expanded to include some previously "variant" genders (binary trans men and women), sexualities (lesbian, gay, and bisexual), and family groupings (monogamous gay and lesbian couples and their children; Allen & Mendez, 2018). However, people whose identities fall under the LGBTQ+ "umbrella" still face identity-based stigma and discrimination and subsequent negative impact on mental and physical health.

In addition to heteronormativity, essential concepts towards understanding the types of discrimination experienced by the LGBTQ+ community include intersectionality theory and the minority stress model (Meyer, 2003; Meyer, 2015). Introduced to the scholarly community by Black feminist author Kimberlé Crenshaw, intersectionality is a framework that allows an understanding of how intersecting systems of oppression (e.g. heteronormativity, cisgenderism, racism) create a unique experience of oppression in persons whose identities are tied to these systems. As herself stated:

> Intersectionality is a lens through which you can see where power comes and collides ... it's not simply that there's a race problem here, a gender problem here, and a class or [LGBTQ+] problem there ...

Thus, taking an intersectional approach to the study of LGBTQ+ communities is essential in order to fully understand risks and opportunities for healing (Mink et al., 2014; Tan et al., 2020).

After Crenshaw noted the importance of intersectionality in understanding legal inequities, Meyer (1995) developed the minority stress model to note the observed mental and physical health inequities experienced by the LGB community.

According to this model, distal or external (e.g. experiencing discrimination) and proximal or internal (e.g. expecting future discrimination experiences) stressors that are unique, identity-based, and emanate from the social/cultural level and have direct impacts on LGB health (Meyer, 2003). This initial model has since been expanded to be inclusive of trans and non-binary (TNB) identities, with unique distal (e.g. non-affirmation of identity) and proximal (e.g. concealment of trans identity) stressors identified in this population (Hendricks & Testa, 2012; Testa et al., 2015; McLemore, 2018). Importantly, the minority stress model and other models, such as the Intersectional Ecology Model (IEM) of LGBTQ+ health, show that the source of stress and subsequent negative impact on health does not lie *within* LGBTQ+ individuals, nor is due to one's LGBTQ+ identity (Mink et al., 2014; Meyer, 2015). Instead, observed health inequities that LGBTQ+ people face are due to social level determinants of health, such as stigma, discrimination, and rejection due to one's identity that does not align with heteronormativity.

2 General Impact of Discrimination on LGBTQ+ Health and Wellbeing

Researchers in public health and psychology have documented a number of detrimental impacts of minority stress and experiences of discrimination in the LGBTQ+ community. Broadly, LGBTQ+ identified peoples' reported rates of mental health disorders such as anxiety and depression (Irish et al., 2019; Plöderl & Tremblay, 2015), disordered eating behaviors (Austin et al., 2009), psychological distress (Kelleher, 2009; Becker et al., 2014), and substance abuse (Bränström & Pachankis, 2018) are elevated in relation to heterosexual persons. Further, some studies have found that LGB-identified individuals are significantly more likely to have comorbid mental health conditions than their same-gender heterosexual peers (e.g. Cochran et al., 2003; Bränström & Pachankis, 2018).

Additionally, suicidal ideation and attempts are a major concern for persons who fall under the LGBTQ+ umbrella, especially for LGBTQ+ youth (Haas et al., 2010; Hottes et al., 2016; Rhoades et al., 2018). Particular types of identity-related stressors faced by the LGB community include law enforcement harassment, threats of bodily harm, barred access to social resources and support, workplace discrimination, housing insecurity, concealment of identity, social isolation, familial rejection, identity disclosure-related stress, subsequent negative emotional experiences such as shame and guilt, and the use of maladaptive coping mechanisms (Mink et al., 2014; DeSouza et al., 2017; Riggle et al., 2017; Kaniuka et al., 2019; Bruce et al., 2015; Pachankis et al., 2015; Mereish et al., 2014; Mallory et al., 2014). Of particular importance, familial rejection (Needham & Austin, 2010) and experiencing conflict between one's religious and sexual minority identity (e.g. Gibbs & Goldbach, 2015) have been identified as predictors of psychiatric distress and negative socioeconomic outcomes such as housing insecurity.

3   Impact of Discrimination on the Health and Wellbeing of LGBTQ+ BIPOC Communities

The scholarship using intersectionality theory to examine the impact of heteronormativity and racism, classism, ageism, adultism, xenophobia, and other interlocking oppressions on LGBTQ+ health is still emerging. Much of the research emerging initially has suggested that being LGBTQ+ and BIPOC (Black, Indigenous, People of Color) increases the likelihood of experiencing racialized forms of heteronormativity, such as unequal access to socioeconomic resources like employment and health insurance, and vicarious or secondary trauma through witnessing violence and rejection (Balsam et al., 2015; Ramirez & Paz Galupo, 2019). For instance, LGBTQ+ BIPOC experience both discrimination and anticipation of rejection from their own racial/ethnic communities *and* from the broader, majority white LGBTQ+ community (Hailey et al., 2020; McConnell et al., 2018; Balsam et al., 2011). These unique distal and proximal stressors create barriers in the access to social capital, such as experiencing a sense of belongingness, connection to community, and the conferral of other community level resources that can buffer the impact of racism and heterosexism.

Rejection and discrimination from within one's own racial/ethnic community can also be experienced as particularly distressing due to the absence of community support in the face of structural and interpersonal racism, and has been postulated as the reason for lower rates of sexual identity disclosure among LGBTQ+ BIPOC (Balsam et al., 2015). However, some studies have shown that despite being exposed to more discrimination and victimization, LGBTQ+ BIPOC show little to no differences in the domains of physical and mental health (e.g. Balsam et al., 2015; Hatzenbuehler, 2009). Scholars have suggested that this pattern of results may in part be due to LGBTQ+ BIPOC resilience and coping processes, perhaps informed by prior exposure to race-based stress in development and the need to cope with and be resilient to racism that then strengthens resistance to racialized heteronormative bias (Bowleg et al., 2003; McConnell et al., 2018).

4   Impact of Discrimination on the Health and Wellbeing of TNB Communities

As previously stated, the specific identity-related minority stressors due to heteronormativity and cisnormativity in society are similar yet distinct processes for members of the TNB community (Hendricks & Testa, 2012; Testa et al. 2015). The scholarship regarding TNB individuals' experiences of discrimination and subsequent impact on mental health has grown over the last few decades, but still lags in important areas such as epidemiology and psychology (Reisner et al., 2016; Valentine & Shipherd, 2018). We do know that TNB people experience highly disparate rates of negative health and wellbeing, as well as high rates of identity-related stigma and victimization, when compared to their cisgender counterparts (Millet et al., 2017; Tan et al., 2020; James et al., 2016). This holds true even when compared to cisgender people who identify as a sexual minority (Sue et al., 2016).

Specific types of minority stressors for TNB individuals include non-affirmation of identity through misgendering or the incorrect use of name and pronouns, discrimination in medical settings, victimization and harassment in public settings like bathrooms, home and family violence, and loss of control over identity disclosure choice due to factors such as stage of medical transition and access to medical care (McLemore, 2018; Testa et al., 2015; Hendricks & Testa, 2012; Cogan et al., 2020; Goldberg et al., 2019). These distal or external stressors also contribute to specific proximal or internal identity based stressors, such as fear of future rejection or victimization, internalized negative beliefs about oneself due to TNB identity, identity concealment, and using subsequent maladaptive coping mechanisms such as isolation, substance abuse and non-suicidal self-harm behaviors to mitigate feelings of shame, fear, and hypervigilance (Dickey et al., 2015; Testa et al., 2017; Sue et al., 2016; Testa et al., 2015; Hendricks & Testa, 2012; Cogan et al., 2020; Rood et al., 2016).

Also of note, the TNB community is itself a community made of up of multiple micro-communities of individuals with varying gender identities such as binary trans people (e.g. trans man), non-binary people (e.g. genderqueer), and people who do not identify with having a gender identity (e.g. gendervoid; Matsuno, 2019). Recent scholarship has shown that non-binary people experience more frequent and pervasive minority stressors and subsequent increased rates of mental health disparities (e.g. Goldberg et al., 2019; Lefevor et al., 2019). More research is desperately needed regarding the unique experiences and needs of non-binary and genderqueer individuals as this literature base is nascent.

While research with the TNB community is growing, there is a dearth in research centering the unique experiences of racialized trans-prejudice in the lives of TNB BIPOC. Additionally, research centering the intersectional impact of other systems of oppression (e.g. classism, religious affiliation) are nascent. However, existing studies have shown that the detrimental impact of living at the intersection of racism and trans-prejudice produces particularly insidious and consistent patterns of exposure to violence, discrimination, and prejudice, with subsequent detrimental impacts on health (James et al., 2016). The deadly impact of racism intersecting with trans-prejudice, and the protective privilege of whiteness, was highlighted in a recent report showing that while overall, TNB individuals were less likely to be murdered than their cisgender counterparts, young Black and Latina transfeminine persons were significantly more likely to be murdered than their cisgender counterparts (Dinno, 2017). Similarly, in 2019, of the 25 reported killings of TNB people, 91% were Black trans women and 81% were younger than 30 (Human Rights Campaign Foundation, 2019). These reported statistics of violence against TNB people also highlight other variables that are salient in the lives of TNB BIPPOC—geographic location and age. For instance, the majority of TNB people murdered are under the age of 30 and live in the South (Human Rights Campaign Foundation, 2019).

In addition to homicide, documented distal stressors against TNB BIPOC include barred access to socioeconomic resources like employment discrimination and subsequent poverty and housing insecurity, emotional abuse, high rates of living with HIV, police harassment, dispirate incarceration rates, high levels of sexual assault and violence, and discrimination within healthcare settings (James et al., 2016; Poteat et al., 2016; James & Salcedo, 2017; Brown & Jones, 2014). Importantly, such experiences of discrimination have been linked to not just one's trans identity, but one's *racialized* trans identity (e.g. Howard et al., 2019). While there have been important methodological questions raised regarding the reported high rates of HIV/AIDS in the TNB community (e.g. Poteat et al., 2016), TNB BIPOC are often forced to engage in survival sex work, an employment strategy which carries with it a high risk for HIV/AIDS, due to factors such as employment discrimination and subsequent poverty, in order to provide for basic needs and access to trans-affirming medical procedures (Poteat et al., 2017; Bith-Melander et al., 2010; Sevelius, 2013). Further investigating unique intersectional structural impacts on experiences of discrimination, Latinx TNB individuals immigrating to the U.S. face unique stressors, such as trauma due to their TNB identity pre-immigration in their home country, and a severe lack of social and structural support post-immigration such as policy-level barriers to accessing resources such as housing, education, and employment (Morales, 2013; Rhodes et al., 2015).

Overall, it is clear that (a) sexual orientation and gender minority stress have real and detrimental impacts on the health and wellbeing of the LGBTQ+ community, (b) different types of minority stress exist within the micro-communities embedded under the LGBTQ+ umbrella, and (c) the impact of interlocking systems of oppression with heteronormativity and cisnormativity compound experiences of unique types of minority stress. Finally, more research is desperately needed that takes an intersectional approach to understanding the impact of discrimination, violence, rejection, and the internalization of these events in the lives of LGBTQ+ people (Fig. 2).

5   LGBTQ+ Coping and Resilience

When research studying the health outcomes of LGBTQ+ people first became prevalent, this scholarship initially focused heavily on what were considered unhealthy behaviors (e.g. substance use, sex work) and experienced violence (Benotsch et al., 2013; Clements-Nolle et al., 2006). However now, the research focus has shifted away from events that happen to LGBTQ+ people, and their "problem behaviors" to how these communities cope with anti-LGBTQ+ bias and build and express resilience (Kwon, 2013; Meyer, 2015; Singh et al., 2014). Research on coping and resilience has started with defining resilience and types of coping and has only recently started to examine how resilience and coping may help reduce the impact of anti-trans bias and improve health outcomes (Budge et al., 2017; Kwon 2013; Meyer, 2015; Singh et al., 2014; White Hughto et al., 2017).

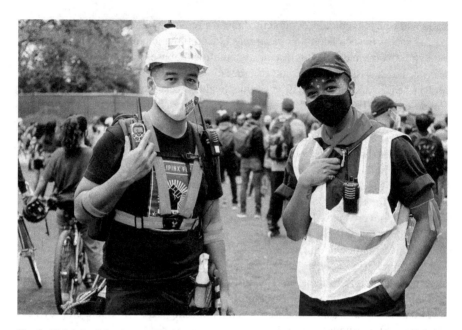

Fig. 2 Kalaya'an Mendoza and Robyn Ayers are members of Across Front Lines—a collective of social justice practitioners who work alongside communities to advocate for justice and equity. Photo Courtesy of Kalaya'an Mendoza

Literature defining the coping strategies among LGBTQ+ people is still scarce. The majority of studies that do exist examine avoidant coping strategies (e.g. substance use, self-harm, ignoring the problem) in response to discrimination and stigma. In line with other coping research, avoidant coping in LGBTQ+ people is associated with more negative mental health outcomes in response to stigma than those who did not endorse avoidant coping mechanisms. Avoidant coping has been associated with higher levels of depression and anxiety in multiple studies (Budge et al., 2013; Kwon, 2013; Mizock & Mueser, 2014; White Hughto et al., 2017). Only in one study was coping clearly defined as the mediator between discrimination and mental health, leaving room for future research (White Hughto et al., 2017).

One study with TNB people examined adaptive strategies mediating the impact of coming out on mental health (Budge et al., 2017). Nine themes of adaptive coping were identified that closely reflect resilience strategies as well. Some themes were: accepting support and seeking support, utilization of agency and increasing protection of self, self-efficacy, and self-acceptance. This study marks the beginning of researchers identifying identity-specific coping strategies and bridging the gap in research between TNB resilience and coping (Budge et al., 2017).

Where there is a dearth in research adaptive coping strategies among TNB people, multiple qualitative studies have examined the themes of resilience among TNB people. Qualitative research has identified seven themes of resilience among transgender and TNB people (Moody et al., 2015; Singh, 2013; Singh et al., 2011; Singh

& McKleroy, 2010; Singh et al., 2014). They are: (1) evolving definition of self, (2) embracing self-worth, (3) awareness of oppressions, (4) connection with a supportive community, (5) cultivating hope for the future, (6) social activism and (7) being a positive role model (Moody et al., 2015; Singh, 2013; Singh et al., 2011; Singh & McKleroy, 2010; Singh et al., 2014).

Another resilience factor that has recently emerged in research is asserting oneself or confrontation (Bry et al., 2017; Budge et al., 2016). Qualitative research with TNB young people has found this factor to be especially important in building confidence and dealing with microaggressions and other forms of discriminatory stress (Bry et al., 2017; Budge et al., 2016). The act of standing up for oneself and expressing one's opinion allowed the participants to feel heard, and feel like they took action, even if it did not result in the person changing their mind (Bry et al., 2017; Budge et al., 2016). This resilience factor combines other previously identified factors, such as self-defining identity and participation in activism/advocacy.

The themes of resilience represent individual processes that exist within the context of a TNB person's community and resources. Resilience, as conceptualized for TNB people in response to minority stress, exists on the community level, where it cannot exist without the presence of the community, and community-based, affirming resources (Meyer, 2015). While to be resilient, the person must take part in individual resilient processes, it is not solely dependent on the processes listed previously, making it different from coping strategies. Additionally, resilience has been described as successful coping (Meyer, 2015). Whereas coping can be adaptive or maladaptive, resilience is by definition adaptive.

The community context of resilience is a key element in TNB resilience and is what differentiates it from the original academic conceptualizations of resilience. Because TNB individuals experience chronic stress and discrimination based on their community identity, it would be unrealistic to claim that the response to the community stress is individualistic (Meyer, 2015). Thinking about resilience on the community level allows for resilience to rely on the presence of resources such as community centers, affirming clinics and other healthcare providers, support groups, networking, and organizations that provide opportunities to both provide advocacy and needed resources (Meyer, 2015; Singh et al., 2014). It is within the context of the community provided resources that individuals can participate in individual resilience processes (Meyer, 2015; Singh et al., 2011).

Current research in the field of resilience among TNB individuals has focused on describing the processes of resilience and providing conceptual and theoretical frameworks. Most studies that examine resilience do not directly tie it to any outcomes other than to hypothesize that it increases survival and decreases mental health issues (Moody et al., 2015; Singh & McKleroy, 2010). However, some researchers have examined how specific components of resilience are associated with health outcomes among TNB people, mainly mental health outcomes (Bockting et al., 2013; Breslow et al., 2015; Budge et al., 2013; Pflum et al., 2015).

Multiple studies found that social (or peer) support moderates the impact of stigma on mental health (Bockting et al., 2013; Breslow et al., 2015; Budge et al., 2013; Pflum et al., 2015). Social support is the resilience theme that has been found most consistently in research to improve the mental health outcomes of TNB people. One key factor about social support is that, while not necessary, social support from other TNB people was especially protective against negative mental health outcomes (Budge et al., 2013; Moody et al., 2015; Pflum et al., 2015). Other resilience themes such as identity pride and activism/advocacy have contradictory findings in terms of their impact on TNB mental health (Breslow et al., 2015). This may come from the lack of a community-specific measurement tool, or from small sample sizes. What is clear from these findings in that more research must be conducted on both adaptive coping strategies and resilience to discrimination so that future interventions and counseling methods can be constructed from clear research-based evidence.

Up to now in this chapter, we have explored the broad experiences of LGBTQ+ discrimination, resilience, and coping. In the next section, we integrate attention to how sexism, classism, immigration, and fatphobia can interlock with the oppressions of anti-LGBTQ+ discrimination and racism. We follow this intersectional case example with implications for practice, policy, and advocacy.

6 Case Example

Pritham is a 66-year old lesbian, cisgender woman who identifies as a Sikh, third-generation South Asian American and U.S. citizen who uses she/her/hers pronouns. She works as an engineer in the southern U.S., where she is Vice-President of her organization. Pritham has struggled the last 2 years with depression that emerged after the death of her partner of 30 years. She is estranged from her immediate siblings who rejected her because of her lesbian identity, although she does have strong relationships with some of her nephews and nieces. Pritham does not believe in counseling, however, she has been having difficulty getting out of bed in the mornings and is starting to miss work a few days a month. She sought counseling at the urging of her friend, who is extremely worried about her overall well-being.

As you work with Pritham, you explore her family history. She shares that her grandfather immigrated to the U.S. to work on the railroad in California. Her grandfather married a Chicana woman, and they had four children together. Her grandparents did not live long due to working in harsh conditions and exposure to toxins as they worked in agriculture in their 30s. Pritham never met her grandparents and does not identify with her Chicana heritage, as her father felt he had to hide this part of himself or be at risk of even more discrimination as a dark-skinned Indian, Sikh person wearing a turban. Pritham shares experiences of racism throughout her life in school and within her job currently, although when asked more about these experiences, she minimizes them.

Pritham shares that she never shared her lesbian identity with her family, as she was fearful that she would not be accepted. She always felt like she was hiding something from them and struggled with feelings of worthlessness. Pritham describes beginning to gain weight in her early 20s and experiencing fatphobia from her South Asian family and friends. She also shares that she felt pressure to "do everything right" and become an "engineer or doctor" to please her family. During college, she was able to explore her sexuality and date cisgender women, and she met her partner in her doctoral studies as an engineer. Her parents were accepting of her relationship, however, her siblings were not accepting, which caused strife throughout the rest of her life, especially as her parents died. Three months after her parents died, her partner died as well. Pritham had been caring for her partner alone, while also interfacing with her siblings and grieving their deaths. She shares that she has nothing to live for anymore, and that she has no community or friends—although she describes that her nieces and nephews ask to spend time with her and were close with her partner. Pritham was recently diagnosed with Multiple Sclerosis, and she has not shared this diagnosis with anyone. She makes a high salary at her job; however, she spent her life savings and sold her house in order to pay for necessary medical care for her partner and parents, so she is struggling with debt as she is also thinking about retirement. Pritham shares she has many questions about her life—whether she should have had children and whether she failed her parents by being a lesbian. Pritham also shares that she has been thinking about her own death and what she might experience as she ages with no partner.

7   Implications for Practice, Policy, and Advocacy

Pritham's case is a complex one. The forces of LGBTQ+ bias and racism are certainly operating on her life and provide context for her depression. However, the interlocking oppressions related to racism, immigration, disability, gender, class, age, and more are also influencing how she is coping in the aftermath of multiple deaths of loved ones. There are multiple implications for practice, policy, and advocacy.

7.1   Practice

With regard to practice, the mental health professional who works with Pritham should have a strong understanding of the history of racism in the U.S., including how racism interlocks with anti-immigrant, anti-Latinx, anti-Sikh, and anti-South Asian discrimination. A first step is of course, validating the multiple grief processes that Pritham is experiencing with the loss of her parents and long-time partner. However, there are other losses as well—loss of complete understanding of her Chicana history, loss of her sibling support, and the losses that come with feeling she had to please her family through becoming an engineer and worrying about whether she would lose connection with her parents as a lesbian. In addition, there may be losses related to her gender and sexism, as there is much to explore about how she experienced patriarchy within her family and within her work as an engineer. There is also the recent grief of knowing Pritham is living with a disability and that she had experienced fatphobia within her community and society that resulted in distrust and not valuing her body. There is also the lived experience of multiple classes statuses—having access to wealth, losing wealth, and still having access to wealth through her job, but not being able to build wealth because of her age and the disappearance of her savings.

As she begins to process these multiple losses, it is important to do a thorough trauma and suicide assessment, and it is also important to assess the resiliencies and coping strategies that Pritham developed over her life. Exploring these strategies will provide insight into Pritham's strengths that she can leverage to address the influence of interlocking areas of discrimination in her life. For instance, the support and desire to connect expressed from her nieces and nephews—and their closeness to her long-time partner—could be possible areas to explore related to not only connection, but the trust that she may need and want to build as she thinks about aging with a physical and mental health disability. There is also the potential resilience and coping related to her religious/spiritual beliefs, as well as the privileges associated with her advanced educational degree, job status as a leader, and her third generation U.S. citizen status.

As Pritham explores her grief in counseling, it is also important that she be validated in her grief. The systems of oppression that have operated on her life—and across generations of her life—have real impacts on her well-being now. Her mental health practitioner should have a strong understanding of what community support resources exist with regard to grief for LGBTQ+ people of color, as well as resources for people living with Multiple Sclerosis and financial stressors. There is also the opportunity to identify to what degree Pritham has internalized the mechanisms of oppression that have operated on her life. For instance, does she feel valuable as a lesbian, as a cisgender woman, as an engineer, and as a person recently learning about her physical disability and also mental health challenges. Assessing these degrees of internalized oppression will be helpful to support her on the journey of valuing herself and knowing she is deserving of support and help during the most stressful time in her life. If LGBTQ+ discrimination and interlocking oppressions are designed to suppress and oppress historically marginalized groups, creating a practice environment where Pritham is able to remember, explore, and value her own resilience, learn about her self-defined interests, and even experience joy and empowerment as a 66-year old, cisgender, lesbian, Sikh, South Asian with Chicana heritage, engineer, person of size, and living with disability is the antidote to these oppressions.

7.2   Advocacy and Policy

Pritham's case has many issues related to advocacy and policy embedded within it. Her mental health provider should have strong skills and knowledge of how to access the culturally-responsive and empowering resources for LGBTQ+ BIPOC

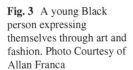

Fig. 3 A young Black person expressing themselves through art and fashion. Photo Courtesy of Allan Franca

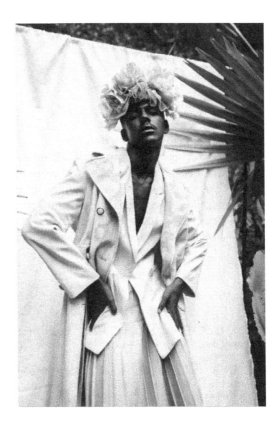

people experiencing grief and be connected with support resources related to mental and physical disability. As this provider shares these resources with Pritham, it is important to vet them beforehand to ensure they are affirming of LGBTQ+ people in all of their diversities; and, to advocate for LGBTQ+ affirming policies and procedures when anti-LGBTQ+ ones are encountered in vetting these resources so that Pritham does not experience further harm.

Because societal anti-LGBTQ+ discrimination and other oppression is so widespread, it will be challenging to refer Pritham to the right ones even as a strong advocate. Therefore, an important aspect of advocacy bridges back to practice, and to ensure that Pritham has the opportunity to role-play and know her rights when she is interfacing with societal institutions and other family and work settings where she needs to advocate for herself. Other policy needs include advocating for universal healthcare and extensive and interdisciplinary support resources for LGBTQ+ BIPOC as they age, while also seeking to counter anti-immigrant and anti-disability policies. For instance, what are the policies that will help and/ or harm Pritham as she experiences more impact on her life as someone living with Multiple Sclerosis? Fatphobia was certainly operating on Pritham's life in many ways, so it is also important to ask how might fatphobic policies in society be challenged and revised? Strong advocacy and policy change can also include demanding that the entire history, her-story, and trans-story of LGBTQ+ communities be more widely known, taught, and affirmed across all societal institutions.

8 Conclusion

As we noted in the opening to this chapter, writing about LGBTQ+ discrimination and interlocking oppressions is a task where we literally grieve as we write. Yet, we in the mental health professions with the power, privilege, and advantage we have can feel this grief and channel it into action every opportunity we can. When we take these actions, we are changing the future possibilities for LGBTQ+ people and communities to experience less harm and less discrimination, which in turns develops environments that are more affirming and more liberating (Fig. 3).

References

Allen, S. H., & Mendez, S. N. (2018). Hegemonic heteronormativity: Toward a new era of queer family theory. *Journal of Family Theory and Review, 10*(1), 70–86. https://doi.org/10.1111/jftr.12241.

American Psychological Association. (2015). Guidelines for psychological practice with transgender and gender nonconforming people. *American Psychologist, 70*(9), 832–864. https://doi.org/10.1037/a003990.

Austin, S. B., Ziyadeh, N. J., Corliss, H. L., Rosario, M., Wypij, D., Haines, J., Camargo, C. A., Jr., & Field, A. E. (2009). Sexual orientation disparities in purging and binge eating from early to late adolescence. *Journal of Adolescent Health, 45*(3), 238–245. https://doi.org/10.1016/j.jadohealth.2009.02.001.

Balsam, K. F., Molina, Y., Beadnell, B., Simoni, J., & Walters, K. (2011). Measuring multiple minority stress: The LGBT people of color microaggressions scale. *Cultural Diversity and Ethnic Minority Psychology, 17*(2), 163–174. https://doi.org/10.1037/a0023244.

Balsam, K. F., Molina, Y., Blayney, J. A., Dillworth, T., Zimmerman, L., & Kaysen, D. (2015). Racial/ethnic differences in identity and mental health outcomes among young sexual minority women. *Cultural Diversity and Ethnic Minority Psychology, 21*(3), 380–390.

Becker, M., Cortina, K. S., Tsai, Y. M., & Eccles, J. S. (2014). Sexual orientation, psychological Well-being, and mental health: A longitudinal analysis from adolescence to young adulthood. *Psychology of Sexual Orientation and Gender Diversity, 1*(2), 132–145. https://doi.org/10.1037/sgd0000038.

Benotsch, E. G., Zimmerman, R., Cathers, L., McNulty, S., Pierce, J., Heck, T., Perrin, P. B., & Snipes, D. (2013). Non-medical use of prescription drugs, polysubstance use, and mental health in transgender adults. *Drug and Alcohol Dependence, 132*(1–2), 391–394. https://doi.org/10.1016/j.drugalcdep.2013.02.027.

Bith-Melander, P., Sheoran, B., Sheth, L., Bermudez, C., Drone, J., Wood, W., & Schroeder, K. (2010). Understanding sociocultural and psychological factors affecting transgender people of color in San Francisco. *Journal of the Association of Nurses in AIDS Care, 21*(3), 207–220. https://doi.org/10.1016/j.jana.2010.01.008.

Bockting, W. O., Miner, M. H., Romine, R. E. S., Hamilton, A., & Coleman, E. (2013). Stigma, mental health, and resilience in an online sample of the US transgender population. *American Journal of Public Health, 103*(5), 943–951. https://doi.org/10.2105/AJPH.2013.301241.

Bowleg, L., Huang, J., Brooks, K., Black, A., & Burkholder, G. (2003). Triple jeopardy and beyond: Multiple minority stress and resilience among Black lesbians. *Journal of Lesbian Studies, 7*(4), 87–108. https://doi.org/10.1300/J155v07n04_06.

Bränström, R., & Pachankis, J. E. (2018). Sexual orientation disparities in the co-occurrence of substance use and psychological distress: A national population-based study (2008–2015). *Social Psychiatry and Psychiatric Epidemiology, 53*(4), 403–412. https://doi.org/10.1007/s00127-018-1491-4.

Breslow, A. S., Brewster, M. E., Velez, B. L., Wong, S., Geiger, E., & Soderstrom, B. (2015). Resilience and collective action: Exploring buffers against minority stress for transgender individuals. *Psychology of Sexual Orientation and Gender Diversity, 2*(3), 253–265. https://doi.org/10.1037/sgd0000117.

Brown, G. R., & Jones, K. T. (2014). Racial health disparities in a cohort of 5,135 transgender veterans. *Journal of Racial and Ethnic Health Disparities, 1*(4), 257–266. https://doi.org/10.1007/s40615-014-0032-4.

Bruce, D., Harper, G. W., & Bauermeister, J. A. (2015). Minority stress, positive identity development, and depressive symptoms: Implications for resilience among sexual minority male youth. *Psychology of Sexual Orientation and Gender Diversity, 2*(3), 287–296. https://doi.org/10.1037/sgd0000128.

Bry, L. J., Mustanski, B., Garofalo, R., Burns, M. N. (2017). Management of a concealable stigmatized identity: A qualitative study of concealment, disclosure, and role flexing among young, resilient sexual and gender minority individuals. *Journal of Homosexuality, 64*, 745–769. https://doi.org/10.1080/00918369.2016.1236574.

Budge, S. L., Adelson, J. L., & Howard, K. A. S. (2013). Anxiety and depression in transgender individuals: The roles of transition status, loss, social support, and coping. *Journal of Consulting and Clinical Psychology, 81*(3), 545–557. https://doi.org/10.1037/a0031774.

Budge, S. L., Thai, J. L., Tebbe, E. A., Howard, K. A. S. (2016). The intersection of race, sexual orientation, socioeconomic status, trans identity, and mental health outcomes. *The Counseling Psychologist, 44*, 1025–1049. https://doi.org/10.1177/0011000015609046.

Budge, S. L., Chin, M. Y., & Minero, L. P. (2017). Trans individuals' facilitative coping: An analysis of internal and external processes. *Journal of Counseling Psychology, 64*(1), 12–25. https://doi.org/10.1037/cou0000178.

Clements-Nolle, K., Marx, R., & Katz, M. (2006). Attempted suicide among transgender persons: The influence of gender-based discrimination and victimization. *Journal of Homosexuality, 51*(3), 53–69. https://doi.org/10.1300/J082v51n03_04.

Cochran, S. D., Sullivan, J. G., & Mays, V. M. (2003). Prevalence of mental disorders, psychological distress, and mental health services use among lesbian, gay, and bisexual adults in the United States. *Journal of Consulting and Clinical Psychology, 71*(1), 53–61. https://doi.org/10.1037/0022-006X.71.1.53.

Cogan, C. M., Scholl, J. A., Lee, J. Y., Cole, H. E., & Davis, J. L. (2020). Sexual violence and suicide risk in the transgender population: The mediating role of proximal stressors. *Psychology & Sexuality*, 1–12. [REI1]. https://doi.org/10.1080/19419899.2020.1729847.

Cooper, B. (2018). *Eloquent rage: A Black feminist discovers her superpower*. New York, NY: St. Martin's Press.

Crenshaw, K. (1991). Mapping the margins: Intersectionality, identity politics, and violence against women of color. *Stanford Law Review, 43*(6), 1241–1299. https://doi.org/10.2307/1229039.

DeSouza, E. R., Wesselmann, E. D., & Ispas, D. (2017). Workplace discrimination against sexual minorities: Subtle and not-so-subtle. *Canadian Journal of Administrative Sciences/Revue Canadienne des Sciences de l'Administration, 34*(2), 121–132. https://doi.org/10.1002/CJAS.1438.

Dickey, L. M., Reisner, S. L., & Juntunen, C. L. (2015). Non-suicidal self-injury in a large online sample of transgender adults. *Professional Psychology: Research and Practice, 46*(1), 3–11. https://doi.org/10.1037/a0038803.

Dinno, A. (2017). Homicide rates of transgender individuals in the United States: 2010–2014. *American Journal of Public Health, 107*(9), 1441–1447. https://doi.org/10.2105/AJPH.2017.303878.

Gibbs, J. J., & Goldbach, J. (2015). Religious conflict, sexual identity, and suicidal behaviors among LGBT young adults. *Archives of Suicide Research, 19*(4), 472–488. https://doi.org/10.1080/13811118.2015.1004476.

Goldberg, A. E., Kuvalanka, K. A., Budge, S. L., Benz, M. B., & Smith, J. Z. (2019). Health care experiences of transgender binary and nonbinary university students. *The Counseling Psychologist, 47*(1), 59–97. https://doi.org/10.1177/0011000019827568.

Haas, A. P., Eliason, M., Mays, V. M., Mathy, R. M., Cochran, S. D., D'Augelli, A. R., et al. (2010). Suicide and suicide risk in lesbian, gay, bisexual, and transgender populations: Review and recommendations. *Journal of Homosexuality, 58*(1), 10–51. https://doi.org/10.1080/00918369.2011.534038.

Hailey, J., Burton, W., & Arscott, J. (2020). We are family: Chosen and created families as a protective factor against racialized trauma and anti-LGBTQ oppression among African American sexual and gender minority youth. *Journal of GLBT Family Studies, 16*(2), 176–191. https://doi.org/10.1080/1550428X.2020.1724133.

Hatzenbuehler, M. L. (2009). How does sexual minority stigma "get under the skin"? A psychological mediation framework. *Psychological Bulletin, 135*(5), 707–730. https://doi.org/10.1037/a0016441.

Hendricks, M. L., & Testa, R. J. (2012). A conceptual framework for clinical work with transgender and gender nonconforming clients: An adaptation of the minority stress model. *Professional Psychology, Research and Practice, 43*(5), 460–467. https://doi.org/10.1037/a0029597.

Hottes, T. S., Bogaert, L., Rhodes, A. E., Brennan, D. J., & Gesink, D. (2016). Lifetime prevalence of suicide attempts among sexual minority adults by study sampling strategies: A systematic review and meta-analysis. *American Journal of Public Health, 106*(5), e1–e12.

Howard, S. D., Lee, K. L., Nathan, A. G., Wenger, H. C., Chin, M. H., & Cook, S. C. (2019). Healthcare experiences of transgender people of color. *Journal of General Internal Medicine, 34*(10), 2068–2074. https://doi.org/10.1007/s11606-019-05179-0.

Human Rights Campaign Foundation (2019). *A national epidemic: Fatal anti-transgender violence in the United States in 2019*. Retrieved from https://assets2.hrc.org/files/assets/resources/Anti-TransViolenceReport2019.pdf

Irish, M., Solmi, F., Mars, B., King, M., Lewis, G., Pearson, R. M., et al. (2019). Depression and self-harm from adolescence to young adulthood in sexual minorities compared with heterosexuals in the UK: A population-based cohort study. *The Lancet Child & Adolescent Health, 3*(2), 91–98. https://doi.org/10.1016/S2352-4642(18)30343-2.

James, S. E., Herman, J. L., Rankin, S., Keisling, M., Mottet, L., & Anafi, M. (2016). *The report of the 2015 U.S. transgender survey*. Washington, DC: National Center for Transgender Equality.

James, S., & Salcedo, B. (2017). 2015 US transgender survey: Report on the experiences of Latino/a respondents.

Kaniuka, A., Pugh, K. C., Jordan, M., Brooks, B., Dodd, J., Mann, A. K., Williams, S. L., & Hirsch, J. K. (2019). Stigma and suicide risk among the LGBTQ population: Are anxiety and depression to blame and can connectedness to the LGBTQ community help? *Journal of Gay & Lesbian Mental Health, 23*(2), 205–220. https://doi.org/10.1080/19359705.2018.1560385.

Kelleher, C. (2009). Minority stress [REI2] and health: Implications for lesbian, gay, bisexual, transgender, and questioning (LGBTQ) young people. *Counselling Psychology Quarterly, 4*, 373–379. https://doi.org/10.1080/09515070903334995.

Knutson, D., Koch, J. M., & Goldbach, C. (2019). Recommended terminology, pronouns, and documentation for work with transgender and non-binary populations. *Practice Innovations, 4*(4), 214–224. https://doi.org/10.1037/pri0000098.

Kwon, P. (2013). Resilience in lesbian, gay, and bisexual indivduals. *Personality and Social Psychology Review, 17*(4), 371–83. https://doi.org/10.1177/1088868313490248.

Lefevor, G. T., Boyd-Rogers, C. C., Sprague, B. M., & Janis, R. A. (2019). Health disparities between genderqueer, transgender, and cisgender individuals: An extension of minority stress theory. *Journal of Counseling Psychology, 66*(4), 385–395. https://doi.org/10.1037/cou0000339.

Mallory, C., Hasenbush, A., & Sears, B. (2014). Addressing harassment and discrimination by law enforcement against LGBT police officers and community members to improve effective policing. *LGBTQ Policy Journal, 5*, 79–87.

Matsuno, E. (2019). Nonbinary-affirming psychological interventions. *Cognitive and Behavioral Practice, 26*(4), 617–628. https://doi.org/10.1016/j.cbpra.2018.09.003.

McConnell, E. A., Janulis, P., Phillips, G., II, Truong, R., & Birkett, M. (2018). Multiple minority stress and LGBT community resilience among sexual minority men. *Psychology of Sexual Orientation and Gender Diversity, 5*(1), 1–12. https://doi.org/10.1037/sgd0000265.

McLemore, K. A. (2018). A minority stress perspective on transgender individuals' experiences with misgendering. *Stigma and Health, 3*(1), 53–64. https://doi.org/10.1037/sah0000070.

Mereish, E. H., O'Cleirigh, C., & Bradford, J. B. (2014). Interrelationships between LGBT-based victimization, suicide, and substance use problems in a diverse sample of sexual and gender minorities. *Psychology, Health & Medicine, 19*(1), 1–13.

Meyer, I. H. (1995). Minority stress and mental health in gay men. *Journal of Health and Socialhavior, 36*(1), 38–56. https://doi.org/10.2307/2137286.

Meyer, I. H. (2003). Prejudice, social stress, and mental health in lesbian, gay and bisexual populations: Conceptual issues and research evidence. *Psychological Bulletin, 129*(5), 674–697. https://doi.org/10.1037/0033-2909.129.5.674.

Meyer, I. H. (2015). Resilience in the study of minority stress and health of sexual and gender minorities. *Psychology of Sexual Orientation and Gender Diversity, 2*(3), 209–213. https://doi.org/10.1037/sgd0000132.

Millet, N., Longworth, J., & Arcelus, J. (2017). Prevalence of anxiety symptoms and disorders in the transgender population: A systematic review of the literature. *International Journal of Transgenderism, 18*(1), 27–38. https://doi.org/10.1080/15532739.2016.1258353.

Mink, M. D., Lindley, L. L., & Weinstein, A. A. (2014). Stress, stigma, and sexual minority status: The intersectional ecology model of LGBTQ health. *Journal of Gay & Lesbian Social Services, 26*(4), 502–521. https://doi.org/10.1080/10538720.2014.953660.

Mizock, L., & Mueser, K. T. (2014). Employment, mental health, internalized stigma, and coping with transphobia among transgender individuals. *Psychology of Sexual Orientation and Gender Diversity, 1*(2), 146–158. https://doi.org/10.1037/sgd0000029.

Moody, C., Fuks, N., Peláez, S., & Smith, N. G. (2015). 'Without this, I would for sure already be dead': A qualitative inquiry regarding suicide protective factors among trans adults. *Psychology of Sexual Orientation and Gender Diversity, 2*(3), 266–280. https://doi.org/10.1037/sgd0000130.

Morales, E. (2013). Latino lesbian, gay, bisexual, and transgender immigrants in the United States. *Journal of LGBT Issues in Counseling, 7*(2), 172–184. https://doi.org/10.1080/1553860 5.2013.785467.

Needham, B. L., & Austin, E. L. (2010). Sexual orientation, parental support, and health during the transition to young adulthood. *Journal of Youth and Adolescence, 39*(10), 1189–1198. https://doi.org/10.1007/s10964-010-9533-6.

Oswald, R., Blume, L., & Marks, S. (2005). Decentering heteronormativity: A proposal for family studies. In V. Bengtson, A. Acock, K. Allen, P. Dilworth-Anderson, & D. Klein (Eds.), *Sourcebook of family theories and methods: An interactive approach* (pp. 143–165). Thousand Oaks, CA: Sage. https://doi.org/10.4135/9781412990172.d32.

Pachankis, J. E., Cochran, S. D., & Mays, V. M. (2015). The mental health of sexual minority adults in and out of the closet: A population-based study. *Journal of Consulting and Clinical Psychology, 83*(5), 890–901. https://doi.org/10.1037/ccp0000047.

Pflum, S. R., Testa, R. J., Balsam, K. F., Goldblum, P. B., & Bongar, B. (2015). Social support, trans community connectedness, and mental health symptoms among transgender and gender nonconforming adults. *Psychology of Sexual Orientation and Gender Diversity, 2*(3), 281–286. https://doi.org/10.1037/sgd0000122.

Plöderl, M., & Tremblay, P. (2015). Mental health of sexual minorities. A systematic review. *International Review of Psychiatry, 27*(5), 367–385. https://doi.org/10.3109/09540261.2015.1083949.

Poteat, T., German, D., & Flynn, C. (2016). The conflation of gender and sex: Gaps and opportunities in HIV data among transgender women and MSM. *Global Public Health, 11*(7–8), 835–848. https://doi.org/10.1080/17441692.2015.1134615.

Poteat, T., Malik, M., Scheim, A., & Elliott, A. (2017). HIV prevention among transgender populations: Knowledge gaps and evidence for action. *Current HIV/AIDS Reports, 14*(4), 141–152. https://doi.org/10.1007/s11904-017-0360-1.

Ramirez, J. L., & Paz Galupo, M. (2019). Multiple minority stress: The role of proximal and distal stress on mental health outcomes among lesbian, gay, and bisexual people of color. *Journal of Gay & Lesbian Mental Health, 23*(2), 145–167. https://doi.org/10.1080/19359705.2019.1568946.

Reisner, S. L., Poteat, T., Keatley, J., Cabral, M., Mothopeng, T., Dunham, E., Holland, C. E., Max, R., & Baral, S. D. (2016). Global health burden and needs of transgender populations: A review. *The Lancet, 388*(10042), 412–436. https://doi.org/10.1016/S0140-6736(16)00684-X.

Rhodes, S. D., Alonzo, J., Mann, L., Simán, F., Garcia, M., Abraham, C., & Sun, C. J. (2015). Using photovoice, Latina transgender women identify priorities in a new immigrant-destination state. *International Journal of Transgenderism, 16*(2), 80–96. https://doi.org/10.1080/15532739.2015.1075928.

Rhoades, H., Rusow, J. A., Bond, D., Lanteigne, A., Fulginiti, A., & Goldbach, J. T. (2018). Homelessness, mental health and suicidality among LGBTQ youth accessing crisis services. *Child Psychiatry and Human Development, 49*(4), 643–651. https://doi.org/10.1007/s10578-018-0780-1.

Riggle, E. D., Rostosky, S. S., Black, W. W., & Rosenkrantz, D. E. (2017). Outness, concealment, and authenticity: Associations with LGB individuals' psychological distress and Well-being. *Psychology of Sexual Orientation and Gender Diversity, 4*(1), 54–62. https://doi.org/10.1037/sgd0000202.

Rood, B. A., Reisner, S. L., Surace, F. I., Puckett, J. A., Maroney, M. R., & Pantalone, D. W. (2016). Expecting rejection: Understanding the minority stress experiences of transgender and gender-nonconforming individuals. *Transgender Health, 1*(1), 151–164. https://doi.org/10.1089/TRGH.2016.0012.

Sevelius, J. M. (2013). Gender affirmation: A framework for conceptualizing risk behavior among transgender women of color. *Sex Roles, 68*(11–12), 675–689. https://doi.org/10.1007/s11199-012-0216-5.

Singh, A. A., Parker, B., Aqil, A., & Thacker, F. (2020). Liberation psychology and LGBTQ+ communities: Naming colonization, uplifting resilience, and reclaiming ancient his-stories, her-stories, and t-stories. In L. Comas-Dias & E. Torres-Rivera (Eds.), *Liberation psychology: Theory, method, practice, and social justice*. Washington, DC: American Psychological Association.

Singh, A. A. (2013). Transgender youth of color and resilience: Negotiating oppression and finding support. *Sex Roles, 68*(11–12), 690–702. https://doi.org/10.1007/s11199-012-0149-z.

Singh, A. A., Hays, D. G., & Watson, L. S. (2011). Strength in the face of adversity: Resilience strategies of transgender individuals. *Journal of Counseling and Development, 89*(1), 20–27. https://doi.org/10.1002/j.1556-6678.2011.tb00057.x.

Singh, A. A., & McKleroy, V. S. (2010). "Just getting out of bed is a revolutionary act": The resilience of transgender people of color who have survived traumatic life events. *Traumatology, 17*(2), 34–44. https://doi.org/10.1177/1534765610369261.

Singh, A. A., Meng, S. E., & Hansen, A. W. (2014). "I am my own gender": Resilience strategies of trans youth. *Journal of Counseling & Development, 92*(2), 208–218. https://doi.org/10.1002/j.1556-6676.2014.00150.x.

Sue, D., Irwin, J. A., Fisher, C., Ramos, A., Kelley, M., Mendoza, D. A. R., & Coleman, J. D. (2016). Mental health disparities within the LGBT population: A comparison between transgender and nontransgender individuals. *Transgender Health, 1*(1), 12–20. https://doi.org/10.1089/trgh.2015.0001.

Tan, K. K. H., Treharne, G. J., Ellis, S. J., Schmidt, J. M., & Veale, J. F. (2020). Gender minority stress: A critical review. *Journal of Homosexuality, 67*(10), 1471–1489. https://doi.org/10.1080/00918369.2019.1591789.

Testa, R. J., Habarth, J., Peta, J., Balsam, K., & Bockting, W. (2015). Development of the gender minority stress and resilience measure. *Psychology of Sexual Orientation and Gender Diversity, 2*(1), 65–77. https://doi.org/10.1037/sgd0000081.

Testa, R. J., Michaels, M. S., Bliss, W., Rogers, M. L., Balsam, K. F., & Joiner, T. (2017). Suicidal ideation in transgender people: Gender minority stress and interpersonal theory factors. *Journal of Abnormal Psychology, 126*(1), 125–136. https://doi.org/10.1037/abn0000234.

Truth, S. (1863). *Ain't I a woman*. Retrieved from https://www.thesojournertruthproject.com

Valentine, S. E., & Shipherd, J. C. (2018). A systematic review of social stress and mental health among transgender and gender non-conforming people in the United States. *Clinical Psychology Review, 66*, 24–38. https://doi.org/10.1016/j.cpr.2018.03.003.

White Hughto, J. M., Pachankis, J. E., Willie, T. C., & Reisner, S. L. (2017). Victimization and depressive symptomology in transgender adults: The mediating role of avoidant coping. *Journal of Counseling Psychology, 64*(1), 41–51. https://doi.org/10.1037/cou0000184.

Queering Psychology Research Methods

Alison Cerezo and Roberto Renteria

1 What Is Research and Why Do We Do It?

Research can be described as a series of small, manageable steps intended to uncover new knowledge for the advancement of society. In the broad field of psychology, research typically falls into two camps: empirical research and non-empirical scholarship. Empirical research involves the collection and interpretation of data whereas non-empirical scholarship includes theoretical, conceptual and methodological writings. Psychological research covers a broad range of scientific inquiry and is commonly centered on understanding and explaining human behavior, emotion, and thought. This includes examinations of the individual, groups and society—and their interactions—with an assumption that personal and cultural lived experience is pertinent to understanding how humans function in the world (Fig. 1).

Empirical research in psychology falls into three main categories: quantitative, qualitative, and mixed methodologies. These methodologies are separated by the types of data used to study a particular phenomenon. In *quantitative research*, data collection and analysis are rooted in positivist theory which asserts that "truth" exists and that via refined methods, researchers have the capacity to uncover and explain these truths. Related to this belief is an assumption that the researcher is objective and therefore does not affect or influence the research under investigation. Many psychology researchers regard investigator objectivity as unachievable; however, it is important to point out that quantitative research is originally rooted in positivist theory and as such, plays a significant role in how researchers engage in

A. Cerezo (✉)
University of California—Santa Barbara, Santa Barbara, CA, USA
e-mail: acerezo@ucsb.edu

R. Renteria
Arizona State University, Tempe, AZ, USA
e-mail: rrenter3@asu.edu

© The Author(s), under exclusive license to Springer Nature
Switzerland AG 2021
K. L. Nadal and M. R. Scharrón-del Río (ed.), *Queer Psychology*,
https://doi.org/10.1007/978-3-030-74146-4_8

139

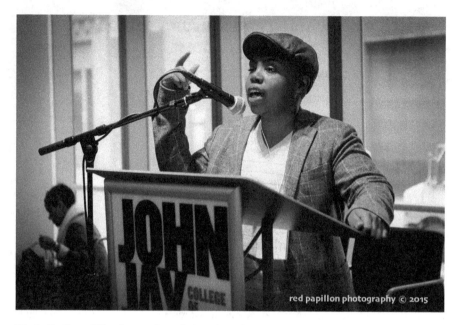

Fig. 1 Professor Riley Snorton is a scholar who writes on racial, sexual and transgender histories and cultural productions. Photo Courtesy of Riya Ortiz/Red Papillon Photography

their work. This includes lack of attention to a researchers' social positions (e.g., gender, race, social class) and how the assumptions tied to those positions inform research questions posed, methods to carry out research and the analysis of data.

Research designs and their accompanying statistical methods in psychology are diverse. Researchers engage in projects that include randomized controlled designs (e.g., testing whether a behavioral intervention improves the uptake of PrEP [Pre-exposure prophylaxis; antiviral drugs used to prevent AIDS among people who are HIV negative], in men who have sex with men as compared to brief consultation about PrEP from one's primary care physician) to descriptive, associational and a multitude of advanced latent growth model designs, among others. Ultimately, myriad research designs and their accompanying analytic methods allow for the exploration and examination of important, timely research that holds the capacity to build new knowledge and make the case for social change.

As a tradition, psychology researchers are commonly trained in the *scientific method*, a six-step process that guides a research project from start to finish that was developed by Sir Frances Bacon (1561–1626). The steps are: (1) identifying the research question and/or topic of study, (2) consulting extant research literature to learn more about the topic of study, (3) constructing a hypothesis about the relationship between the key variables of the study, (4) carrying out the study (experimental or non-experimental designs), (5) analyzing data to draw a conclusion about the relationship between the key variables of the study, and (6) reporting of results. The scientific method has provided a useful system to guide research in psychology and related fields. That said, the scientific method is not devoid of limitations. Related to culture, the scientific method does not explicitly name how culture plays a key role in all areas of research, from assumptions the researcher brings in step 1 when devising their research question (e.g., that discrimination is experienced by many; that discrimination is negatively associated with positive mental health outcomes) to step 2 where the assumptions that previous researchers brought to their studies are used to shape how a certain topic area is understood and studied (i.e., psychometric measures). Another example is in step 4 where the researcher is collecting data and/or running an experiment to test a hypothesis. For many psychology researchers, step four relies on existing psychometric instruments with an assumption that the mechanisms by which researchers assess the topic under study (e.g., discrimination or coping) is commonly understood and/or experienced across the sample of their study. In reality, the overwhelming majority of psychometric instruments have been validated among *W*estern, *E*ducated, and from *I*ndustrialized, *R*ich and *D*emocratic countries (WEIRD) which makes them invalid for diverse communities in the US and around the world. Thus, the surveys and instruments by which researchers and the general public have come to understand common psychological phenomena, like resilience, have been shaped by participants with limited diversity in social position and lived experience.

Starkly different from quantitative research is *qualitative research*, which has become more widely used in psychology research. Qualitative research is rooted in constructivist theory which asserts that individuals construct meaning of the world based on their own personal epistemology. In other words, qualitative researchers work from the premise that what is known as "truth" or as knowledge is processed through one's own personal experience in the world. As such, qualitative researchers typically employ open-ended methods of data collection via interviews and focus groups as a means to capture data on a topic area that is driven by participants' own experiences with the phenomenon under investigation. For example, a researcher may be interested in exploring how recent policies under the 45th presidential administration, such as *Remain in Mexico*, has impacted immigrants' mental health and sense of hope. Introduced in January 2019, Migrant Protection Protocols, also known as *Remain in Mexico*, have impacted over 60,000 asylum seekers who are required to remain in México while they await an appointment with US immigration courts (see Pierce, 2019). In this type of project, the questions posed to participants are open-ended and are more concerned with *why* and *how* participants' mental health has been impacted—versus whether or not (i.e., hypothesis testing)—*Remain in Mexico* is associated with psychological distress or some other psychological outcome.

Psychology researchers employ a wide range of approaches to carry out qualitative projects. Common approaches include phenomenology, grounded theory, narrative and case study, with numerous variations within each of these major domains (e.g., Interpretative phenomenological analysis; Critical Instance Case Studies). In qualitative research, as a general rule, phenomena are explored in an open-ended manner with the assumption that individuals construct their own reality and describe phenomena based on that reality. For example, *Remain in Mexico*, a policy enacted in 2019, is relatively new and little is known about its impact on mental health. A researcher may therefore employ a qualitative approach in studying the impact of this policy; participants' narratives of their experiences would illuminate key factors tied to stress and mental health that would inform future research, particularly studies driven by hypothesis testing (i.e., quantitative studies).

The third major type of research in psychology is *mixed methodologies* (mixed methods). Psychology researchers often use mixed methods as a means to better understand a research problem that neither quantitative or qualitative research can answer on their own. Just as the name implies, mixed methods are a combination of quantitative and qualitative research. It is important to note that there is no particular standard for choosing the order of approaches (i.e., collecting quantitative and qualitative data concurrently or sequentially) or about the magnitude or size of either approach (e.g., mostly qualitative). Rather, researchers approach mixed methods with the goal of carrying out either an explanatory or exploratory design. In explanatory mixed methods, a researcher may choose to compare data that are quantitative and qualitative research to arrive at a deeper understanding of the phenomenon under study. For example, in an explanatory mixed methods study, a researcher running an experiment/intervention to reduce bullying in a local middle school may collect data at baseline (prior to the start of the intervention) and post-test (at the culmination of the intervention) via psychometric instruments. These data are quantitative with the goal of assessing shifts in attitudes toward bullying—hopefully a reduction in the acceptance of bullying—from before and after students take part in the intervention. The researcher may then collect qualitative data at the end of the intervention to gather data on *how* and *why* the intervention reduced the acceptance of bullying in students. These data may explain *why* and *how* particular elements of the intervention were impactful (or not) and/or particular elements of the school environment that were not captured in the psychometric instruments.

2   Why Queering Psychology Research Matters

At the beginning of this chapter we described research as a "series of small, manageable steps" intended to uncover new knowledge for the advancement of society. With that overarching goal in mind, research has the capacity to advance knowledge and improve psychological health outcomes for general society as well as for historically marginalized groups that have been long disserved by the field of psychology. We would be remiss not to mention that psychology and the general health sciences have mistreated several groups that include women, persons of color, the sexual and gender diverse community, among others.

2.1   Ethics in Psychology Research

In the late 1990's President Clinton introduced several important initiatives in the realm of research. These included providing a public acknowledgement and apology for the atrocities carried out against African American men and their families during the Tuskegee Syphilis Study in addition to introducing legislation to address ongoing health disparities among people of color in the US via improved funding for biomedical and behavioral health research. These acts made significant headway in addressing health disparities among historically disenfranchised groups tied to structural inequalities weaved into US social, economic and health systems. In 2012, the US Department of Health and Human Services (2012) released "Healthy People 2020" in which lesbian, gay, bisexual, and transgender (LGBT) people were for the first time identified as an "at risk" population that warranted research focus in US health priorities.

The Tuskegee Study of Untreated Syphilis in the Negro Male was carried out from 1932 to 1972 and was the longest non-therapeutic experiment on human beings in medicine and public health (see CDC, n.d.-a, n.d.-b). A sample of 600 Black men (399 with syphilis, 201 who did not have the disease) were enrolled into a study under the guise that researchers were studying "bad blood." The study was carried out by The Public Health Service in partnership with the Tuskegee Institute. An important fact that must be highlighted is that the study was not discontinued in 1945 when penicillin became a known effective treatment of syphilis. Instead, the study carried on for another 30 years to examine how syphilis affects the human body long-term. The decision to continue the study was made by the Centers for Disease Control and Prevention (CDC) with the support of the American Medical Association and National Medical Association. These actions make clear that the US government, and national medical associations, did not protect its own Black citizens and instead used them as pawns in the name of scientific inquiry. On May 16, 1997, President Clinton issued the first ever formal apology to participants, their families and the larger African American community for the atrocities done in their communities in the name of American medical science.

The Tuskegee Syphilis Study continues to negatively impact public perceptions of research, particularly among communities of color. When researchers were demanded to stop the study, they moved it to Central America and purposefully infected soldiers, sex workers, prisoners and patients in a psychiatric facility without their knowledge or consent (see Rodriguez & Garcia, 2013). Another famous ethical violation in US research includes the Puerto Rican Pill Trial of the 1950s, the first ever widespread study that assessed side effects of a birth control pill (see PBS, n.d.). Three women died during the course of the study. US researchers specifically targeted low-income women of color in Puerto Rico and again participants had no knowledge of the study nor provided consent to participate in the study.

A review of US research ethics makes clear that certain lives are valued more so than others and that these values are often associated with race, gender, sexual orientation, and social class (among other factors). The AIDS epidemic is another example of a delayed response in engaging research to protect citizens. The CDC, and other medical entities, were slow to respond to the growing AIDS epidemic among men who have sex with men. Many critics attribute this delay to the federal governments' disregard of the gay community. Recent data from 2018 show that Black and Latinx men who have sex with men are the hardest hit demographic groups when it comes to HIV (see CDC, n.d.-a, n.d.-b). These communities continue to face a number of barriers that contribute to disparate rates of HIV that include poverty, stigma related to sexual orientation and lack of access to health supports--these include access to condoms, education about safe sex practices, and contact with health providers who can alert men about their HIV status.

2.2 Health Disparities

The National Institutes of Health define health disparities as, "differences in the incidence, prevalence, mortality, and burden of diseases and other adverse health conditions that exist among specific population groups in the United States." The movement to prioritize and fund health disparities research gained traction in the 1990's with eventual formalization of The National Center on Minority Health and Health Disparities as an Institute in 2010. In 2012, the National Institutes of Health included language on "sexual and gender minorities" as a classified group that faced barriers to health equity. Under this charge, federal funding began to be more intentionally distributed to improve research knowledge on the health of sexual and gender diverse individuals. In 2011, the Institute of Medicine (IOM, n.d.) released a report concerning health research on sexual and gender diverse individuals and argued that much remains unknown about the specific health conditions and needs of sexual and gender diverse communities of color. In 2019, the National Institutes of Health highlighted the need for research that considers intersectional experiences related to stigma and discrimination and how those experiences are associated with health disparities (see Flowers, 2019).

2.3 Health Equity

Many psychology and other health researchers have begun to approach their work from a health equity lens. From this perspective, research is used as a social justice tool that both illuminates disparities in our communities as well as honors the "voice" of community members via the adoption of methodologies that are collaborative in nature and therefore responsive to community needs. Many theoretical tools guide health equity researchers working in sexual and gender diverse communities, particularly those that honor the intersectional nature of LGBTQ+ lives. These theories include Critical Race Theory (CRT), Queer Theory, and Intersectionality.

Critical Race Theory (CRT) emerged from legal scholarship in the post-Civil Rights movement (Delgado & Stefancic, 2017). The central tenets of CRT proposed that legal and judicial positionality that adopts a "color-blind" approach is inherently racist in denying the structural racism embedded in existing laws. CRT seeks to acknowledge that the sociopolitical systems in the United States are constructed to benefit White populations and systemically disempower Black, Indigenous, and people of color (BIPOC). Thus, one of the goals of CRT was to apply methods to identify how legal and judicial procedures enable and perpetuate racism in U.S. society. A particular innovative feature of CRT within legal scholarship was the emphasis and focus on turning to the "voice of color" to advance its epistemology. CRT scholars rejected the assumptions made by traditional legal scholarship that stated that "objective legal reasoning" resulted in objective public policy. CRT thus applied an epistemology that utilized personal narrative and storytelling to hear the "voice of color" and better understand the experiences among marginalized communities.

Researchers working from a *Queer Theory* perspective approach their work from the premise that there is no neutral viewpoint; researchers hold bias and assumptions that informs their work. Naming institutional bias, particularly related to heterosexism, is part of the research process. Foucalt (1978) is commonly regarded as introducing the original writings that fueled what is considered today as queer theory. The premise of Foucalt's work was an understanding that power is a relational process wherein resistance and struggle is required as a means for minoritized individuals to gain access to power in systems and institutions that serve to marginalize, exclude and in some cases intentionally harm them.

Resistance lays at the heart of the queer community as evidenced by Pride, the Stonewall Riot, Compton Riot and major efforts connected to the AIDS epidemic. These regular, ongoing events reaffirm the role of resistance in the sexual and gender diverse community. When applied to research, queer theory functions as a process to critique and thereby expand how sexual and gender diverse people are considered in research. Researchers whose work is guided by queer theory can study topics that include identity formation, how educational, healthcare and other systems represent SGD individuals' lived experiences and the consequent connection to health outcomes.

Researchers engaged in queering their scholarship are more commonly embracing *Intersectionality* as a conceptual framework. *Intersectionality* emerged from Black feminist spaces in the US with the traiblazing work of Beale (1969), Bambara (1970), The Combahee River Collective (1977) and bell hooks (1981). The theory gained widespread attention in the social sciences when Crenshaw (1991) published "Mapping the Margins" to highlight how women of color face unique and amplified barriers to social, health, economic resources at the intersection of race, gender, social class and other critical social positions. A key element to Crenshaw's work was a focus on how structural and political intersectionality have severe, chronic impacts on women's lives. It is important to point out that intersectionality emerged in the late 1960's, at a time when Black women faced marginalized from the larger Civil Rights and Feminist movements. Black feminist groups developed intersectionality as a way to shed light on synergistic experiences of oppression; how being both Black and a woman were singularly and intersectionality tied to lived experience, including one's ability to live a healthy life.

Intersectionality has begun to be more actively integrated into psychology research in recent years. Feminist psychologists have written seminal pieces on the incorporation of intersectionality in psychology research that includes deep-level discussions of the theory itself and deliverables related to methodology and data analyses. (see Bowleg, 2008; Cole, 2009; Else-Quest & Hyde, 2016a, b). Bowleg

(2008) argued that intersectionality should be considered at every level of the research process. This includes how measurement, analysis, and interpretation and interpretation of data are responsive to intersections of social experience, particularly experiences tied to minoritized positions.

3 Approaching Research Via a Queer Lens

In this next section we present a real-world vignette that calls for a community rooted research approach. Next, we present four different methods for carrying out a study in response to the identified community need. The four methods presented are purposefully diverse as a means to provide myriad opportunities to address a community need through research. The four methods include: (1) constructivist grounded theory, (2) explanatory mixed methods, (3) a cross-sectional survey design, and (4) repeated measures via daily diaries.

Vignette
María (she/her/hers), a fourth year doctoral student in a Counseling Psychology program, is gearing up to run a research project to examine whether social support buffers the impact of intersectional stigma (across gender, race, and sexual orientation) on depression among Latinx sexual and gender diverse individuals residing in Arizona. María is partnering with a community-based organization in Arizona on this project. Recently, there has been a number of mental health crises, including suicidal attempts, among the Latinx sexual and gender diverse community in the region of Arizona where María attends graduate school. María has been charged with providing several examples of different kinds of projects she and the organization can carry out to better understand the needs of the community and to identify intervention points for health promotion.

3.1 Qualitative and Quantitative Data Collection

A critical step in empirical research is determining the sample of interest and developing a recruitment strategy. To develop an appropriate recruitment strategy, a researcher needs to clarify the population of relevance to ensure recruitment is culturally-relevant and appropriate. For example, in the case of Maria, recruiting Latinx sexual and gender diverse individuals may require understanding the cultural and social values of those communities. For example, considerations could include whether recruitment advertisements should be in English and in Spanish. Additionally, where should advertisements be placed in the community? Should online advertisements be used as well? To answer these questions, it would be necessary for the researcher to have some understanding and knowledge of the community. Similarly, working with a community-based organization can be an effective approach to involve community members in the recruitment process. Lastly, an important consideration in the planning of the recruitment process is to estimate the desired sample size. As will be discussed in the following, this decision depends on the research question driving the study and whether the team is using a qualitative and/or quantitative approach.

A particular strength of qualitative research as an epistemology is the focus on the *how* and *why* of psychological mechanisms. This is a defining characteristic of qualitative data; in contrast to quantitative methods that seek to understand mechanisms in a "representative" sample of the population, qualitative data instead seeks to understand the experiences of a specific group. Therefore, qualitative research tends to obtain relatively smaller sample sizes compared to quantitative. However, it would be a critical mistake to assume that qualitative research is overall less arduous.

The selection of participants has a great impact on the knowledge that is obtained from the semi-structured interviews. It is critical that prior to beginning interviewing participants, the specific eligibility criteria has been set in congruence with the research questions that wished to be answered. In the case of sexual and gender diverse populations, for example, it would be a different type of sample if the topic of interest was "experiences of sexual identity development" versus "experiences of gender identity development." Purposive sampling, for example, is the approach of specifically seeking participants who meet the purpose of the research question. This facilitates in-depth empirical knowledge on severely understudied populations. As was mentioned previously in this chapter, many theoretical perspectives outside of psychology propose the use of qualitative artifacts (e.g., interviews, story-telling, etc.) to raise the experiences of historically marginalized individuals.

In the case of quantitative analysis, researchers usually need to recruit a large enough sample size to ensure obtaining enough statistical power to identify associations between variables. This is its own challenge with sexual and gender diverse communities where various factors make this community hard to reach (e.g., fears of publicly identifying as sexual and/or gender diverse, lack of culturally-sensitive and inclusive research materials, high-burden research participation with little to no incentive) (see Deblaere et al., 2010). These challenges are especially difficult for graduate students and early career researchers who typically have fewer resources for large-scale data recruitment methods.

One strategic approach is the use of online surveys to expand the reach of recruitment that can garner a large enough sample to run more complex statistical techniques. Online survey recruitment may have certain benefits over in-person sampling (e.g., at LGBT Pride events; bars/nightclubs) with respect to anonymity and privacy (Moradi et al., 2009) but at the same time, online research often yields overly White and college-educated samples (Grov et al., 2016). That said, some research supports that internet studies provide findings that are consistent with those obtained from traditional interviewing methods (Gosling et al., 2004; Kosinski et al., 2015) and should not be ruled out when carrying out community-based research.

3.2   Method Example #1: Constructivist Grounded Theory

The overarching goal of grounded theory research is to develop a "process" theory that explains phenomenon, actions, interactions, etc. that occur over time. Many researchers employ grounded theory when extant theories are ill fit to explain the phenomenon under study. Constructivist Grounded Theory is a branch under the larger umbrella of Grounded Theory and is rooted in an interactive process that involves the researcher and participant coming together to construct a shared reality. Qualitative research that explores phenomena across race, gender, and sexual orientation (among other critical demographic domains) often demands a constructivist approach; previous research has rarely centered the voices and lived experiences of sexual and gender diverse persons of color.

María has a unique opportunity to center the voices and needs of the Arizona residents in her community facing a mental health crisis. As described in the previous section on qualitative research, María's approach should be open-ended with the goal of creating a space where she can work with participants to co-construct a reality of the phenomenon at hand, including the language used to address and understand participants' lived experiences. The topic María is addressing involves how social support buffers the impact of intersectional stigma on participants' depression, particularly in the context of being a Latinx sexual and gender diverse person. We recommend that María use a semi-structured individual interview with an approximate sample of 12–20 participants. Before starting the recruitment process, María should explore with her community partner which members of the community should be included in the study, particularly those members that are often ignored in research (e.g., immigrants, trans and non-binary Latinxs). María should also work with her community partner on the interview protocol to ensure that the question prompts are aligned with the knowledge needs of the community. The language in the vignette suggests a focus on social support. It will be important for María to ascertain the types of support that should be explicitly asked about (e.g., family or religious community) during the individual interviews.

In this study, constructivist grounded theory is being used in the development of a process theory to explain *how* social support buffers the impact of intersectional stigma on depression. María should continuously assess whether her original interview questions and prompts are yielding the kinds of data that allow her to develop a process theory rooted in her data. She should transcribe interviews during the course of the study—versus at the end of the study—to explore terms, themes, interactions, etc. that are emerging in the data. Emerging themes should inform the continued collection of data. María should work toward achieving saturation (see Saunders et al., 2018), which involves reaching a threshold in data collection where new interviews are unlikely to yield new discoveries about the phenomenon under study. Saturation may occur after interview 8 or well after interview 20; the goal is to be confident that new interviews would not yield new discoveries that will impact the culmination of a process theory. Creswell et al. (2007) provides recommendations for carrying out data analysis for constructivist grounded theory that should be referenced, including open, axial and selective coding. Researchers typically employ reflexive practices throughout data collection and analysis (e.g., member checks, memoing) as a means to achieve rigor and trustworthiness in their research process.

María's interview process could encompass prompts to ascertain participants' conceptualizations of their social support, discrimination and mental health, particularly the intersectional nature of being Latinx and a sexual and gender diverse person. Interviews can start with, *"You volunteered to participate in this study to discuss your experiences with mental health and social support. To start, can you tell me about the key individuals in your life that you rely on for support?"* Other prompts may include, *"Can you tell me about the kinds of support you seek when faced with a challenge related to being Latinx and/or LGBTQ+? What is helpful or unhelpful about the support that you've received during these challenges?"* Ultimately, via Constructivist Grounded Theory (Charmaz, 2014), María and the participants in her study will arrive at a shared understanding of the process by which participants rely on social support to reduce the negative impact of intersectional stigma on their mental health. By engaging in a collaborative, co-constructing process, María is sharing the power in the research process—a key element of research grounded in a queer, intersectional lens.

3.3   Method Example #2: Mixed Methods, Explanatory

In the previous example, María employed a qualitative research approach to uncover an underlying mechanism—the power of social support—to buffer against the negative impact of intersectional stigma on mental health. It may be the case that María and her community partner want to expand their study to also examine whether particular types of support are more effective and/or whether certain types of individuals (e.g., cisgender men vs. transgender women) benefit greater from social support. In this type of scenario, a mixed methods explanatory design provides a great platform to explore the phenomenon from a couple of different angles (Fig. 2).

In this particular example, María is relying on a two-step process that begins with a qualitative portion followed by a quantitative portion. The goal is to first explore the topic; second, to test for associations that emerged in the first leg of the research study. Let's imagine that María employed constructivist grounded theory in step 1, interviewing 20 participants to uncover how social support buffers against the negative impact of intersectional stigma on mental health. María discovers that having access to emotional support from (a) LGBTQ+ peers and (b) strangers online is especially helpful to participants. Based on this data, María and her community partner set out to sample another 200 individuals in Arizona to learn whether emotional support from LGBTQ+ peers, in-person and on-line, significantly reduces (mediates) the relation between intersectional stigma and mental health. Further, the researchers want to explore whether this is particularly true for certain segments of the community (e.g., bisexual participants).

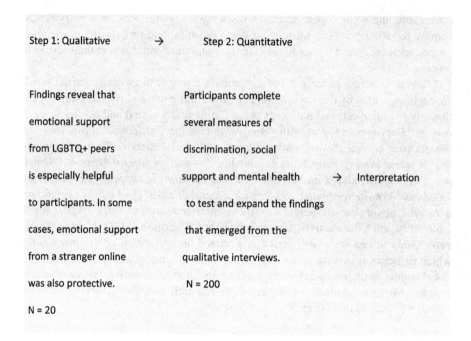

Step 1: Qualitative	→	Step 2: Quantitative		
Findings reveal that		Participants complete		
emotional support		several measures of		
from LGBTQ+ peers		discrimination, social		
is especially helpful		support and mental health	→	Interpretation
to participants. In some		to test and expand the findings		
cases, emotional support		that emerged from the		
from a stranger online		qualitative interviews.		
was also protective.		N = 200		
N = 20				

Fig. 2 Mixed methods explanatory design

In the design above, María has an opportunity to engage collaboratively through-out the process, working with her community partner to determine emergent themes in the data and the relationship between the variables of interest. By working with her community partner in a collaborative manner, María is co-constructing the methodology used to explore the topic in a deep manner and is shifting the power from solely being held by the researcher.

3.4   Method Example #3: Cross-Sectional Research Designs

A variety of research questions can be answered using statistical methods with a cross-sectional sample. Cross-sectional samples are collected at one time; meaning, there are no repeats in data collection. Data will therefore reflect participants' expe-riences of discrimination, social support and mental health on the specific day they completed the study measures. There are limitations with cross-sectional designs; participants may have experienced a particularly challenging event prior to com-pleting the study measures that make their responses on that particular day more extreme than is usual for them. That said, researchers can examine whether there are outliers in the data and also test for skewness of the data to address any threats to the assumptions of the statistical tests they are running.

María has been tasked with examining whether social support buffers the impact of intersectional stigma (race and sexual orientation) on depression among Latinx sexual and gender diverse individuals residing in Arizona. We recommend that she recruit a mid-size sample ($N = 400$) to ensure statistical power. As previously described, the scientific method requires the preemptive review of literature to determine current theoretical frameworks that would inform the research design. María may utilize an intersectional framework (Cole, 2009; Else-Quest & Hyde, 2016a, b) with stigma/minority stress theory (Hatzenbuehler, 2009; Meyer, 1995, 2003) to design a research survey that includes measures of depression and experiences of discrimination relevant to the Latinx LGBTQ+ community (e.g., racism and heterosexism).

It is important to also note that María's sample is described as "sexual and gender diverse" so the measures used to capture stigma should capture a holistic experience; many measures solely ask about heterosexist discrimination with no attention given to race, ethnicity, or gender identity. María should therefore include a measure on sexism for those participants that self-identify as women as well as a measure of transphobic discrimination for those participants that self-identify as transgender and/or nonbinary. In this section we will describe how María can employ (a) multiple regression, (b) mediation and moderation models, (c) path analysis, and (d) structural equation modeling to support her community driven research topic.

3.4.1 Multiple Regression Analysis

Multiple regression is an extension of simple linear regression that allows for researchers to test the value of an outcome variable (e.g., depression) based on two or more predictor variables (e.g., age, perceived discrimination). Multiple regression is an umbrella term that includes several commonly used analyses like simultaneous, stepwise, hierarchical and logistic regression, among others. Below we run through two examples of applying multiple regression to María's research: simultaneous and hierarchical regression.

María and her community partner decide that while they are most interested in examining whether age, income, and discrimination tied to (a) race and (b) sexual orientation discrimination predict depression, they do not have a particular order in which they hypothesize these variables to impact depression. Thus, their question is exploratory and can be answered using *simultaneous multiple regression*. The variables of age, income, race-based and sexual orientation-based discrimination are entered into the model simultaneously as predictors; there is no assumed order of strength of the predictors on the outcome variable of depression (Fig. 3).

Imagine if the community-based organization wanted to know if experiences of discrimination were stronger predictors of depression than other demographic variables (e.g., age, income). A *hierarchical multiple regression* model would allow María to answer this question. First, María could include survey items inquiring about important demographic characteristics and carry out a 2-step regression model. Step 1 would include the demographic variables and step 2 would include

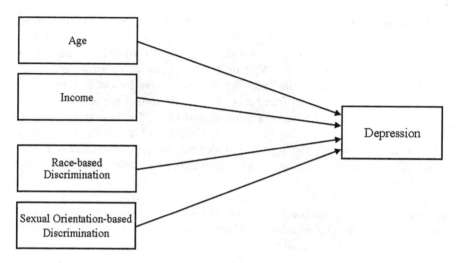

Fig. 3 Simultaneous multiple regression

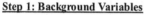

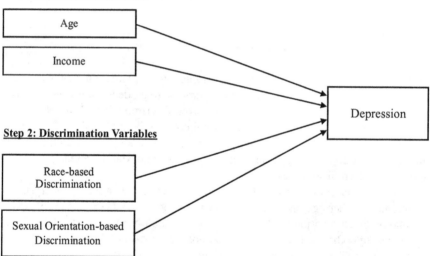

Fig. 4 Hierarchical multiple regression

the discrimination variables. The overall model and individual predictor effect sizes would allow us to evaluate whether experiences of discrimination predict depression even after accounting for gender, socioeconomic status, and education level (Fig. 4).

3.5   Hierarchical Multiple Regression

Moderation analysis is another common tool that can answer interesting research questions. The community partner María is collaborating with might want to allow explore whether social support *protects* against the effects of discrimination on depression among Latinx LGBTQ+ communities. A research question such as this could be answered by carrying out a moderation analysis. Essentially, the community organization is asking whether the association between discrimination and depression *changes* across different levels of social support. Note that prior language asked if social support protects against the effects of discrimination. This language suggests that experiencing an increased rate of discrimination predicts higher depression scores but only for individuals reporting lower levels of social support. In this case, a social support measure would also be included in the survey and María would carry out a moderation test to examine if levels of social support *change the association* between discrimination and depression.

3.6   Moderation Analysis

Structural Equation Modeling (SEM) is a statistical analytical technique that allows to test for a more complex model of pathways between multiple variables. That is, SEM allows for testing a *structure* of theory-informed associations between variables to assess whether the proposed structural model adequately fits the sample data. This is particularly useful given the complexity of human behavior and experience, especially for sexual and gender diverse communities. Individuals with intra- and interpersonal psychological mechanisms that occur within multiple overlapping sociopolitical ecosystems. Of course, even SEM as a statistical tool is insufficient in explaining the full reality of individuals' lived experience. Yet, SEM allows for far more complex models relative to multiple regression.

Psychological science on sexual and gender diverse populations has posited various complex theoretical models to understand health disparities (minority stress model; Meyer, 1995, 2003), models of sexual identity development (Dillon et al., 2011), gender identity development (Bockting, 2014), health and comorbidity (syndemic theory; Wilson et al., 2014), to name a few. Path analysis and structural equation models provide a quantitative tool to test these complex models and further our understanding of the lived experiences among sexual and diverse individuals, identify risk and protective factors related to health, and inform the development of interventions to promote well-being.

María may propose a *path analysis* that tests a theoretical model of mental health among Latinx LGBTQ+. For example, an intersectional structural model may propose pathways of various discrimination variables predicting various mental health outcomes (e.g., depression, anxiety, suicidality). According to minority stress theory, coping behaviors (e.g., social, cognitive, affective) may function as mediators

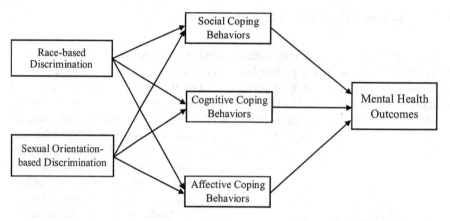

Fig. 5 Path analyses

in these pathways. María may then be able to test if a theory-informed model of mental health is effective in explaining the variance and association in a sample of Latinx sexual and gender diverse individuals. This method would then provide empirical evidence that informs the utility of the theoretical model in this sample while also providing effect sizes for the specific pathways and associations between those variables (Fig. 5).

3.7 Method Example #4: Repeated Measures Via Daily Diaries

Researchers studying discriminatory effects on health and well-being are turning to *ecological momentary assessment* (EMA) to capture data in real time and in participants' natural environments. Data collection in EMA is diverse; participants are commonly asked to complete a brief set of items on a daily schedule and in some cases, multiple times per day. One example of EMA is daily diaries where researchers ask participants to report events, behaviors, cognitions and moods. Many researchers employ daily diaries for a series of days or weeks to track patterns in participants' experiences and consequent behaviors (see Heron et al., 2019; Mereish et al., 2018).

María and her community partner can employ daily diaries to study the daily effects of discrimination on mental health and other important variables like exercise, eating and substance use. We recommend that every participant be asked to complete baseline measures that include a demographic questionnaire, measures related to stigma and discrimination, social support, and coping. Baseline measures will allow María and her community partner to test for mediators and moderators. Next, participants are asked to complete a daily diary for 14 days that involves a series of questions that take about 5–15 min to complete. These items should be specific to discrimination events, mood/mental health, coping behaviors and

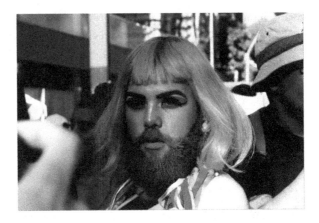

Fig. 6 For many trans and queer people, gender is a difficult concept to measure with traditional research methods. Photo Courtesy of Matteus Bernardes

anything else the team wants to explore. At the end of the 14 days, participants complete a follow-up measure about their experiences altogether and are provided with an opportunity to share feedback to María and her community partner. For example, participants may share that the time they were asked to complete the diary was too early in the day or that a paper copy of the diary was a preferred method to an online diary. Providing participants with an opportunity to share their feedback is immensely helpful; certain persons and communities respond to methods differently based on cultural norms and other social and environmental factors. Assuming every participant would respond to methods in the same way will lead to inequity in whose voice is included in important research that informs policy and practice.

Generalized Linear Mixed Modeling (GLMM) is a common statistical method used for repeated measures—in this case, daily diaries. GLMM allows for researchers to assess both within-person and across-person variability. In other words, if María is assessing discrimination events and depression scores on a daily basis, she can test for how these scores vary over the 14 days for a particular participant (within-person) or between a number of participants (across-person). GLMM also allows for more sophisticated analysis and would give María and her community partner the opportunity to assess important, nuanced associations between discrimination and depression and to do so in real time and in the participant's real-world context (Fig. 6).

4   Conclusion

Psychology research has a long history of being rooted in theories and practices that assume objectivity and neutrality and as such, function to uphold the status quo. Researchers have become increasingly interested in queering the methods employed to explore important research questions affecting the psychological health of sexual and gender diverse communities and more so than ever, centering the lived experiences and needs of BIPOC who have paved the way on civil rights issues at the intersection of race, gender and sexual orientation. In this chapter we presented a vignette that explores how to address a community health need from four different research approaches. The overarching goal was to demonstrate how research can be used to engage in social justice work and in doing so, center the voices of those individuals disparately impacted by societal oppression.

References

Bambara, T. C. (1970). *The black woman: An anthology*. New York: New American Library.

Beale, F. (1969). Double jeopardy: To be black and female. In T. Cade (Ed.), *The black woman: An anthology* (pp. 90–100). New York: Signet.

Bockting, W. (2014). The impact of stigma on transgender identity development and mental health. In *Gender dysphoria and disorders of sex development* (pp. 319–330). Boston, MA: Springer.

Bowleg, L. (2008). When black + lesbian + woman ≠ black lesbian woman: The methodological challenges of qualitative and quantitative intersectionality research. *Sex Roles: A Journal of Research, 59*, 312–325. https://doi.org/10.1007/s11199-008-9400-z.

Broadcasting Service. (n.d.). *The Puerto Rico pill trials*. Retrieved from https://www.pbs.org/wgbh/americanexperience/features/pill-puerto-rico-pill-trials/

Centers for Disease Control and Prevention. (n.d.-a). *The Tuskegee timeline*. Retrieved from https://www.cdc.gov/tuskegee/timeline.htm

Centers for Disease Control and Prevention. (n.d.-b). *HIV and African Americans*. Retrieved from https://www.cdc.gov/hiv/group/racialethnic/africanamericans/index.html

Charmaz, K. (2014). *Constructing grounded theory* (2nd ed.). Sage.

Cole, E. R. (2009). Intersectionality and research in psychology. *American Psychologist, 64*, 170–180. https://doi.org/10.1037/a0014564.

Combahee River Collective. (1977). *The Combahee River collective statement*. Retrieved from https://combaheerivercollective.weebly.com/

Crenshaw, K. (1991). Mapping the margins: Intersectionality, identity politics, and violence against women of color. *Stanford Law Review, 43*, 1241–1299. https://doi.org/10.2307/1229039.

Creswell, J. W., Hanson, W. E., Clark Plano, V. L., & Morales, A. (2007). Qualitative research designs: Selection and implementation. *The Counseling Psychologist, 35*(2), 236–264.

Deblaere, C., Brewster, M. E., Sarkees, A. M., & Moradi, B. (2010). Conducting research with LGB people of color: Methodological challenges and strategies. *The Counseling Psychologist, 38*, 331–362. https://doi.org/10.1177/0011000009335257.

Delgado, R., & Stefancic, J. (2017). *Critical race theory: An introduction* (3rd ed.). New York: New York University Press.

Dillon, F. R., Worthington, R. L., & Moradi, B. (2011). Sexual identity as a universal process. In *Handbook of identity theory and research* (pp. 649–670). New York, NY: Springer.

Else-Quest, N. M., & Hyde, J. S. (2016a). Intersectionality in quantitative psychological research: I. Theoretical and epistemological issues. *Psychology of Women Quarterly, 40*, 155–170. https://doi.org/10.1177/0361684316629797.

Else-Quest, N. M., & Hyde, J. S. (2016b). Intersectionality in quantitative psychological research: II. Methods and techniques. *Psychology of Women Quarterly, 40*, 319–336. https://doi.org/10.1177/0361684316647953.

Flowers, H. (2019). *Intersectionality part one: Intersectionality defined*. Retrieved from https://www.edi.nih.gov/blog/communities/intersectionality-part-one-intersectionality-defined

Foucalt, M. (1978). *The history of sexuality: An introduction*. New York: Pantheon Books.

Gosling, S. D., Vazire, S., Srivastava, S., & John, O. P. (2004). Should we trust web-based? A comparative analysis of six preconceptions about internet questionnaires. *Studies American Psychologist, 59*(2), 93–104. https://doi.org/10.1037/0003-066X.59.2.93.

Grov, C., Cain, D., Whitfield, T. H., Rendina, H. J., Pawson, M., Ventuneac, A., & Parsons, J. T. (2016). Recruiting a US national sample of HIV-negative gay and bisexual men to complete at-home self-administered HIV/STI testing and surveys: Challenges and opportunities. *Sexuality Research and Social Policy, 13*(1), 1–21.

Hatzenbuehler, M. L. (2009). How does sexual minority stigma "get under the skin"? A psychological mediation framework. *Psychological Bulletin, 135*, 707–730. https://doi.org/10.1037/a0016441.

Heron, K. E., Lewis, R. J., Shappie, A. T., Dawson, C. A., Amerson, R., Braitman, A. L., Winstead, B. A., & Kelley, M. L. (2019). Rationale and design of a remote web-based daily diary study examining sexual minority stress, relationship factors, and alcohol use in same-sex female couples across the United States: Study protocol of project relate. *JMIR Research Protocols, 8*(2), 1–23. https://doi.org/10.2196/11718.

Hooks, B. (1981). *Ain't I a woman: Black women and feminism*. Chicago, IL: Pluto Press.

Institute of Medicine (IOM). (n.d.). *Committee on lesbian gay bisexual and transgender health issues and research gaps and opportunities. The health of lesbian, gay, bisexual, and transgender people: Building a foundation for better understanding*. Washington, DC: National Academies Press.

Kosinski, M., Matz, S. C., Gosling, S. D., Popov, V., & Stillwell, D. (2015). Facebook as a research tool for the social sciences: Opportunities, challenges, ethical considerations, and practical guidelines. *American Psychologist, 70*(6), 543–556. https://doi.org/10.1037/a0039210.

Mereish, E. A., Kuerbis, A., & Morgenstern, J. (2018). A daily diary study of stressful and positive events, alcohol use, and addiction severity among heavy drinking sexual minority men. *Drug and Alcohol Dependence, 187*, 149–154. https://doi.org/10.1016/j.drugalcdep.2018.03.003.

Meyer, I. H. (1995). Minority stress and mental health in gay men. *Journal of Health and Social Behavior, 36*, 38–56. https://doi.org/10.2307/2137286.

Meyer, I. H. (2003). Prejudice, social stress, and mental health in lesbian, gay, and bisexual populations: Conceptual issues and research evidence. *Psychological Bulletin, 129*, 674–697. https://doi.org/10.1037/0033-2909.129.5.674.

Moradi, B., Mohr, J. J., Worthington, R. L., & Fassinger, R. E. (2009). Counseling psychology research on sexual (orientation) minority issues: Conceptual and methodological challenges and opportunities. *Journal of Counseling Psychology, 56*(1), 5–22. https://doi.org/10.1037/a0014572.

Pierce, S. (2019). *Immigration-related policy changes in the first two years of the Trump administration*. Washington, DC: Migration Policy Institute. Retrieved from www.migrationpolicy.org/research/immigration-policy-changes-two-years-trumpadministrationPublic.

Rodriguez, M. A., & Garcia, R. (2013). First, do no harm: The US sexually transmitted disease experiments in Guatemala. *American Journal of Public Health, 103*(12), 2122–2126. https://www.ncbi.nlm.nih.gov/pmc/articles/PMC3828982/pdf/AJPH.2013.301520.pdf.

Saunders, B., Sim, J., Kingstone, T., Baker, S., Waterfield, J., Bartlam, B., Burroughs, H., & Jinks, C. (2018). Saturation in qualitative research: exploring its conceptualization and operationalization. *Quality & Quantity, 52*(4), 1893–1907.

U.S. Department of Health and Human Services (2012). *Healthy people 2020 objectives*. Retrieved from http://www.healthypeople.gov/2020/topicsobjectives2020/default.aspx

Wilson, P. A., Nanin, J., Amesty, S., Wallace, S., Cherenack, E. M., & Fullilove, R. (2014). Using syndemic theory to understand vulnerability to HIV infection among Black and Latino men in New York City. *Journal of Urban Health, 91*(5), 983–998.

Beyond LGBTQ-Affirmative Therapy: Fostering Growth and Healing Through Intersectionality

Darren J. Freeman-Coppadge and Khashayar Farhadi Langroudi

1 Clinical Issues Among LGBTQ Communities

Evidence has consistently shown that lesbian, gay, bi+, trans+, and queer (LGBTQ) people generally experience greater mental health disparities and tend to utilize mental health services at higher rates than cisgendered heterosexual people do (Cochran et al., 2017; Filice & Meyer, 2018). Such higher rates of utilization are due to the accumulated, multilayered effects of minority stress (Meyer, 2013) and not because of innate dysfunction or pathology. Nonetheless, therapeutic modalities traditionally have not been designed with LGBTQ people in mind, but under assumptions that these modalities are universal and equally efficacious for all people (Dominguez, 2017). In the past few decades, however, these assumptions have been challenged, and growing evidence has demonstrated that therapy adapted for specific cultures and peoples are more beneficial and less harmful (Pachankis, 2018). Through decentering Western White hegemony, culturally adapted therapies to meet the needs of various groups have proliferated, including those adapted for the LGBTQ community, collectively known as LGBTQ-affirmative therapies (Fig. 1).

For the most part, LGBTQ-affirmative therapy is not conceptualized as a distinct orientation of therapy (like CBT), but rather adaptations of existing evidence-based practices (O'Shaughnessy & Speir, 2018). Moreover, empirical evidence has not fully elucidated if, when, or how to adapt therapies to LGBTQ people, though preliminary efficacy findings on these emerging practices seem promising (Pachankis, 2018). What is most needed at this time are evidence-based practices that utilize intersectional and social justice lenses to apply to sexual and gender minorities

D. J. Freeman-Coppadge (✉)
Coppadge, Congruence Counseling & Psychology, LLC, Glen Burnie, MD, USA

K. F. Langroudi
Private Practice, San Francisco, CA, USA

© The Author(s), under exclusive license to Springer Nature
Switzerland AG 2021
K. L. Nadal and M. R. Scharrón-del Río (ed.), *Queer Psychology*,
https://doi.org/10.1007/978-3-030-74146-4_9

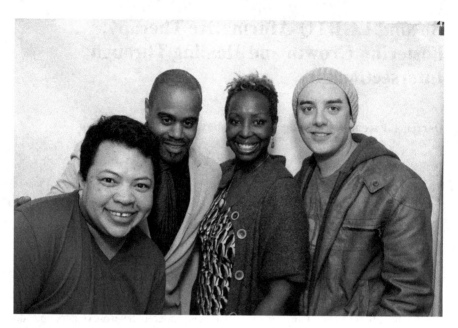

Fig. 1 A group of friends attending the LGBTQ Scholars of Color Conference. Photo Courtesy of Kevin Nadal

(SGMs) with multiple marginalized identities at individual, interpersonal, and institutional levels. In this chapter, we highlight some of the extant research and how it applies to LGBTQ in general, and those with multiple interlocking oppressions specifically, based upon our clinical experiences as queer practitioners who work with a broad array of queer clients.

1.1 Common Presenting Problems for LGBTQ People

LGBTQ people tend to first seek therapy with concerns that are consistent with those of the general population, such as depression, anxiety, relationship problems, etc. (American Psychological Association [APA], 2012; 2015). Nonetheless, there are certain psychosocial and experiential developmental factors affecting many LGBTQ people that can impact therapy (such as minority stress, voluntary and forced identity disclosure, effects of identity concealment.). Conversely, therapists must be careful not to assume that an SGM client's presenting concerns are necessarily related to their queer identity, as research has consistently shown how such assumptions can be damaging to the therapeutic alliance and therapy outcomes (Filice & Meyer, 2018; O'Shaughnessy & Speir, 2018). Thus, therapists must not only possess familiarity with community and systemic issues related to LGBTQ people but must also adeptly implement that knowledge clinically at the right time in the right way (O'Shaughnessy & Speir, 2018). Striking this delicate balance is likely best facilitated by developing cultural competence and humility.

1.1.1 Minority Stress, Stigma, and Discrimination

Professional psychologist consensus guidelines (APA, 2012; 2015) have described various common themes arising in therapy specifically with SGMs. Many such issues emanate from minority stress-related stigma, discrimination, victimization, and microaggressions that SGMs face throughout the lifespan, such as bullying in early childhood through college-age, workplace discrimination and harassment in adulthood, or abuse and neglect in care settings for older adults. Minority stress has been associated with new and/or exacerbated mental distress (anxiety, depression, suicidality, etc.) and physical health problems (pain, cardiovascular problems, infections, etc.; Bockting et al., 2013; Mereish & Poteat, 2015). Moreover, the perpetual devaluing of queer identities and lives causes many to internalize stigma (homonegativity, transnegativity, binegativity, etc.) which has also been associated with negative mental health effects (Puckett et al., 2018).

Given the shame and trauma experienced personally and vicariously because of their SGM identities, it is unsurprising that many conceal their identities, or even seek to change them through sexual orientation and gender identity change efforts (SOGICE). It is imperative that psychologists/therapists avoid colluding with client requests for SOGICE as these methods consistently have been shown to be ineffective and place individuals at significant risk of serious harm according to APA resolutions (APA, 2021a, 2021b) and the consensus of a plethora of mental and medical health organizations. Overwhelming empirical evidence suggests that LGBTQ-affirmative therapy be utilized instead.

1.1.2 Identity Development and Conflict

There are a number of common issues related to identity development that may arise in therapy with SGMs which clinicians should be appropriately trained to encounter. First, therapists must have a good understanding of coming out, including recognition that coming out is not a single event, but an ongoing process that affects LGBTQ people throughout their lives. For instance, a trans woman who has been healthy, independent, and very open about her trans identity most of her adult life may find herself going back into the closet upon entering a nursing home later in life for fear of discrimination, abuse, and neglect at a vulnerable stage of life (Porter et al., 2016). Every new environment or social context LGBTQ people encounter requires a complex calculation about if, when, and how to come out—a perennial issue that may arise multiple times throughout the course of therapy with long-term clients. Clinicians should also be familiar with the risks and benefits of coming out, recognizing that it is not always advisable nor safe to do so. They must hold a strong working knowledge of identity development models for various SGM identities, while understanding the myriad ways in which LGBTQ people come to understand their sexuality and/or gender and how they affect their lives and relationships.

Perhaps the most crucial identity-related issues that therapists can aid clients in resolving is the dissonance that results from attempting to live in two (or more) worlds that are perceived as being incompatible. One of the more common areas addressed in therapy is conflict with religious or spiritual worldviews. LGBTQ religious people who are part of religious/spiritual communities that do not affirm them can either pursue integration of their identities, or attempt to suppress some aspect of themselves, but such suppression can be detrimental to their health and well-being. Identity integration strategies often involve helping clients minimize negative messages about their identity through connection with sects of their religious tradition that can provide affirmation, support, and appropriate resources (such as affirming interpretations of sacred texts). While many religious groups encourage congregants to pursue SOGICE, some have tacitly accepted the potential harms of such approaches and have promoted celibacy instead for sexual minorities. Yet emerging evidence suggests that there are harms associated with suppressing sexuality for the sake of religious identity (Freeman-Coppadge & Horne, 2019). Identity integration has consistently shown to be the healthiest option for SGMs who consider their spirituality to be a crucial aspect of their identity (e.g., Rodriguez et al., 2019).

Identity conflicts are not restricted to religious/spiritual concerns; they can occur for any number of salient identities for a client, including race/ethnicity, culture, or family values. When any such conflicts occur, it is important to recognize that social relationships are at risk for the client who has not resolved their conflict. Research has shown how crucial family and social support is to the health and well-being of LGBTQ people (Filice & Meyer, 2018; Ryan et al., 2010). Thus, therapists are encouraged to help clients reconcile with families when appropriate and/or be familiar with affirming community resources to which they can connect their clients as they build families of choice (FoC) in light of family and community destabilization or rejection.

1.1.3 Relationships and Family

While stigma and discrimination have effects on attachments styles and romantic relationships among LGBTQ people, emerging research has described the benefits and strengths of queer relationships. For instance, queer relationships tend to be more inclusive (of sexualities and identities), open in form and structure, and sex-positive in ways that meet needs for connection and community not afforded by traditional, heterononormative relationships (Hammack et al., 2019). Moreover, perhaps because many queer relationships are not beholden to traditional gender-based power structures, they manifest other strengths like mutual respect and appreciation; use of healthy communication to navigate disagreements in the relationship and resolving conflicts; use of humor and spirituality as sources of support; and more egalitarian relationships with equal division of labor (Rostosky & Riggle, 2017).

The landscape for LGBTQ relationships and families is not all positive, unfortunately. Stigma and discrimination affect queer people's ability to form, grow, and maintain healthy families and relationships. For instance, LGBTQ families have a long history of being harmed through societal and legal delegitimization, discrimination, and denigration which provide structural barriers to adoption, surrogacy, foster care and other forms of child rearing (Haines et al., 2018). Further, intimate partner violence is common among queer and trans people, but most laws only codify heteronormative domestic violence; SGMs are often retraumatized by law enforcement and medical/social service providers, and thus do not always seek nor receive appropriate resources (Nadal, 2020). It is imperative that clinicians understand the systemic, interpersonal, and individual-level factors that contribute to mental health concerns affecting SGM relationships and families. Competency requires therapists to exhibit non-judgmental, non-pathologizing, positive attitudes about SGM sex and relationships—including kink culture and consensual non-monogamous relationships structures, which are often clinically neglected to the detriment of a substantial portion of the LGBTQ community (Schechinger et al., 2018).

In therapy, clients may present with a variety of ways to approach both the queer and normative aspects of their relationships (Hammack et al., 2019). There may be numerous reasons SGMs seek normativity in their relationships, such as conforming or assimilating for the sake of minimizing stigma and discrimination. Clinicians must maintain openness to both the queering and normativity inclinations, attending to assisting clients with discovering their respective benefits and challenges. This is especially important when working with clients who are in mixed orientation relationships (e.g., a bisexual man and a heterosexual woman, or a bisexual woman and a lesbian), whether intentionally or unbeknownst to one or both partners prior to starting the relationship (Vencill & Wiljamaa, 2016).

1.1.4 Queer Erasure: Neglected Identities in Clinical Practice

Another issue that affects the broader LGBTQ community is the persistent, insidious cultural centralization of heterosexism, monosexism, and cisgenderism, leading to erasure of certain queer identities. Thus, many SGMs—trans, nonbinary, bisexual, pansexual, and ace/asexual identities, among others—struggle to find vital acceptance and support due to discrimination from society, as well as neglect by and oppression from those within the LGBTQ community who have relatively more sociopolitical power. Identity erasure is not without consequence. Non-monosexual people (e.g., bisexuals, pansexuals) are commonly assumed to be heterosexual if they are in "opposite gender" relationships, accused of being in denial about their sexuality, and considered to be promiscuous and incapable of being in long-term relationships, all of which may contribute to higher rates of substance abuse as well as sexual and mental health problems compared to other sexual minorities (Feinstein

& Dyar, 2017). People on the asexual spectrum (e.g., asexuals, demisexuals) often have their sexual and romantic lives framed as medical or psychopathological problems, leading to high rates of perceived discrimination and subsequent mental health problems at least on par with, if not worse than, other sexual minorities (Rothblum et al., 2020). Trans and nonbinary (TNB) people have been pathologized in Western society for centuries—in both general society and within SGM communities (Nadal, 2020).

The persistent institutionalized medicalization of gender dysphoria places psychologists in the uncomfortable role of being "gatekeepers" who possess inordinate power over trans bodies, with the ability to approve or deny gender confirmation procedures (Singh & Burnes, 2010). It can be extremely humiliating for TNB people to place their bodies and self-actualization into the hands of healthcare professionals. Requests for letters for gender affirming procedures therefore should be handled with utmost care, especially in the case of children and adolescents where further knowledge about potential development trajectories should be considered carefully with clients and their families as appropriate (APA, 2015). Moreover, finding caring clinicians can be incredibly difficult for TNB individuals, so it is important for clinicians to advertise their services appropriately. If a provider has not received training in writing individualized letters, does not know gender affirming physicians in their area who provide care (e.g., surgeries, hormone treatments, gynecological care), or isn't familiar with the challenges TNB people face during the transition process, then it may be considered disingenuous to advertise themselves as a trans-competent or an LGBTQ-competent practitioner.

TNB individuals seek services for a wide variety of concerns, and may not need support for transitioning per se. At a minimum, all clinicians should be aware of the differences between sexual orientation and gender identity/expression; be familiar with the overwhelming evidence demonstrating how gender confirmation leads to significant improvements in mental, emotional, social, physical, and spiritual health; and understand some of the unique stigma that gender minorities experience throughout their lives.

1.1.5   Applying LGBTQ-Affirmative Therapy

LGBTQ-affirmative therapy is largely geared toward mitigating the detrimental effects of the systemic and internalized processes described by Minority Stress Theory. Therapists should seek appropriate training in affirmative therapy given the chances of encountering LGBTQ clients in their practice, as training has been shown to be effective in helping therapists improve their cultural competence (Pepping et al., 2018). Numerous evidence-based practices have been adapted to meet the needs of SGMs based on the issues they uniquely face. For instance, several studies have utilized cognitive behavioral therapies (Pachankis et al., 2015), interpersonal therapy (Budge, 2013), attachment-based family therapy (Diamond et al., 2013), acceptance and commitment therapy (Yadavaia & Hayes, 2012), and couples therapy (relationship education; Pepping et al., 2020). Some novel approaches, such as online interventions to reduce internalized stigma, have also been devised (Lin et al., 2019; Israel et al., 2019). These treatments help SGMs understand that their sexuality and gender variations are normal, healthy, and beautiful, and to counteract the mental health distress that comes from years of being told otherwise.

Some evidence-based aims of LGBTQ-affirmative therapy include helping clients to focus on resilience and strengths; empowering clients through assertive communication; connecting SGMs with vital community support and resources; and decreasing emotional avoidance behaviors while enhancing abilities to regulate their emotions through awareness, acceptance, and transformation (Proujansky & Pachankis, 2014). Many therapeutic interventions, informed by intimate knowledge about LGBTQ people generally and individual clients specifically, can be employed to reach these goals through attending to minority stressors. For instance, decentering (the ability to view thoughts and feelings as distinct from the self) has been shown to mitigate the distress associated with internalized heterosexism (Puckett et al., 2018). Decentering and its related constructs can be facilitated by multiple modalities such as cognitive and mindfulness based (e.g., CBT, ACT, DBT), emotion focused, and psychodynamic therapies, among others. As applied to LGBTQ clients, decentering helps them to recognize that the views that they have about themselves, their sexuality, their gender norms, etc. are distortions based upon systemic oppression rather than truths that define them.

1.2 Intersectional Considerations in Clinical Work

From an intersectional identity standpoint, there are additional considerations to be made regarding appropriate care for LGBTQ people that are not always addressed by existing affirmative therapy research and clinical applications. First, the overwhelming literature on queer psychology has focused on data and narratives for and about Western, White, cisgender, LGB, middle- to upper-middle-class, highly educated, able-bodied individuals. Religion and spirituality studies of LGBTQ populations largely center on Christian sects, with much less attention to Judaism, even less to Islam, and still less to other spiritualities (Buddhism, Sikhism, earth-spirited faiths, etc.). Thus, little is empirically known about LGBTQ people with other marginalized intersectional identities such as race, ethnicity, class, ability, religion/spirituality, nationality, and culture, often leaving these individuals with the heavy burden of educating the very therapists they've enlisted to help them address their problems. In the process of educating their therapists, they often endure microaggressions from them, which has the potential to disrupt rapport, lead to early termination, and worsen therapy outcomes (Filice & Meyer, 2018; O'Shaughnessy & Speir, 2018), all of which foment further distrust of mental health and medical fields within marginalized communities.

Clinicians must understand how multiple-marginalized identities affect their clients, starting with acknowledging that LGBTQ clinical competence is not synonymous with intersectional LGBTQ clinical competence. Therapists should endeavor to learn the complex history of gender constructs and their functional nuances within the LGBTQ community, all of which have implications for identity, self-empowerment, connection, and safety (Levitt, 2019). Consistently across studies, sexist themes of masculine dominance (androcentrism) and feminine inferiority exist within the LGBTQ community. Navigating and transgressing gendered norms can feel dangerous but can also be empowering and liberating. The process of supporting a client's gender experimentation and discovery requires adroit clinical skills, especially when working with SGMs with multiple interlocking marginalized identities.

It is essential for therapists to become comfortable with understanding and discussing racism, particularly how it may impact queer Black, Indigenous, and People of Color (QBIPOC). For instance, QBIPOC may feel conflicted between their allegiance to their racial/ethnic context that prejudices their SGM status, and the broader LGBTQ community that exhibits racism (e.g., Sarno et al., 2015). QBIPOC may suffer with internalized racism—seeing themselves and their identities as inferior to White people—compounding their negative self-view as SGMs rejected by White-dominated society and their cultural communities. Within the Black community specifically, this can be partially explained by Post Traumatic Slave Syndrome, whereby the compounded effects of multigenerational trauma from slavery and continued oppression through systematic disenfranchisement produce patterns of behavior that lower self-esteem, produce anger, and perpetuate Black inferiority through adoption of the White master's view of Black people (DeGruy, 2017). It is easy to conceive of how similar experiences of minority stress among other racial/ethnic minorities leads to corresponding internalized oppressive attitudes that interact powerfully with internalized views of queer inferiority. What results for QBIPOC is a unique form of inferiority that differs from the inferiority of their constitutive identities alone.

Furthermore, the impacts of class on the intersections of race, gender, and sexuality are not well studied. Clinical assumptions about the wealth of LGBTQ clients may overlook QBIPOC's (and White lower SES individual's) experiences with poorer health, health disparities, and incidents of more severe stigma compared to those with more economically privileged backgrounds (Shangani et al., 2020). Assumptions that overlook the impacts of age and ability status can produce similar problems clinically, causing therapists to misunderstand the uniqueness of their clients' experiences. For instance, studies on age-based cohorts of sexual minorities suggest that the eras in which they were socialized influences health and sexual identity development; younger SGMs who have dealt with relatively less stigma have tended to accept themselves earlier in life and at a faster pace than those in older generations (Bishop et al., 2020). Recent literature supports that QBIPOC may come out earlier in life than their White counterparts, perhaps because coping with racial stigma provides a framework for better understanding and accepting themselves as sexual minorities (Bishop et al., 2020).

SGMs with disabilities—whether related to physical attributes, sensory functioning, somatic health, intellectual or learning capacities, emotional regulation, or otherwise—face similar dual stigmas as many QBIPOC: rejection or neglect of their disability within the LGBTQ community and their SGM identity within the disabled community. They experience being pathologized by the medical community through conflation of their sexuality and/or gender with their disability; being denied institutional supports necessary for their success in school, the workplace, and society at large; and being desexualized with sparse attention to their romantic, sexual, and relationship needs (Duke, 2011). Inadequate training on these matters only perpetuates the discrimination and suffering they routinely encounter.

1.2.1   Best Practices for Whom?

Common "best practices" in the culturally competent care of LGBTQ individuals may prove ineffectual, or even harmful, to LGBTQ people with multiple marginalized identities. For example, encouraging clients to embrace their gay identity and come out is culturally, and often therapeutically, considered the *sine qua non* process for healthy development and well-being. However, coming out in various cultural contexts (at family and community levels) can be psychologically, emotionally, and/or physically dangerous to some clients with multiple oppressions. Healthy internal integration and external compartmentalization strategies may be preferred ways of assisting such clients in their identity development.

For QBIPOC, connection to family, local community, and religion/spirituality may be more salient than for White SGMs, thus coming out may risk important aspects of self-identification and connection to their ethnic, family, and religious roots which can be destabilizing (Lassiter, 2014; Potoczniak et al., 2009). QBIPOC may be less likely than their White counterparts to come out to their parents; for example, Filipino American queer people tend to struggle with religious (Catholicism) and cultural barriers to coming out, as well as bringing shame to their families in the process (Nadal & Corpus, 2013). At the same time, cultural values like collectivism and closeness of family (e.g., *familismo* within Latin@ culture) can provide strengths for helping families of QBIPOC to accept their SGM loved ones (Boe et al., 2018; Potoczniak et al., 2009).

Clinicians therefore should be careful to factor in these important cultural considerations when working with QBIPOC and not assume that disclosure to loved ones is necessarily beneficial. There is a difference between nondisclosure of SGM identity in particular environments, which is not thought to impact mental health, and the shame-based concealment of identity that does negatively affect well-being (Jackson & Mohr, 2016). Nor should a therapist assume that coming out to a racial/ethnic minority family will be disastrous, as many such communities exhibit fewer long-term rejections of their QBIPOC family members than do White families. Moreover, emerging evidence suggests that resilience is just as important as coming out and garnering social support; QBIPOC may be able to mitigate psychosocial distress through developing a greater sense of agency and adaptive ways of coping with stressors rather than coming out to family (Follins et al., 2014).

With regard to critical analysis of best practices, consider also transgender people of color in the transition process who are sometimes not adequately prepared to face the interlocking oppressions of certain identities. As an example, a Black transman who was accustomed to objectification and minimization projected by racist and genderist discrimination (when living as the gender assigned to them at birth), may have a hard time adjusting to the aspersions more often accorded to Black men as violent, and the subsequent aggressive treatment by other men in response (de Vries, 2015). Thus, it would behoove clinicians to determine when, how, and with whom to apply LGBTQ-affirming best practices when treating clients with intersectional identities (Fig. 2).

1.2.2   Intersectional LGBTQ-Affirmative Therapy

While LGBTQ-affirmative therapeutic practices have been increasing, we believe there are additional clinical considerations to be made when working with clients possessing multiple marginalized identities. A therapist with a solid case conceptualization will be able to explore, understand, and shape a treatment plan that includes all the aspects of the client's life. Various aspects of intersectionality may be highlighted or may emerge in treatment based on different environments or contexts. For example, a gay Muslim person from Jordan moving to the U.S. might notice how their ethnicity is perceived differently in the U.S. or how certain sexual identities are projected on them (e.g., "Arab men are only tops"). These microaggressions may take priority at the beginning of therapy rather than working on their queer identity development.

We hypothesize that a contextual behavioral framework can encompass a variety of theoretical techniques and evidence-based skills. Adapting evidenced-based tools in a flexible way can help to overcome limits of protocols, which might address the needs of QBIPOC. One of the common themes in psychotherapy with QBIPOC is targeting internalized stigma regarding race and/or sexual differences. For example, an LGBTQ-affirmative therapist attuned to intersectionality is cognizant of the

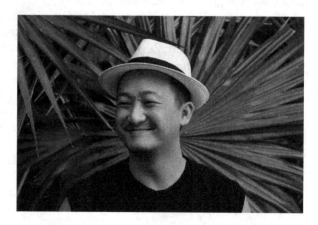

Fig. 2 Dennis Chin is a community organizer who demonstrates the importance of self-care. Photo Courtesy of Marcia Liu

negative impacts of acculturation in the U.S. Thus, a contextual behavioral therapist would try to target internalized stigma by validating the QBIPOC experience. This approach helps the client verbalize their own valued life, while expressing their identity through committed actions.

Healing relies on resiliency and surpasses individual impact. It aims for growth of a community through acceptance, change, and compassion. For instance, French et al. (2020) articulated a radical healing for POC that seeks to position dysfunction as a matter of systemic oppression vs. individual deficiency, and in parallel fashion to transform communities rather than individuals. These aims are accomplished through developing a *critical consciousness* about the causes of oppression and the possibility of changing them; relying on *radical hope* that such changes can and will occur; embodying *strength and resistance* to oppression through joyful living; embracing *cultural authenticity and self-knowledge* by reclaiming and valuing ancestral wisdom vs. prioritizing Western knowledge; and achieving liberation by relying on the community interdependence of *collectivism* (French et al., 2020).

Radical healing models of treatment are trauma-informed practices that are in response to historical and transgenerational trauma born of the conquest, colonization, enslavement, and oppression of BIPOC. The theoretical underpinnings of racial healing included intersectionality, liberation psychology, Black psychology, and other Indigenous psychologies (Comas-Díaz et al., 2019). Relatedly, Indigenous interventions, initiated and maintained by the communities that need them *for* the communities that need them, integrate holistic traditional healing approaches with wisdom from other arenas which may or may not include modern medicine and psychology. Indigenous psychologies emanating from trauma and cultural psychology offer hope for culturally relevant healing that might not otherwise be accepted by Indigenous communities, nor as effective for them as standard Western psychotherapeutic interventions (Hill et al., 2010). Through centering Indigenous LGBTQ concerns and peoples, there is hope for Western LGBTQ-affirmative therapy to be dramatically improved through collaboration with transnational queer psychologies (Horne et al., 2019), and thereby to transform the lives of LGBTQ people in the U.S. who are not defined (solely) by Western queer constructs.

Unfortunately, a common mistake in treatment and working toward healing is made through reductionist models that only acknowledge one part of the behavior or identity and therefore avoid contextual factors. Further, due to the current U.S. composition of psychologists, it is likely that QBIPOC individuals seeking therapy will work with a White therapist. While this might seem problematic at first glance, it also provides an impetus for deep racial and sexual healing. A therapist who understands their own intersectionality, power, and privileges—and how they interact in the therapist-client dyad—has an opportunity to create and foster a safe space to transform both clinician and client. We hypothesize that this process requires:

(a) Confronting implicit and explicit biases through self-awareness, therapeutic conversations with the client, consultation with colleagues, and careful honest examination of power and privilege;

(b) Thinking beyond symptom reduction and moving toward healing through incorporating culturally appropriate techniques to the therapy room;
(c) Observing intersectional identities as a source of resilience and a unique way of being; and
(d) Welcoming behavioral change as a compassionate contribution to the individual and/or the community.

Moreover, psychologists in clinical practice who are committed to social justice and intersectionality will necessarily have to apply these lenses to the individuals, couples, and small groups that they encounter in therapy, as the therapist-client relationship has historically been the primary focus of the field. At the same time, intersectionality, as grounded in its Black feminist roots, should inspire therapists to think and engage beyond the therapeutic space, and to actively undermine social inequality at the systemic level (Collins & Bilge, 2016). Intersectionality-oriented applied psychologists can work toward healing through actions such as political and institutional advocacy, grassroots community organization and support, and collaborative (vs. savior-oriented) engagement with Indigenous or marginalized communities.

1.3   Cultural Competence and Cultural Humility: How to Provide Affirmative Care

Over the past 30 years, multicultural counseling competence (MCC) has become an essential component in the pedagogy and training of psychology researchers and practitioners, and there has been abundant research demonstrating its benefits in therapy (Soto et al., 2018). MCC has traditionally focused on the awareness, knowledge, and skills necessary to become a culturally competent practitioner, with more recent attention aimed at social-justice-oriented action (Ratts et al., 2016). However, MCC has been criticized for conceptual limitations in that "competence" implies that there is some "destination" a practitioner can arrive at whereby they have attained a concrete level of awareness, knowledge, and skill to have objectively learned all that they need to know about client cultures (Buchanan et al., 2020). Such a posture positions the practitioner as superior, expert, and powerful, while framing their learning process as one that can be sufficient, finalized, or complete— a contrast to the ever-shifting, dynamic contexts of power and privilege described by intersectionality (Collins & Bilge, 2016).

Multicultural orientation (MCO) has been suggested as a more comprehensive framework for understanding and assessing the multicultural underpinnings of the complex interpersonal relationship between therapists and clients. MCO has been described as the therapist's "way of being" in the therapeutic space, such as their attunement to cultural factors related to themselves or their clients, whereas MCC is a "way of doing" therapy, in terms of how well the therapist exercises their multicultural skills (Owen et al., 2011). MCO involves at least three components: cultural humility, cultural opportunities (moments when a therapist can engage a client's culture in therapy), and cultural comfort (ease with which the therapist can bring up cultural discussions in therapy; Davis et al., 2018). The most studied component of MCO, cultural humility, has been defined as holding an other-focused, non-superior, respectful interpersonal stance about client cultural matters (Hook et al., 2013). Unlike MCC, cultural humility stresses an open, ongoing journey or process of learning how to respond to limitations of knowledge and awareness in light of both the therapist's and client's cultures, a posture that coheres well with intersectionality (Buchanan et al., 2020).

Literature and research on intersectional cultural humility is steadily growing, including a focus on SGM populations (e.g., Davis et al., 2021). A review of MCO (Davis et al., 2018) summarized evidence demonstrating how embodying cultural humility in therapy is associated with better outcomes for clients, improved therapeutic alliance, reduced risk of early client termination, fewer and less severe microaggressions perceived by the client, and less negative impact of microaggressions and/or missed opportunities to engage cultural issues when they occurred. Some literature has illustrated how healthcare practitioners can aid queer people with multiple oppressed intersectional identities in finding greater self-efficacy well-being despite systems of power and oppression that cause their emotional, mental, spiritual, and physical suffering (e.g., Adames et al., 2018). Themes that consistently emerge in this literature are the need for therapists to accept their missteps, cultural missed opportunities, and blind spots. Additionally, therapists must be willing to adopt the *other-centered self-growth* that characterizes intersectional cultural humility (Davis et al., 2021) by consistently (re-)educating themselves, interrogating biases, challenging assumptions, requesting feedback from clients and colleagues, broaching the sometimes uncomfortable topics of power and oppression within and outside the therapeutic space, and decentering normalized but deleterious hegemonic narratives (heterocentrism, ciscentrism, Whiteness, etc.) Only through a humble approach to competence can such aims be achieved. The aforementioned evidence demonstrates how well clients respond and grow from—and how systems can be impacted by—the multicultural, social-justice-focused, competent actions of the intersectionally-informed, culturally humble therapist.

1.4   Case Study

Devon is a 26yo, single, cisgender, Black, gay, Christian-identified man from an urban mid-Atlantic city. He presented to his college's counseling center with significant anxiety, depression, and academic stress. Devon had been in school for several years and had a pattern of starting semesters well, faltering mid-semester, and often failing courses that necessitated him retaking them. Additionally, he complained of poor self-esteem related to his ability to finish school; his body image; and about conflicts between his culture (paternal Nigerian heritage), sexuality, and religious views. Devon has always felt that he was too feminine, so he has worked hard to cover his gender nonconforming behaviors. He also acknowledged that at a young age he began "talking White" and adopting other culturally nonconforming manner-isms both to survive in the mostly White high school he attended and because he felt rejected by the Black community, thus he resisted many cultural connections to his heritage.

At intake, Devon revealed that he was born several weeks premature and had numerous health problems from infancy to early childhood. His parents divorced when he was a toddler, and the family has always struggled financially. He came out to himself around the age of 18 when he had his first boyfriend, but he experienced interpersonal violence for the 2-year duration of the relationship. He explained that he stayed with his boyfriend for so long because he never felt that he could do any better. Only after a serious injury did he leave the relationship, but he developed significant PTSD as a result of his abuse.

Because he was lonely he desperately sought connections, but struggled to find anything meaningful. He tried using gay dating apps, but found many of the men near campus to discriminate against him as a Black man, and there were few QBIPOC men in his rural college town using the app. Because he was an older student, he found it hard to relate to the younger, mostly White undergrads he was surrounded by. Moreover, he was afraid to come out to his family or his church and was therefore unable to rely on two communities that helped define him. His social isolation and loneliness caused him to sometimes put himself in compromising positions with sexual partners, including having unsafe sex with multiple people at once. He generally felt intense guilt and shame after these experiences.

Devon had been to another therapist, a cis Black woman, whom he found ini-tially helpful, but he ended the relationship after a few sessions when she labeled him a sex addict and focused treatment on his sexual behavior. Likewise, a psychia-trist diagnosed him with bipolar disorder and prescribed mood stabilizers. The cli-ent had a poor reaction to the diagnosis and never picked up the medication from the pharmacy.

1.4.1 Case Discussion

This is a complex case involving multiple oppressions and multiple rejections. Unfortunately, many elements of the case are all too common to us as queer men of color who practice with many QBIPOC clients (Dr. Freeman-Coppadge identifies as a cis, Black, gay person of faith, and Dr. Farhadi Langroudi identifies as a non-Binary [masculine presentation], Persian, Queer Muslim). The initial case concep-tualization and treatment plan must be embarked upon carefully not only because of the intersectional factors involved indicating that this client has experienced signifi-cant minority stress, but also because he has endured painful microaggressions from another therapist. His previous therapist likely did not possess adequate training in LGBTQ-affirmative therapy or use adequate intersectional lenses to understand Devon, resulting (understandably) in premature termination and other potential harms to his well-being. Devon has several marginalized identities as a Black, sexual minority man from an economically disadvantaged background. Additionally, several other interweaving factors need to be investigated to determine if they are exacerbating his stigma. Devon may have a disability (e.g., a neurodiverse diagnosis like ADHD or learning disorder) given his prematurity and difficulties in college, as well as his age in college which operates as a form of othering for him. Finally, Devon's identity conflict related to sexuality, spirituality, and race/ethnicity/culture will likely need some attention.

With complex cases like these, it can be difficult to know where to begin with treatment, but client-centered approaches to therapy would indicate working collaboratively with Devon to determine that after clarifying the client's history. What is most important is conveying understanding and validation to the client given his presenting problems and employing cultural humility to help him explore his concerns. Aiding him in situating his suffering in systemic oppression may be easy for him to conceptually grasp given his experiences of discrimination, but there are also signs of significant internalized homonegativity and internalized racism that may take time to improve. In our clinical experience, the shame that can be associated with these internalized processes is often quite persistent. Mindfulness, a focus on his many strengths and talents (e.g., highlighting how far he has gotten in life with so little aid and support), and attunement to his resilience are key to Devon building a positive sense of self. Drawing on ways in which he has thrived in the midst of racial discrimination can be expanded upon to provide resistance to and liberation from other intersectional oppressions.

Finally, Devon will most certainly need connection to a community of support. Many college campuses boast LGBTQ student services, but those spaces are not often perceived as friendly to or accepting of people of color, disabled, or socioeconomically challenged queer people (among many others). They may also not be comfortable spaces for those who are struggling to accept themselves because of identity conflicts or lack of self-acceptance.

1.4.2 Treatment Outcomes

Devon was seen for 2 years by his psychologist at his college counseling center before being referred off-campus for further psychotherapy. It became clear to his psychologist early on that the symptoms seen by other providers as sex addiction and bipolar disorder were really manifestations of his emotional and behavioral responses to trauma (relational violence, racism, heterosexism) and neurocognitive struggles. Given Devon's financial challenges, he could not afford the neurocognitive testing his therapist hoped for, but the college did offer some low-cost testing services which confirmed a diagnosis of ADHD with profound impairments in processing speed. The therapist connected the client to the disability office to get accommodations, and to a psychiatrist in the health center whom the therapist knew was competent in providing affirmative pharmacotherapeutic care. Over the course of his first year in therapy, Devon partially responded to an anxiolytic/antidepressant medication that improved his anxiety and depression symptoms, and a stimulant which marginally improved his focus. Devon still struggled with keeping up with a demanding course load; the therapist worked with the disability office to reduce his coarse load to two courses a semester while maintaining full-time student status.

Much of Devon's course of therapy was practical management of his symptoms and a focus on distinct academic resources he had been deprived of his whole life because of institutional failures that disadvantaged him. The therapist contextualized Devon's problems as being rooted in oppressive systems, not Devon himself. As his self-efficacy in academics progressed, the focus of therapy turned toward some of Devon's internalized "isms." This was arduous work because of the necessary defensive walls that Devon had built over the years in order to survive. In our experience, it can take months or even years to establish adequate rapport with clients to reach a level of vulnerability that allows for meaningful transformation of isms.

QBIPOC who have developed strong avoidance and distancing behaviors must learn to see how those techniques are now working against their stated goals of developing a whole, integrated sense of self and establishing better relationships through constructing a family of choice. Patience, persistence, and gentle challenging through trust and culturally sensitive/humble care on the part of the clinician is crucial for realizing such aims in therapy. His therapist, for instance—who was a queer-identified provider—had to engage in the tough internal work of cultural humility by managing his negative reactions when Devon expressed offensive statements about "girly gay guys" (related to internalized homonegativity and stigma around his own gender nonconforming behaviors). His therapist engaged in the equally difficult external work of cultural humility by gently confronting such behaviors and honestly sharing his reactions to them in a collaborative exercise of healing for them both. Through continually reminding Devon of his strength, beauty, and value, these more positive images slowly began to be internalized. He became better able to accept and feel his emotions and recognize that the negative voices in his head were not reflections of who he truly was.

To aid in his journey, the client was referred to an ADHD group and a short-term anxiety workshop to learn basic mindfulness and coping skills; the lessons learned were broadened in therapy to maximal effectiveness through adapting them to his unique circumstances as a student with multiple marginalized identities. To promote healing from trauma, he was also referred to an LGBTQ support group on campus that happened to have been created and run by his therapist. Because the group was carefully created and advertised, there were a number of QBIPOC in the group for him to relate to. The group offered a space for Devon to begin seeing himself as a part of an empowered community of people with similar struggles—an opportunity previously never afforded to him—and the ability to practice some of the vulnerability he was learning in individual sessions with his therapist. Through his time in the group, Devon began to care for other members, and he later became more engaged with activism on campus that related to the oppressions that members of the group discussed.

Intersectional affirming care can be most effective when clients have deep connections to a healing group. Referral to such groups is recommended whenever possible, whether through strengths-based groups that incorporate trauma-informed, Indigenous, and intersectionally-oriented treatments, or to appropriate community centers or organizations. Through his connections to the group and his efforts to build a family of choice, Devon was eventually able to integrate his Black, gay, and Christian identities—seeing them in harmony with (not opposition to) one another. He began attending a Black church nearby that welcomed LGBTQ people and came out to some members of his family who did not reject him, though some of them struggled for some time with their own religious views in learning how to embrace Devon.

College counseling centers, because of their institutional settings, give clinicians opportunities to make systemic changes that can promote social justice. Devon's therapist was able to coordinate services across campus for the client and was able to connect him to needed community. The therapist was able to co-construct (with colleagues, mentors, and students) a brave space for QBIPOC because of his position on the campus, and his outreach to campus offices and administrators. Clinicians in private practice may find it more difficult to intervene at institutional or systemic levels, though through connections to professional and social justice organizations, such change is possible. Additionally, private practitioners can offer pro bono services for individual and group clients, or they can land their services and expertise to legislative or judicial efforts that affect people with multiple marginalized identities. In doing so, they demonstrate that they do all that they can to advocate for their clients – many who may not have other resources or advocates to help them to do so (Fig. 3).

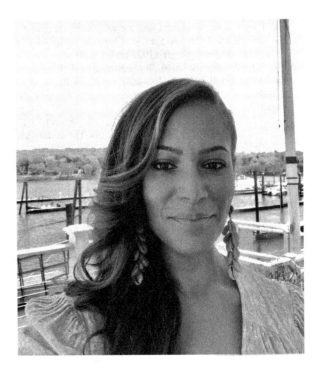

Fig. 3 Risë Nelson—the Dean of the Afro American Cultural Center at Yale University—is a fierce advocate for mental health and wellness, particularly for queer and trans BIPOC students. Photo Courtesy of Kevin Nadal

References

Adames, H. Y., Chavez-Dueñas, N. Y., Sharma, S., & La Roche, M. J. (2018). Intersectionality in psychotherapy: The experiences of an AfroLatinx queer immigrant. *Psychotherapy, 55*(1), 73–79. https://doi.org/10.1037/pst0000152.

American Psychological Association. (2012). Guidelines for psychological practice with lesbian, gay, and bisexual clients. *American Psychologist, 67*(1), 10–42. https://doi.org/10.1037/a0024659.

American Psychological Association. (2015). Guidelines for psychological practice with transgender and gender nonconforming people. *American Psychologist, 70*(9), 832–864. https://doi.org/10.1037/a0039906.

American Psychological Association. (2021a). APA resolution on gender identity change efforts. https://www.apa.org/about/policy/resolution-gender-identity-change-efforts.pdf.

American Psychological Association. (2021b). APA resolution on sexual orientation change efforts. https://www.apa.org/about/policy/resolution-sexual-orientation-change-efforts.pdf.

Bishop, M. D., Fish, J. N., Hammack, P. L., & Russell, S. T. (2020). Sexual identity development milestones in three generations of sexual minority people: A national probability sample. *Developmental Psychology, 56*(11), 2177–2193. https://doi.org/10.1037/dev0001105.

Bockting, W. O., Miner, M. H., Romine, R. E. S., Hamilton, A., & Coleman, E. (2013). Stigma, mental health, and resilience in an online sample of the US transgender population. *American Journal of Public Health, 103*(5), 943–951. https://doi.org/10.2105/AJPH.2013.301241.

Boe, J. L., Maxey, V. A., & Bermudez, J. M. (2018). Is the closet a closet? Decolonizing the coming out process with Latin@ adolescents and families. *Journal of Feminist Family Therapy: An International Forum, 30*(2), 90–108. https://doi.org/10.1080/08952833.2018.1427931.

Buchanan, N. T., Rios, D., & Case, K. A. (2020). Intersectional cultural humility: Critical inquiry and praxis in psychology. *Women & Therapy, 34*(3–4), 235–243. https://doi.org/10.1080/02703149.2020.1729469.

Budge, S. L. (2013). Interpersonal psychotherapy with transgender clients. *Psychotherapy, 50*(3), 356–359. https://doi.org/10.1037/a0032194.

Cochran, S. D., Björkenstam, C., & Mays, V. M. (2017). Sexual orientation differences in functional limitations, disability, and mental health services use: Results from the 2013–2014 National Health Interview Survey. *Journal of Consulting and Clinical Psychology, 85*(12), 1111–1121. https://doi.org/10.1037/ccp0000243.

Collins, P. H., & Bilge, S. (2016). Intersectionality. Polity Press.

Comas-Díaz, L., Hall, G. N., & Neville, H. A. (2019). Racial trauma: Theory, research, and healing: Introduction to the special issue. *American Psychologist, 74*(1), 1–5. https://doi.org/10.1037/amp0000442.

Davis, D. E., DeBlaere, C., Owen, J., Hook, J. N., Rivera, D. P., Choe, E., Van Tongeren, D. R., Worthington, J. R., Jr., & Placeres, V. (2018). The multicultural orientation framework: A narrative review. *Psychotherapy, 55*(1), 89–100. https://doi.org/10.1037/pst0000160.

Davis, E. B., Plante, T. G., Grey, M. J., Kim, C. L., Freeman-Coppadge, D., Lefevor, G. T., Paulez, J. A., Giwa, S., Lasser, J., Stratton, S. P., Deneke, E., & Glowiak, K. J. (2021). The role of civility and cultural humility in navigating controversial areas in psychology. Spirituality in Clinical Practice, 8(2), 79–97. https://doi.org/10.1037/scp0000236.

de Vries, K. M. (2015). Transgender people of color at the center: Conceptualizing a new intersectional model. *Ethnicities, 15*(1), 3–27. https://doi.org/10.1177/1468796814547058.

DeGruy, J. (2017). *Post traumatic slave syndrome*. Portland, OR: Joy DeGruy Publications.

Diamond, G. M., Diamond, G. S., Levy, S., Closs, C., Ladipo, T., & Siqueland, L. (2013). Attachment-based family therapy for suicidal lesbian, gay, and bisexual adolescents: A treatment development study and open trial with preliminary findings. *Psychology of Sexual Orientation and Gender Diversity, 1*(S), 91–100. https://doi.org/10.1037/2329-0382.1.S.91.

Dominguez, M. L. (2017). LGBTQIA people of color: Utilizing the cultural psychology model as a guide for the mental health assessment and treatment of patients with diverse identities.

Journal of Gay & Lesbian Mental Health, 21(3), 203–220. https://doi.org/10.1080/1935970 5.2017.1320755.

Duke, T. S. (2011). Lesbian, gay, bisexual, and transgender youth with disabilities: A meta-synthesis. *Journal of LGBT Youth, 8*(1), 1–52. https://doi.org/10.1080/19361653.2011.519181.

Feinstein, B. A., & Dyar, C. (2017). Bisexuality, minority stress, and health. *Current Sexual Health Reports, 9*(1), 42–49. https://doi.org/10.1007/s11930-017-0096-3.

Filice, E., & Meyer, S. B. (2018). Patterns, predictors, and outcomes of mental health service utilization among lesbians, gay men, and bisexuals: A scoping review. *Journal of Gay & Lesbian Mental Health, 22*(2), 162–195. https://doi.org/10.1080/19359705.2017.1418468.

Follins, L. D., Walker, J. J., & Lewis, M. K. (2014). Resilience in black lesbian, gay, bisexual, and transgender individuals: A critical review of the literature. *Journal of Gay & Lesbian Mental Health, 18*(2), 190–212. https://doi.org/10.1080/19359705.2013.828343.

Freeman-Coppadge, D. J., & Horne, S. G. (2019). "What happens if the cross falls and crushes me?": Psychological and spiritual promises and perils of lesbian and gay Christian celibacy. *Psychology of Sexual Orientation and Gender Diversity, 6*(4), 486–497. https://doi.org/10.1037/sgd0000341.

French, B. H., Lewis, J. A., Mosley, D. V., Adames, H. Y., Chavez-Dueñas, N. Y., Chen, G. A., & Neville, H. A. (2020). Toward a psychological framework of radical healing in communities of color. *The Counseling Psychologist, 48*(1), 14–46. https://doi.org/10.1177/0011000019843506.

Haines, K. M., Boyer, C. R., Giovanazzi, C., & Galupo, M. P. (2018). "Not a real family": Microaggressions directed toward LGBTQ families. *Journal of Homosexuality, 65*(9), 1138–1151. https://doi.org/10.1080/00918369.2017.1406217.

Hammack, P. L., Frost, D. M., & Hughes, S. D. (2019). Queer intimacies: A new paradigm for the study of relationship diversity. *Journal of Sex Research, 56*(4–5), 556–592. https://doi.org/1 0.1080/00224499.2018.1531281.

Hill, J. S., Lau, M. Y., & Sue, D. W. (2010). Integrating trauma psychology and cultural psychology: Indigenous perspectives on theory, research, and practice. *Traumatology, 16*(4), 39–47. https://doi.org/10.1177/1534765610388303.

Hook, J. N., Davis, D. E., Owen, J., Worthington, E. L., Jr., & Utsey, S. O. (2013). Cultural humility: Measuring openness to culturally diverse clients. *Journal of Counseling Psychology, 60*(3), 353–366. https://doi.org/10.1037/a0032595.

Horne, S. G., Maroney, M. R., Nel, J. A., Chaparro, R. A., & Manalastas, E. J. (2019). Emergence of a transnational LGBTI psychology: Commonalities and challenges in advocacy and activism. American Psychologist, 74(8), 967–986. https://doi.org/10.1037/amp0000561.

Israel, T., Choi, A. Y., Goodman, J. A., Matsuno, E., Lin, Y.-J., Kary, K. G., & Merrill, C. R. S. (2019). Reducing internalized binegativity: Development and efficacy of an online intervention. *Psychology of Sexual Orientation and Gender Diversity, 6*(2), 149–159. https://doi.org/10.1037/sgd0000314.

Jackson, S. D., & Mohr, J. J. (2016). Conceptualizing the closet: Differentiating stigma concealment and nondisclosure processes. *Psychology of Sexual Orientation and Gender Diversity, 3*(1), 80–92. https://doi.org/10.1037/sgd0000147.

Lassiter, J. M. (2014). Extracting dirt from water: A strengths-based approach to religion for African American same-gender-loving men. *Journal of Religion and Health, 53*, 178–189. https://doi.org/10.1007/s10943-012-9668-8.

Levitt, H. M. (2019). A psychosocial genealogy of LGBTQ+ gender: An empirically based theory of gender and gender identity cultures. *Psychology of Women Quarterly, 43*(3), 275–297. https://doi.org/10.1177/0361684319834641.

Lin, Y.-J., Israel, T., & Ryan, W. S. (2019). Releasing internalized stigma for empowerment: Development of theory-driven interventions for sexual and gender minorities. *Journal of LGBT Issues in Counseling, 13*(4), 276–292. https://doi.org/10.1080/15538605.2019.1662358.

Mereish, E. H., & Poteat, V. P. (2015). A relational model of sexual minority mental and physical health: The negative effects of shame on relationships, loneliness, and health. *Journal of Counseling Psychology, 62*(3), 425–437. https://doi.org/10.1037/cou0000088.

Meyer, I. H. (2013). Prejudice, social stress, and mental health in lesbian, gay, and bisexual populations: Conceptual issues and research evidence. *Psychology of Sexual Orientation and Gender Diversity, 1*(S), 3–26. https://doi.org/10.1037/2329-0382.1.S.3.

Nadal, K. L. (2020). Queering law and order: LGBTQ communities and the criminal justice system. Lexington.

Nadal, K. L., & Corpus, M. J. H. (2013). "Tomboys" and "baklas": Experiences of lesbian and gay Filipino Americans. *Asian American Journal of Psychology, 4*(3), 166–175. https://doi.org/10.1037/a0030168.

O'Shaughnessy, T., & Speir, Z. (2018). The state of LGBQ affirmative therapy clinical research: A mixed-methods systematic synthesis. *Psychology of Sexual Orientation and Gender Diversity, 5*(1), 82–98. https://doi.org/10.1037/sgd0000259.

Owen, J. J., Tao, K., Leach, M. M., & Rodolfa, E. (2011). Clients' perceptions of their psychotherapists' multicultural orientation. *Psychotherapy, 48*(3), 274–282. https://doi.org/10.1037/a0022065.

Pachankis, J. E. (2018). The scientific pursuit of sexual and gender minority mental health treatments: Toward evidence-based affirmative practice. *American Psychologist, 73*(9), 1207–1219. https://doi.org/10.1037/amp0000357.

Pachankis, J. E., Hatzenbuehler, M. L., Rendina, H. J., Safren, S. A., & Parsons, J. T. (2015). LGB-affirmative cognitive-behavioral therapy for young adult gay and bisexual men: A randomized controlled trial of a transdiagnostic minority stress approach. *Journal of Consulting and Clinical Psychology, 83*(5), 875–889. https://doi.org/10.1037/ccp0000037.

Pepping, C. A., Halford, W. K., Cronin, T. J., & Lyons, A. (2020). Couple relationship education for same-sex couples: A preliminary evaluation of rainbow CoupleCARE. *Journal of Couple & Relationship Therapy, 19*(3), 230–249. https://doi.org/10.1080/15332691.2020.1746458.

Pepping, C. A., Lyons, A., & Morris, E. M. J. (2018). Affirmative LGBT psychotherapy: Outcomes of a therapist training protocol. *Psychotherapy, 55*(1), 52–62. https://doi.org/10.1037/pst0000149.

Porter, K. E., Brennan-Ing, M., Chang, S. C., Dickey, L. M., Singh, A. A., Bower, K. L., & Witten, T. M. (2016). Providing competent and affirming services for transgender and gender nonconforming older adults. *Clinical Gerontologist: The Journal of Aging and Mental Health, 39*(5), 366–388. https://doi.org/10.1080/07317115.2016.1203383.

Potocznik, D., Crosbie-Burnett, M., & Saltzburg, N. (2009). Experiences regarding coming out to parents among African American, Hispanic, and White gay, lesbian, bisexual, transgender, and questioning adolescents. *Journal of Gay & Lesbian Social Services: Issues in Practice, Policy & Research, 21*(2–3), 189–205. https://doi.org/10.1080/10538720902772063.

Proujansky, R. A., & Pachankis, J. E. (2014). Toward formulating evidence-based principles of LGB-affirmative psychotherapy. *Pragmatic Case Studies in Psychotherapy, 10*(2), 117–131.

Puckett, J. A., Mereish, E. H., Levitt, H. M., Horne, S. G., & Hayes-Skelton, S. A. (2018). Internalized heterosexism and psychological distress: The moderating effects of decentering. *Stigma and Health, 3*(1), 9–15. https://doi.org/10.1037/sah0000065.

Ratts, M. J., Singh, A. A., Nassar-McMillan, S., Butler, S. K., & McCullough, J. R. (2016). Multicultural and social justice counseling competencies: Guidelines for the counseling profession. *Journal of Multicultural Counseling and Development, 44*(1), 28–48. https://doi.org/10.1002/jmcd.12035.

Rodriguez, E. M., Etengoff, C., & Vaughan, M. D. (2019). A quantitative examination of identity integration in gay, lesbian, and bisexual people of faith. *Journal of Homosexuality, 66*(1), 77–99. https://doi.org/10.1080/00918369.2017.1395259.

Rostosky, S. S., & Riggle, E. D. B. (2017). Same-sex couple relationship strengths: A review and synthesis of the empirical literature (2000–2016). *Psychology of Sexual Orientation and Gender Diversity, 4*(1), 1–13. https://doi.org/10.1037/sgd0000216.

Rothblum, E. D., Krueger, E. A., Kittle, K. R., & Meyer, I. H. (2020). Asexual and non-asexual respondents from a U.S. population-based study of sexual minorities. *Archives of Sexual Behavior, 49*, 757–767. https://doi.org/10.1007/s10508-019-01485-0.

Ryan, C., Russell, S. T., Huebner, D., Diaz, R., & Sanchez, J. (2010). Family acceptance in adolescence and the health of LGBT young adults. *Journal of Child and Adolescent Psychiatric Nursing, 23*(4), 205–213. https://doi.org/10.1111/j.1744-6171.2010.00246.x.

Sarno, E. L., Mohr, J. J., Jackson, S. D., & Fassinger, R. E. (2015). When identities collide: Conflicts in allegiances among LGB people of color. *Cultural Diversity and Ethnic Minority Psychology, 21*(4), 550–559. https://doi.org/10.1037/cdp0000026.

Schechinger, H. A., Sakaluk, J. K., & Moors, A. C. (2018). Harmful and helpful therapy practices with consensually non-monogamous clients: Toward an inclusive framework. *Journal of Consulting and Clinical Psychology, 86*(11), 879–891. https://doi.org/10.1037/ccp0000349.

Shangani, S., Gamarel, K. E., Ogunbajo, A., Cai, J., & Operario, D. (2020). Intersectional minority stress disparities among sexual minority adults in the USA: The role of race/ethnicity and socioeconomic status. *Culture, Health & Sexuality, 22*(4), 398–412. https://doi.org/10.108 0/13691058.2019.1604994.

Singh, A. A., & Burnes, T. R. (2010). Shifting the counselor role from gatekeeping to advocacy: Ten strategies for using the competencies for counseling with transgender clients for individual and social change. *Journal of LGBT Issues in Counseling, 4*(3–4), 241–255. https://doi.org/1 0.1080/15538605.2010.525455.

Soto, A., Smith, T. B., Griner, D., Domenech Rodríguez, M., & Bernal, G. (2018). Cultural adaptations and therapist multicultural competence: Two meta-analytic reviews. *Journal of Clinical Psychology, 74*, 1907–1923. https://doi.org/10.1002/jclp.22679.

Vencill, J. A., & Wiljamaa, S. J. (2016). From MOM to MORE: Emerging research on mixed orientation relationships. *Current Sexual Health Reports, 8*, 206–212. https://doi.org/10.1007/ s11930-016-0081-2.

Yadavaia, J. E., & Hayes, S. C. (2012). Acceptance and commitment therapy for self-stigma around sexual orientation: A multiple baseline evaluation. *Cognitive and Behavioral Practice, 19*(4), 545–559. https://doi.org/10.1016/j.cbpra.2011.09.002.

Queering Sex and Romance: Considerations of Gender Diversity, Sex, and Relationships

G. Nic Rider, Jieyi Cai, and Leonardo Candelario-Pérez

People of color, women, and trans and gender diverse (TGD) people have often been overlooked in the literature on queer relationships. Eurocentric and heteronormative biases of sexuality have contributed to various forms of intimacy among marginalized communities being rendered invisible throughout history (Fassinger & Israel, 2010; Greene & Boyd-Franklin, 1996). Research on TGD people of color is generally lacking, particularly research on transgender men of color (Barnett et al., 2019). However, the existing research on transgender women of color, much like the research on cisgender queer men of color, focuses largely on HIV/STI risk and prevention. This chapter will begin with an overview of research on LGBQ+ people of color's sexual romantic relationships (albeit much of the literature is on men who have sex with men), and then shift to focus on TGD individuals' sexual and romantic relationships as a way of exploring issues in relationships for populations that have been historically marginalized even in the literature on queer relationships (Fig. 1).

The original version of this chapter was revised. The correction to this chapter is available at https://doi.org/10.1007/978-3-030-74146-4_18

G. N. Rider (✉) · J. Cai · L. Candelario-Pérez
Institute for Sexual and Gender Health, Department of Family Medicine and Community
Health, University of Minnesota Medical School, Minneapolis, MN, USA
e-mail: gnrider@umn.edu; cai00058@umn.edu;
Leonardo.E.CandelarioPerez@healthpartners.com

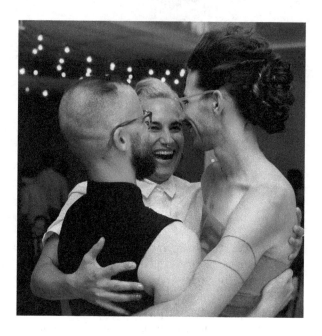

Fig. 1 A moment of queer love and friendship between a couple and their officiant at their wedding. Photo Courtesy of Yana Calou/Sean Fader

1   Sexual and Romantic Relationships for LGBQ People of Color

Some authors have discussed the particular challenges queer people of color face in navigating romantic and sexual relationships. Fassinger and Israel (2010) argue that heterosexism in communities of color must be seen in the context of systematic racism, which casts these communities as inferior and thus places them under great external pressure to absorb the heterosexist and patriarchal norms of the mainstream society. Greene et al. (2013) posit that these norms may be more strictly enforced in communities of color, specifically African American communities. Due to being stereotyped as hypersexual, degenerate, and dangerous, Black people must police their own sexualities to conform with dominant White morality. Black people who do not conform to this sexual morality, such as LGBTQ individuals, are then "scapegoated" because of their potential use as an example of Black moral degeneracy and therefore an excuse to marginalize Black communities at large.

Greene et al. (2013) suggest that internalized racism manifesting in the policing of one's own sexuality and that of the members of one's community, combined with internalized heterosexism (from one's own community and mainstream society) creates a sense in many Black LGBQ individuals that they do not deserve love or will never be able to have a successful relationship. These beliefs can then harm any relationships these individuals enter into, and may be compounded by a lack of visible models for successful, queer Black relationships. Black men and women also must contend with racialized and gendered sexual stereotypes. Gay Black men may thus feel caught in a dichotomy in which they are hypermasculinized under white supremacy and feminized within their own racial community. Further, within their own queer community, they are also hypersexualized, exoticized, or both. Meanwhile, Black lesbians may find that they are stereotyped as masculine and seen as "defective women" both because they are Black and because they are lesbian. Previous studies also indicate that women of color, including queer women of color, experience sexual objectification and exoticization by heterosexual men based on racially gendered stereotypes such as Asian American women being perceived as sexually submissive, Latinas being perceived as feisty, and African American women perceived as Jezebels (Nadal, 2013; Nadal et al., 2012; Rivera et al., 2010; Sue et al., 2008, 2009).

Sexual stereotypes point to ways in which Black LGBQ individuals and other LGBQ people of color often face racism within White-dominated LGBQ communities (Greene et al., 2013; Han & Choi, 2018; Wade & Harper, 2019). This racism is encountered in romantic or sexual partner-seeking in the form of a) race-based exclusion, or b) fetishization of particular racial identities. The specific form of racism encountered in the context of sexual or romantic partner-seeking has been termed "sexual racism" or "racialized sexual discrimination" (Greene, 1996; Wade & Harper, 2019). Research in this area has primarily focused on men who have sex with men.

Much race-based exclusion of certain people from a pool of potential partners is based on racist stereotypes, both sexual and non-sexual; for example, that Black men are uneducated or "thugs," while Asian men are "effeminate" (Han, 2007; Hidalgo et al., 2013; Wade & Harper, 2019). On the other side of the same coin is race-based fetishization and objectification: men of color also encounter men whose interest in them is driven by these same denigrating stereotypes. Latino men may find themselves desired because of beliefs that they are "sexually insatiable," while Black men are often the object of beliefs about hypermasculinity, sexual aggression, or penis size (Han, 2007; Hidalgo et al., 2013). Meanwhile, Asian men may be sought out because of beliefs that they are submissive, or out of desire for an exotic "other" (Han, 2007; Paul et al., 2010). In Paul et al.'s (2010) study, Asian men in particular reported receiving attention from older White men, implying a power dynamic in which the younger Asian "boy" would serve as a sexual object. Such experiences of sexual racism has been associated with depression, anxiety, stress, self-esteem concerns, body-image concerns, suicidal ideation with a plan, non-suicidal self-injury, and higher risk for substance use (Bhambhani et al., 2019, 2020; Hidalgo et al., 2020; Newcomb et al., 2015; Thai, 2020).

2 Transgender and Gender Diverse (TGD) People's Sexual and Romantic Relationships

Although scholarly work on TGD people continues to expand, research focusing on TGD people's romantic and sexual relationships to date is limited (Moradi et al., 2016). TGD individuals are stigmatized and oppressed based on their gender identities and expressions as well as other social and/or perceived identities they have (e.g., race and ethnicity, sexual orientation, ability status, etc.). This is a community that is erotically marginalized, or "at risk of being pathologized and oppressed both outside and inside the clinical setting due to their sexual identities, orientations and practices" (Constantinides et al., 2019, p. 1). With the medicalization of TGD identities even in the field of psychology, TGD people have been simultaneously treated as hypersexual deviants and as desexualized beings not imagined to seek and experience sexual intimacy (Lev, 2014). These external messages can contribute to internalized beliefs of being unlovable, not worthy of intimate (sexual and non-sexual) relationships, and/or only valued as sexual objects. These dehumanizing and harmful ways TGD people are perceived are examples of how erotic marginalization can intersect with transphobia.

Further, within some medical treatment protocols (that are often considered to be based in anti-trans theory), the legitimacy of a TGD person's gender identity was questioned if they experienced any sexual attraction to or sexual engagement with someone of the same identified gender (Doorduin & van Berlo, 2014; Lev, 2014). Attempts to delegitimize and invalidate TGD people's experiences is not uncommon. This view conflates gender and sexual orientation (at least from a Western understanding where these concepts are considered separate but related) and assumes that in order for a trans person's gender to be legitimate, they must exhibit heteronormative attraction.

The categorization of sexual orientation (e.g. using labels such as straight, gay, bisexual, etc.) tends to be predicated on the relationship between one's own gender(s) and the gender(s) of the people to whom one is attracted. The labels used to describe sexual orientation may change as a person transitions because they now occupy a different gender relative to the people they are attracted to, or because they find their attraction to others has changed. Despite heteronormative assumptions that a person must be heterosexual in order to "really" be transgender, research has shown that TGD people often endorse multiple labels for their sexual orientation and find that conventional labels do not fit them neatly. Some also choose to not label their sexual orientation at all. In a study by Galupo et al. (2016), transgender participants reported that the perceptions of others and designations associated with their genitalia factored into their choice of descriptors, and highlighted the complexity of labeling themselves in the context of dominant understandings of sex and gender as binary and biological. Some participants chose to describe their sexuality only in terms of who they were attracted to rather than using conventional labels, removing the need to reference their own gender in the description (Fig. 2).

Fig. 2 A QTPOC couple showing their love and affection for each other. Photo Courtesy of Rodnae Productions

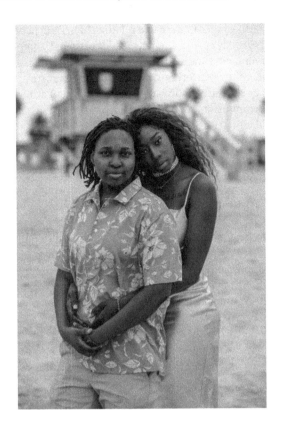

2.1 Transgender People Can and Do Have Sexual and Romantic Relationships

Contrary to early beliefs that trans people could not have relationships (or at least could not have healthy ones), Iantaffi and Bockting (2011) found that 62.9% of transmasculine participants and 54.1% of transfeminine participants in their study were currently in primary romantic relationships. In Meier et al.'s (2013) study of trans men, 51% reported currently being in a relationship. Meier et al.'s findings also suggest that relationships confer similar health benefits to trans people as they do to other populations, as those in relationships reported fewer symptoms of depression than those who were not in relationships. Platt and Bolland's (2017) study reflected how trans people navigate normative dynamics and challenges in maintaining healthy, long-term relationships. However, trans people also face particular relationship issues related to their identities.

In a heteronormative and cissexist society, it can be difficult for trans people to find partners who embrace their transness. For trans people with cisgender partners, having to explain their transness may become burdensome (Duran & Nicolazzo, 2017). In addition to the gendered and binary role expectations that cisgender partners might bring to a relationship, TGD people may experience cissexist micro-aggressions from their cisgender partner. Examples might include the partner under-mining the authenticity of or simply failing to understand the TGD partner's gender identity, interfering with the TGD partner's transition, or respecting the TGD part-ner's identity in private but not in public. Partners of TGD people may struggle with the implications of their partner's gender identity or transition for their own sexual identity (Pulice-Farrow et al., 2017, 2019b). Pulice-Farrow et al. (2019a), however, also outline ways in which TGD people feel affirmed by their partners, including cisgender partners validating their gender expression, helping them process their identity, using gender-affirming language, and acknowledging and leveraging their own cisgender privilege.

Unwillingness to face the social stigma that may accompany having a TGD part-ner can contribute to the ending of a relationship following one partner coming out or beginning their gender transition (Platt & Bolland, 2017, 2018). Gamarel et al. (2014) examined the effect of gender minority stress on mental health and relation-ship quality for trans women and their cisgender male partners. They found that discrimination and relationship stigma were correlated with increased depressive distress for both partners. Additionally, for trans women, greater self-reported and partner-reported relationship stigma was associated with lower relationship quality, whereas for the cisgender men, only partner-reported relationship stigma was asso-ciated with lower relationship quality. These results point to the importance of not only examining the effect of minority stress on TGD individuals but also on their relationships and partners.

2.2 Heterosexism and Cissexism

Though TGD people have transgressed conventional bounds of binary gender, research demonstrates how TGD people's relationships are still shaped by dominant gender and sexual discourses (Iantaffi & Bockting, 2011). Dominant sexual and romantic scripts in the US are predicated on a system of binary gender and hetero-normativity. Even in queer relationships, roles may be assigned based on a binary of masculinity and femininity in gender expression, and sexual and gender fluidity can be erased in favor of a dichotomy of straight versus gay (Jourian, 2018; Platt & Bolland, 2017). Gender essentialism, or equating of gender with certain anatomical features, is still prevalent among queer communities, and TGD people may encoun-ter gendered prescriptions of what roles they can or cannot take based on their anatomies (e.g. "you can't be a top because you don't have a dick"; Jourian, 2018 p. 366).

As TGD people socially transition, they must negotiate their relationship to the roles socially assigned to men and women. In addition to exploring their own gen-der, they must also contend with the gendered expectations of partners or potential partners in accordance with sexual and romantic scripts (Platt & Bolland, 2017). TGD people may feel compelled to adhere to binary gender and heterosexual norms as a way of affirming their gender to themselves and in the eyes of others. However, Iantaffi and Bockting (2011) found that greater endorsement of normative gender ideology correlated with greater internalized transphobia, which in turn correlated with lower self-esteem, suggesting that adherence to gender and heterosexual norms may ultimately be detrimental to trans people's well-being. TGD individuals may instead benefit from embracing fluidity in their roles and focusing on personal authenticity, rather than assuming roles out of obligation or gendered assignment. Some may explore and participate in Bondage/Discipline, Dominance/Submission, Sadism/Masochism (BDSM) to express themselves and to experience pleasure that is not solely focused on "penis-in-vagina" sex (Jacobs, 2019).

2.3   BDSM

TGD people often have complex relationships with their bodies and may find it difficult to feel desirable or sexual in their own bodies. Engaging in BDSM (which includes sexual and non-sexual practices) is often seen as resistance against society pressures to conform, marginalize, and stigmatize. As described by Laura Jacobs (2019),

> Within [BDSM and consensual non-monogamous] subcultures we can find safety, trust happiness, empowerment, and shared joyful experiences otherwise absent. Our unconventional bodies, which may limit us in mainstream settings, are often accepted and constructively fetishized in BDSM and non-monogamy communities. Further, while transness is often understood in part as an issue of the body, we rarely discuss *becoming embodied;* yet through non-judgmental exploration we can more fully inhabit the entirety of our physical selves. Also these subcultures offer pleasure outside "penis-in-vagina" sex. Seeking other ways to eroticize the body, genitals may no longer be the primary locus of sex or sexuality; we might … instead concentrate on almost any other area as a source of arousal … for many trans identity, BDSM, and consensual non-monogamy all incorporate politicization of the body and desire as well as an intentional disruption of heteronormativity. (94–95)

Jozifkova (2013) described that the process of ongoing communication and consent throughout BDSM activities is important for demonstrating a commitment to respect and consensual practices as well as for negotiating power dynamics being played out. People engaged in these subcultures may find healing and pleasure in that fact that they are able to assert boundaries (e.g., saying no; stopping the activity) and assume control in various consensual scenarios. The disempowerment that TGD individuals often experience as a result of societal oppression can be made visible, disrupted, and confronted while engaging in BDSM (Jacobs, 2019; Weiss, 2006). TGD individuals are also able to resist sociocultural expectations prescribed to them based on sex assigned at birth or their body parts (Stryker, 2008) and are able to renegotiate and explore identities, roles, and learn/relearn their bodies (Jacobs, 2019). In doing so, some TGD individuals may also gain a sense of choice and agency (Stryker, 2008). Some TGD individuals may also find community or feel a sense of belonging in these subcultures' structured environments and secure spaces, particularly for those who feel isolated in other areas of their lives (Jacobs, 2019).

2.4 Gender Dysphoria, Sex, and Sexual Relationships

Several studies have investigated how gender dysphoria affects TGD individuals' experience of sex and sexual relationships. Some (not all) TGD people experience discomfort with their genitalia or other body parts that they perceive as incongruent with their gender identity. These feelings may be exacerbated during sex and negatively affect sexual pleasure and arousal (Doorduin & van Berlo, 2014; Platt & Bolland, 2017). Other challenges center around how TGD people's bodies are perceived by their sexual partners and how their sexual partners react to their bodies. TGD people have a variety of strategies for coping with this incongruence, including avoiding sex altogether, avoiding certain sexual behaviors or not touching certain areas, or imagining themselves with a different body (which has historically been pathologized as "autogynephilia"). Other strategies involve a "reinterpreting" or "remapping" of the body, meaning a trans person may change their gendered conceptualization of and the language they use for their anatomy (Doorduin & van Berlo, 2014; Lev, 2014), e.g. clitoris = dick or rectum = pussy. In resisting social norms and moving towards "queering the phallus", some may interpret a dildo as "a queer cock, dick, or piece of hardwood, pink, purple, or polka-dotted, and possibly even mechanically enhanced … an object deserving of veneration, not for its conformity but specifically for its otherness" (Jacobs, 2019, p. 102).

As a trans person medically transitions, they must also navigate physiological changes related to their sexuality, such as changes in sex drive, hormonal or surgical changes in genitalia and other body parts, and the experience of having sex in a changing body (Doorduin & van Berlo, 2014; Schilt & Windsor, 2014). Despite prevalent assumptions that all trans people must feel disgust with their genitalia and want genital surgery, TGD people have a wide array of relationships with their bodies, including their genitalia. Many TGD people do not feel that genital surgery is necessary for them. For some trans men and transmasculine people in particular, the cost and complications following phalloplasty either make surgery an unrealistic goal or an intervention they decide to forgo. Of note, many trans men are comfortable with their existing genitalia and reject notions that "the penis makes the man," and/or feel satisfied with the use of prosthetic penises and sex toys instead (Schilt & Windsor, 2014). Additionally, for many TGD people, the experience of navigating all these changes provides an opportunity to be more in touch with their own sexual wants and needs, to communicate about those wants and needs more openly, and to feel more freedom from conventional sexual restrictions (Jourian, 2018; Lev, 2014).

2.5   Other Challenges in Dating

2.5.1   Trans Exclusion in Dating

Given the dominance of binary and essentialist notions of gender, it comes as no surprise that TGD people face a variety of barriers in dating and seeking romantic partners. These challenges start with TGD people often not even being considered viable dating partners. Blair and Hoskin (2019) found that in a sample of 958 straight and LGBTQ people, 87.5% reported that they would not consider dating a trans person. Results indicated that heterosexual cisgender men and women were the most likely to exclude trans people, but over three-quarters of gay and lesbian participants also indicated they would not consider dating a trans person. Participants who identified as bisexual, queer, or two-spirit were most likely to consider dating a trans person (55.2%). Furthermore, participants' indications of willingness to date trans people reflected a preference for trans men over trans women, and participants often indicated willingness to date trans people of genders incongruent to their stated sexual orientation (e.g. a lesbian woman indicating willingness to date trans men but not trans women). These results demonstrate not only widespread exclusion of trans people from dating pools, but also that cissexism and transmisogyny are prevalent even in LGBQ people's dating preferences. The findings also reflect the difficulties trans people face in trying to fit themselves into the gendered and binarist scripts that dictate sexual and romantic interaction (Duran & Nicolazzo, 2017; Jourian, 2018; Platt & Bolland, 2017).

2.5.2   Disclosure of Trans Identity

A significant question TGD people face in any relationship is if, when, and how to disclose their gender identity. As transphobic violence is an ever-present threat, safety is a primary concern for TGD people in their decisions around disclosure. With widespread exclusion of TGD people from dating, TGD people must also navigate fears of rejection on the basis of their gender identities. They may therefore wish to wait before disclosing their TGD identity to avoid immediate dismissal as a potential romantic partner; however, if they wait, they risk being accused of "deceiving" the other person. In Platt and Bolland's (2017) study about relationship experiences of trans individuals, almost all participants recounted negative experiences and rejection resulting from disclosure of their gender identities. Participants described the constant rejection and fears of rejection as being very discouraging in dating.

Given the prevalence of transmisogynistic stigma, fears of rejection or violence may disproportionately affect trans women. In Iantaffi and Bockting's (2011) study, the vast majority of participants reported that their partners knew that they were trans. However, transfeminine participants were three times more likely to have not disclosed their trans identity to their partners and reported more fear of rejection resulting from disclosure than transmasculine participants. Many TGD people have turned to online dating as a way to work around some of these concerns, as dating profiles often offer the opportunity to indicate gender identity. This, however, also increases the possibility of TGD people being fetishized or objectified by potential partners (Platt & Bolland, 2017).

2.6 Gaps in Research/Future Directions

These recent studies have provided new insight into the sexual and romantic experiences of TGD people, moving away from the pathologizing perspective that has historically dominated psychology research on TGD people. However, the current research is thus far limited. Research on TGD people's relationships is lacking in racial and socioeconomic diversity (Lev, 2014); most of the studies reviewed above are based in the US and have samples that are over three-quarters white. Research is also complicated by the frequent conflation of sexual orientation and gender identity, as well as binary or otherwise limited categorization of gender, which often excludes non-binary and other gender diverse people (Galupo et al., 2016; Iantaffi & Bockting, 2011; Pulice-Farrow et al., 2019b). Future research should address these gaps while moving forward in its focus on TGD people's experiences from TGD people's perspectives. More strengths-based research, rather than pathologizing or deficit-focused research, as has been the norm in the study of TGD people, would help build deeper, more complex knowledge of TGD people's experiences (Moradi et al., 2016; Platt & Bolland, 2017, 2019a).

3 Case Study

The following case is a composite of many clients and individuals with whom we are honored to have worked with and known. Viviana is a 39-year-old Guatemalan trans woman who uses she/her pronouns and has been living in the United States for two decades with her maternal aunt in government subsidized housing. She is currently a resident of the US, not a citizen.

Viviana was born in Ciudad de Guatemala (Guatemala City). She was the middle child born into a Catholic, lower middle class family made up of her father, mother and two sisters. By early adolescence, Viviana had become aware that she was "different" and had received several messages from her uncles that she needed to be like the other cisgender boys and men in her family. For example, as a younger child, one of her uncles aggressively pulled her to the side by her arm while playing with her sisters, saying, "Ya es hora de que pares de jugar así con las nenas. Los hombres no corren así ni hacen esos sonidos mientras juegan!" ("It is about time you stopped playing with girls like that. Men do not run that way nor do they make those noises when they play!"). Viviana became increasingly hyperfocused on her behaviors and put forth much effort to conform to social and cultural norms.

She was well-liked in school and had many friends, albeit mostly girls. She would often proclaim some of these girls to be her "novia", especially to her mother and father, as a means of showing her masculinity. As she entered adolescence, she also found herself attracted to cisgender boys and having fantasies about having dates and relationships with them. She did not tell anyone about her attractions and fantasies at this age.

Titi Isa, her maternal aunt, was a special person in Viviana's life, given that she was the only one who would show comfort and kindness to Viviana and would provide respite from the disapproving faces of her father and uncles at times when she behaved or did something seen as feminine. She would also make statements about the treatment of gay and lesbian people that would make Viviana feel like she was accepting or at least tolerant of people who were different.

Viviana had started dressing in her mother's and sisters' clothing when she was home alone. One day, her sister caught her and told her parents. Viviana ran to Titi Isa and explained what happened. Her aunt took a deep breath, hugged her and assured her that she was safe for the time being. Soon after, Viviana's father, two uncles and mother appeared at the home. When her father and uncles found her, they began hitting her, saying "No hay maricones en esta familia! Te voy a hacer un macho aunque sea la última cosa que haga en mi vida!" ("There are no faggots in this family! I will make you a man if it is the last thing I do in my life!") Her mother asked "Por qué harías algo tan horrible? Sabes que esas son cosas del diablo!"(Why would you do something so horrible? You know those things are the devils work!").

Over time, Viviana started to experience traumatic stressor reactions, and she started to isolate herself from others. Although she did not have many friends, she was able to make friends with a boy named David. Viviana and David had shared their mutual liking of each other and began sexually exploring for about a year. As Viviana's relationship with her immediate family became increasingly distant over the years, her mother's need to know what Viviana was up to also increased. Viviana's mother began following Viviana once she left school. One day, while Viviana and David were seated talking in a secluded part of a park holding hands and kissing, Viviana's mother saw them and told her father and priest. After being forced to divulge her actions to the priest, Viviana's father told her that she was disowned from the family.

Due to the nature of what happened, both Viviana and her Titi Isa did not initially seek professional medical help. They feared being in further danger from medical institutions due to ongoing discrimination within Guatemala. In supporting Viviana, Titi Isa had also been ostracized from the family. Viviana and Titi Isa had talked about going to the US. Between Guatemala's increasing socio-political problems and both Viviana and Isa not being welcomed by their family, this was seen as their best option. Viviana quit high school and began the process of crossing the Mexican Border and eventually the US border. It took Viviana approximately 24 months to reach Texas. In that time, she had survived by engaging in sex work to pay for lodging along the way. Through her sex work, Viviana began re-exploring her gender (which she hadn't done since she was an adolescent). She found the attention she would get from clients as a woman very positive. She would later in life better understand that this was due to the gender-affirming nature of these interactions.

Viviana crossed the Texas border at the age of 17, which made her eligible for an immigrant youth program for minors who had crossed the border without parents. She had been placed back in school and graduated high school a few years later. Her focus turned to finding a consistent paying job in order to save money to get Titi Isa to come live with her in the US.

As a young adult, while in general Viviana lived a very private and simple life with access to the internet and social media through her smartphone that she could now afford, she began talking to men online. With the little money she would keep for herself, she began getting clothing coded as feminine, wigs, and makeup. This was followed by her creating accounts on social media platforms where she would present herself as a woman. Through these means, she would talk to men who were interested in her. These encounters sometimes led to meeting up in person. While she was never sexually assaulted, she quickly learned that most of the men she would interact with were seeking only sexual encounters with her and nothing more. While this was disheartening to her and left her feeling more alone, she had internalized messages resulting in her feeling objectified, unworthy of love, and as if she deserves to be treated in this manner due to being "different."

In her need to expedite getting her aunt to the US, Viviana began doing sex work again. This increase in income allowed her to begin bringing her aunt from Guatemala for 3–4 weeks at a time and get support and services from a lawyer who helped with legalities around immigration and bringing family. Soon after, her aunt was able to move to the US and she felt proud to help her aunt.

4   Clinical Considerations from Case Study

While at first glance Viviana's story may appear to be an extraordinary one, many aspects of her life are all too common for Latinx gender diverse individuals. Mental health providers should incorporate intersectionality as a framework in their considerations for case conceptualization, treatment planning, and therapeutic services with TGD individuals. For example, Viviana's background as Guatemalan, lower middle class, and Christian, and her assigned sex at birth and associated gender roles in her family, have an important and unmistakable impact on the messages she received regarding gender and sexuality as well as how her identity development processes unfolded. As Viviana is a client who may be interested in gender services and/or relationship and sex therapy, providers should receive specializing training and be aware of available resources that would be helpful to clients like her.

Language is an important consideration in Viviana's case. Helping clients find the words to describe their experiences can be healing in and of itself. Viviana's first language is Spanish, a language that is highly gendered. Language shapes and forms how people understand and navigate gender and sexuality. From a clinical perspective, providers may want to explore Viviana's understanding of her gender, through an intersectional lens which includes the impact of language. Some clinical questions might include: How does Viviana understand masculinity and femininity? Do words like "maricon" have a gender implication that is unique to Spanish speaking people? What did it mean for her to hear her father state that he would make her a "macho"? As Viviana explores her gender, questions about how to label her own gender and sexual orientation will likely become salient and may change her understanding of herself.

Viviana's experience is also characterized by individual- and systemic-level oppression. Providers should have transparent conversations about oppression and discrimination, both historical and contemporary, that continue to impact the lives of TGD people, particularly transgender women of color. The process of naming, analyzing, and taking blame off of the individual can be transformative. Clinicians should work with clients to understand what messages clients have received about what romantic and sexual relationships should look like, what bodies should look like, what types of sex people should have, and the meanings that people should apply to sexual encounters. Clients may have internalized some of these messages, which then influence their understanding, decisions, and experiences regarding sex and relationships.

Normalizing experiences of gender affirmation during sex work can be empowering for some people. For TGD individuals, sex work can provide an opportunity to explore and express their gender expression in ways that feel more congruent to their identities and engage in behaviors (sexual and not) that help with being more embodied. However, individuals who engage in sex work are often stigmatized and marginalized in society, including in healthcare settings. A transgender woman of color who is also a sex worker may have concerns based on the intersections of her race, gender, sexuality, and engagement in sex work when trying to access therapeutic services, which can contribute to hesitancy or avoidance of accessing services. As such, it is critical that providers practice cultural humility (Tervalon & Murray-Garcia, 1998) in order to engage in an ongoing learning process, examine their own biases, assumptions, experiences, and values that impact therapeutic encounters, and challenge power imbalances by collaborating and approaching care as a reciprocal knowledge-sharing interaction. Cultural humility extends beyond the self to partnering with other people and groups in order to advocate for system-level change (Greene-Moton & Minkler, 2020; Tervalon & Murray-Garcia, 1998).

Lastly, Palazzolo et al. (2016) noted that documentation or asylum status can have a significant impact on the sexual and romantic relationships of transgender Latina women (i.e. by providing a sense of power and control in their relationships as well as access to social services). Precarity in immigration status can leave trans women of color without access to basic necessities and social services, which then may compel them to stay in violent or unhealthy relationships and places them at higher risk for HIV. For clients like Viviana who do present for services, providers are given the opportunity to emphasize the client's strengths such as agency, self-determination, resourcefulness, challenging the status quo (if seen as a strength), and maintaining a sense of connectedness (such as between Viviana and her Titi

Fig. 3 Two men of color demonstrate the beauty of intimacy among same-sex couples. Photo Courtesy of Marcelo Chagas

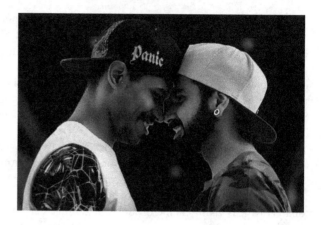

Isa). In providing care and support for people experiencing similar and parallel experiences to someone like Viviana, it is important to be considerate of not only overt intersecting factors, but also to be curious about how subtle and nuanced factors may impact a person's life. In Viviana's case, navigating sex and relationships is most certainly compounded by where she came from as well as her aspirations (Fig. 3).

References

Barnett, A. P., del Río-González, A. M., Parchem, B., Pinho, V., Aguayo-Romero, R., Nakamura, N., Calabrese, S. K., Poppen, P. J., & Zea, M. C. (2019). Content analysis of psychological research with lesbian, gay, bisexual, and transgender people of color in the United States: 1969-2018. *American Psychologist, 74*(8), 898–911. https://doi.org/10.1037/amp0000562.

Bhambhani, Y., Flynn, M. K., Kellum, K. K., & Wilson, K. G. (2019). Examining sexual racism and body dissatisfaction among men of color who have sex with men: The moderating role of body image inflexibility. *Body Image, 28*, 142–148. https://doi.org/10.1016/j.bodyim.2019.01.007.

Bhambhani, Y., Flynn, M. K., Kellum, K. K., & Wilson, K. G. (2020). The role of psychological flexibility as a mediator between experienced sexual racism and psychological distress among men of color who have sex with men. *Archives of Sexual Behavior, 49*, 711–720. https://doi.org/10.1007/s10508-018-1269-5.

Blair, K. L., & Hoskin, R. A. (2019). Transgender exclusion from the world of dating: Patterns of acceptance and rejection of hypothetical trans dating partners as a function of sexual and gender identity. *Journal of Social and Personal Relationships, 36*(7), 2074–2095. https://doi.org/10.1177/0265407518779139.

Constantinides, D. M., Sennott, S. L., & Chandler, D. (2019). *Sex therapy with erotically marginalized clients: Nine principles of clinical support.* New York: Routledge.

Doorduin, T., & van Berlo, W. (2014). Trans people's experience of sexuality in the Netherlands: A pilot study. *Journal of Homosexuality, 61*(5), 654–672. https://doi.org/10.1080/00918369.2014.865482.

Duran, A., & Nicolazzo, Z. (2017). Exploring the ways trans* collegians navigate academic, romantic, and social relationships. *Journal of College Student Development, 58*(4), 526–544. https://doi.org/10.1353/csd.2017.0041.

Fassinger, R. E., & Israel, T. (2010). Sanctioning sexuality within cultural contexts: Same-sex relationships for women of color. In H. Landrine & N. F. Russo (Eds.), *Handbook of diversity in feminist psychology* (pp. 211–231). New York: Springer Publishing Company.

Galupo, M. P., Henise, S. B., & Mercer, N. L. (2016). "The labels don't work very well": Transgender individuals' conceptualizations of sexual orientation and sexual identity. *International Journal of Transgenderism, 17*(2), 93–104. https://doi.org/10.1080/15532739.2016.1189373.

Gamarel, K. E., Reisner, S. L., Laurenceau, J. P., Nemoto, T., & Operario, D. (2014). Gender minority stress, mental health, and relationship quality: A dyadic investigation of transgender women and their cisgender male partners. *Journal of Family Psychology, 28*(4), 437–447. https://doi.org/10.1037/a0037171.

Greene, B. (1996). Lesbian women of color: Triple jeopardy. *Journal of Lesbian Studies, 1*(1), 109–147. https://doi.org/10.1300/J155v01n01_09.

Greene, B., & Boyd-Franklin, N. (1996). African American lesbian couples: Ethnocultural considerations in psychotherapy. *Women & Therapy, 19*, 49–60. https://doi.org/10.1300/J015v19n03_06.

Greene, B., Boyd-Franklin, N., & Spivey, P. B. (2013). African American lesbians and gay men in couples' relationships: Threats to intimacy and considerations in couples' psychotherapy. In K. M. Helm & J. Carlson (Eds.), *Love, intimacy, and the African American couple* (pp. 560–569). New York: Routledge.

Greene-Moton, E., & Minkler, M. (2020). Cultural competence or cultural humility? Moving beyond the debate. *Health Promotion Practice, 21*, 142–145. https://doi.org/10.1177/1524839919884912.

Han, C., & Choi, K. H. (2018). Very few people say "no whites": Gay men of color and the racial politics of desire. *Sociological Spectrum, 38*(3), 145–161. https://doi.org/10.1080/02732173.2018.1469444.

Han, C. S. (2007). They don't want to cruise your type: Gay men of color and the racial politics of exclusion. *Social Identities, 13*(1), 51–67. https://doi.org/10.1080/13504630601163379.

Hidalgo, M. A., Cotten, C., Johnson, A., Kuhns, L. M., & Garofalo, R. (2013). "Yes, I am more than just that": Gay/bisexual young men residing in the United States discuss the influence of minority stress on their sexual risk behavior prior to HIV infection. *International Journal of Sexual Health, 25*(4), 291–304. https://doi.org/10.1080/19317611.2013.818086.

Hidalgo, M. A., Layland, E., Kubicek, K., & Kipke, M. (2020). Sexual racism, psychological symptoms, and mindfulness among ethnically/racially diverse young men who have sex with men: A moderation analysis. *Mindfulness, 11*, 452–461. https://doi.org/10.1007/s12671-019-01278-5.

Iantaffi, A., & Bockting, W. O. (2011). Views from both sides of the bridge? Gender, sexual legitimacy and transgender people's experiences of relationships. *Culture, Health & Sexuality, 13*(3), 355–370. https://doi.org/10.1080/13691058.2010.537770.

Jacobs, L. A. (2019). Hormones and handcuffs: The intersection of transgender identities, BDSM, and polyamory. In G. J. Jacobson, J. C. Niemira, & K. J. Violeta (Eds.), *Sex, sexuality, and trans identities: clinical guidance for psychotherapists and counselors* (pp. 91–108). Philadelphia, PA: Jessica Kingsley Publishers.

Jourian, T. J. (2018). Sexua-romanticised pathways of transmasculine college students in the USA. *Sex Education, 18*(4), 360–375. https://doi.org/10.1080/14681811.2017.1407305.

Jozifkova, E. (2013). Consensual sadomasochistic sex (BDSM): The roots, the risks, and the distinctions between BDSM and violence. *Current Psychiatry Reports, 15*, 8. https://doi.org/10.1007/s11920-013-0392-1.

Lev, A. I. (2014). Understanding transgender identities and exploring sexuality and desire. In G. H. Allez (Ed.), *Sexual diversity and sexual offending: Research, assessment, and clinical treatment in psychosexual therapy* (pp. 45–64). New York: Karnac Books.

Meier, S. C., Sharp, C., Michonski, J., Babcock, J. C., & Fitzgerald, K. (2013). Romantic relationships of female-to-male trans men: A descriptive study. *International Journal of Transgenderism, 14*(2), 75–85. https://doi.org/10.1080/15532739.2013.791651.

Moradi, B., Tebbe, E. A., Brewster, M. E., Budge, S. L., Lenzen, A., Ege, E., Schuch, E., Arango, S., Angelone, N., Mender, E., Hiner, D. L., Huscher, K., Painter, J., & Flores, M. J. (2016).

A content analysis of literature on trans people and issues: 2002-2012. *The Counseling Psychologist, 44*, 960–995. https://doi.org/10.1177/0011000015609044.

Nadal, K. L. (2013). *That's so gay!: Microaggressions and the lesbian, gay, bisexual, and transgender community.* Washington, DC: American Psychological Association.

Nadal, K. L., Escobar, K. M., Prado, G., David, E. J. R., & Haynes, K. (2012). Racial microaggressions and the Filipino American experience: Recommendations for counseling and development. *Journal of Multicultural Counseling and Development, 40*(3), 156–173. https://doi.org/10.1002/j.2161-1912.2012.00015.x.

Newcomb, M. E., Ryan, D. T., Garofalo, R., & Mustanski, B. (2015). Race-based sexual stereotypes and their effects on sexual risk behavior in racially-diverse young men who have sex with men. *Archives of Sexual Behavior, 44*(7), 1959–1968. https://doi.org/10.1007/s10508-015-0495-3.

Palazzolo, S. L., Yamanis, T. J., De Jesus, M., Maguire-Marshall, M., & Barker, S. (2016). Documentation status as a contextual determinant of HIV risk among young transgender Latinas. *LGBT Health, 3*, 132–138. https://doi.org/10.1089/lgbt.2015.0133.

Paul, J. P., Ayala, G., & Choi, K. H. (2010). Internet sex ads for MSM and partner selection criteria: The potency of race/ethnicity online. *Journal of Sex Research, 47*(6), 528–538. https://doi.org/10.1080/00224490903244575.

Platt, L. F., & Bolland, K. S. (2017). Trans* partner relationships: A qualitative exploration. *Journal of GLBT Family Studies, 13*(2), 163–185. https://doi.org/10.1080/1550428X.2016.1195713.

Platt, L. F., & Bolland, K. S. (2018). Relationship partners of transgender individuals: A qualitative exploration. *Journal of Social and Personal Relationships, 35*(9), 1251–1272. https://doi.org/10.1177/0265407517709360.

Pulice-Farrow, L., Bravo, A., & Galupo, M. P. (2019a). "Your gender is valid": Microaffirmations in the romantic relationships of transgender individuals. *Journal of LGBT Issues in Counseling, 13*(1), 45–66. https://doi.org/10.1080/15538605.2019.1565799.

Pulice-Farrow, L., Brown, T. D., & Galupo, M. P. (2017). Transgender microaggressions in the context of romantic relationships. *Psychology of Sexual Orientation and Gender Diversity, 4*(3), 362–373. https://doi.org/10.1037/sgd0000238.

Pulice-Farrow, L., McNary, S. B., & Galupo, M. P. (2019b). "Bigender is just a Tumblr thing": Microaggressions in the romantic relationships of gender non-conforming and agender transgender individuals. *Sexual and Relationship Therapy*, 1–20. https://doi.org/10.1080/1468199 4.2018.1533245.

Rivera, D. P., Forquer, E. E., & Rangel, R. (2010). Microaggressions and the life experience of Latina/o Americans. In D. W. Sue (Ed.), *Microaggressions and marginality: Manifestation, dynamics, and impact* (pp. 59–84). Hoboken, NJ: John Wiley & Sons.

Schilt, K., & Windsor, E. (2014). The sexual habitus of transgender men: Negotiating sexuality through gender. *Journal of Homosexuality, 61*, 732–748. https://doi.org/10.1080/0091836 9.2014.870444.

Stryker, S. (2008). Dungeon intimacies: The poetics of transsexual sadomasochism. *Parallax, 14*, 36–47. https://doi.org/10.1080/13534640701781362.

Sue, D. W., Bucceri, J., Lin, A. I., Nadal, K. L., & Torino, G. C. (2009). Racial microaggressions and the Asian American experience. *Asian American Journal of Psychology, 13*(1), 88–101. https://doi.org/10.1037/1948-1985.S.1.88.

Sue, D. W., Nadal, K. L., Capodilupo, C. M., Lin, A. I., Torino, G. C., & Rivera, D. P. (2008). Racial microaggressions against black Americans: Implications for counseling. *Journal of Counseling and Development, 86*(3), 330–338. https://doi.org/10.1002/j.1556-6678.2008.tb00517.x.

Tervalon, M., & Murray-Garcia, J. (1998). Cultural humility versus cultural competence: A critical distinction in defining physician training outcomes in multicultural education. *Journal of Health Care for the Poor and Underserved, 9*, 117–125. https://doi.org/10.1353/hpu.2010.0233.

Thai, M. (2020). Sexual racism is associated with lower self-esteem and life satisfaction in men who have sex with men. *Archives of Sexual Behavior, 49*, 347–353. https://doi.org/10.1007/s10508-019-1456-z.

Wade, R. M., & Harper, G. W. (2019). Racialized sexual discrimination (RSD) in the age of online sexual networking: Are young black gay/bisexual men (YBGBM) at elevated risk for adverse psychological health? *American Journal of Community Psychology, 65*, 1–20. https://doi.org/10.1002/ajcp.12401.

Weiss, M. D. (2006). Working at play: BDSM sexuality in the San Francisco Bay Area. *Anthropologica, 48*(2), 229–245.

LGBTQ Parenting: Building Families on the Margins

Jan E. Estrellado, Lou Collette S. Felipe, Nadine Nakamura, and Amanda B. Breen

Approximately 37% of LGBTQ adults, across the lifespan, are parents (Gates, 2013). There are between 2 and 3.7 million LGBTQ individuals raising children under the age of 18, and approximately six million individuals have LGBTQ parents in the United States (Gates, 2015). LGBTQ people form families in a variety of ways, including previous relationships, fostering, adoption, and assisted reproduction. Much of the research on LGBTQ families compares same-sex couples to different-sex couples, which ignores the experiences of parents who are not in couple relationships. In addition, this focus on same versus different-sex couples leads to erasure of bi+ persons who actually represent the largest segment of the LGBTQ population of parents (Bartlet et al., 2017). Another shortcoming of the literature on LGBTQ parents is that samples tend to be overrepresented by white participants whereas parenting is more common among LGBTQ people of color. While 17% of white same-sex couples were raising children, these numbers were higher for racial and ethnic minorities with 33% of Latinx, 33% of Native Hawaiian/Pacific Islander, 29% of Native American, 25% of African American, and 25% of Asian American same-sex relationships raising children (Gates, 2012). LGBTQ individuals raising children are three times more likely to be living in poverty

J. E. Estrellado (✉)
Alliant University, California School of Professional Psychology, San Diego, CA, USA
e-mail: jestrellado@alliant.edu

L. C. S. Felipe
University of Colorado, Anschutz Medical Campus, Aurora, CO, USA

N. Nakamura
Alliant University, California School of Professional Psychology, San Diego, CA, USA
e-mail: nadine.nakamura@alliant.edu

A. B. Breen
Neumann University, Aston, PA, USA
e-mail: breena@neumann.edu

199

compared with their heterosexual counterparts and same-sex couples raising children are twice as likely to be living in poverty compared to their different-sex counterparts (Gates, 2013).

Decades of research have examined outcomes on children raised by LGBTQ parents. Sexual minority parents have not been found to differ in their parenting approaches or efficacy as compared with heterosexual parents (Fedewa et al., 2015; Goldberg & Sweeney, 2019; Patterson, 2017). Research indicates that children of sexual minority parents develop in healthy and typical ways in terms of academic achievement, peer relationships, behavioral adjustment, and emotional well-being when compared to children raised by heterosexual parents (Patterson, 2017).

Families with LGBTQ parents face discrimination, and this is further compounded for families of color who also experience racism (American Psychological Association, 2021). In addition, LGBTQ parents may not have support from their families of origin in the same way that their heterosexual and cisgender counterparts do. Despite these challenges, children with LGBTQ parents report feeling positively about their families and demonstrate resilience (Farr et al., 2017; van Gelderen et al., 2012). In addition, same-sex couples tend to be more egalitarian than different-sex couples in terms of childcare, housework, and employment as compared to different-sex couples (Goldberg et al., 2014). While developmental outcomes for children raised by sexual minority parents tend to be positive, LGBTQ parents often face interpersonal and systemic discrimination. LGBTQ parents experience lower well-being when they have less support from their families of origin and work supervisors, live in states that do not offer legal protections, and when they have more internalized homonegativity (Goldberg et al., 2014).

When examining the experiences of parents and families, it is necessary to not only consider the contexts of sexual orientation and gender identity, but how these

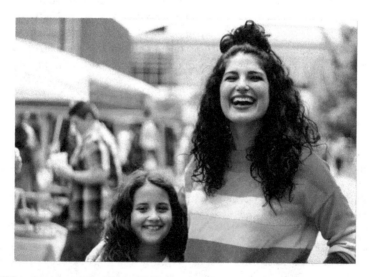

A LGBTQ parent takes their child to a Pride Parade. Photo by Rosemary Ketchum

intersect with race and ethnicity, socio-economic status, disability, immigration status, and spirituality and religion, among others (American Psychological Association, 2021). These identities not only complicate LGBTQ families' daily lived experiences (Fattoracci et al., 2020), but can adversely affect their access to resources (Jeong et al., 2016; Paceley et al., 2019), risk for negative health outcomes (Mays et al., 2018), and even life chances (Clark et al., 2017). Building on the research of Black feminist scholars (see Collins, 1990; Crenshaw, 1991; Lorde, 1984), this chapter utilizes an intersectional framework to identify the disproportionate impact of systemic oppression on marginalized communities within broader LGBTQ communities.

1   Parenting and Diverse Identities

1.1   Gender Identity

There are approximately 1.4 million adults who identify as transgender in the United States (Flores et al., 2016). In a review of 51 studies on transgender parents, Stotzer et al. (2014) found that beween one-quarter and one-half of transgender and non-binary people in the U.S. identify as parents. Trans and non-binary parents face a number of issues particular to gender identity, including transitioning while parenting, having limited access to services, developing new models for parental gender socialization, and experiencing gender identity-based discrimination (Pfeffer & Jones, 2020). A systematic review of the literature suggests that trans and non-binary parents are often left out of the traditional LGB parenting discourse and that their needs are often overlooked (Hafford-Letchfield et al., 2019).

Trans and non-binary parents may have realized their gender identity prior to parenthood, during child-rearing, or after their children were adults. Parents who transition during child-rearing years may consider various factors that may affect the transition process, such as the age of the children and the acceptance or rejection of the partner or spouse (Dierckx et al., 2017). In a study of 50 trans parents and their partners, Haines et al. (2014) found that trans parents often balance their transitions with parenting responsibilities, their children's well-being, and the maintenance of positive relationships with their children and families. Trans parents also reported a lack of institutional support for their families from the legal system, mental health professionals and education systems (Haines et al., 2014).

The internalization of gender expectations can be complex for trans and non-binary parents, and thus, they must often create their own models around gender and parenting (Estrellado & Moore, in press). In a study of 163 predominantly white (88%) trans and non-binary parents, Tornello (2020) found that unpaid household and childcare labor was divided in an egalitarian manner, irrespective of gender expression or identity. Despite the challenges that trans and non-binary parents face, they may also demonstrate strengths related to flexibility and fluidity about gender,

gender role expectations and sexual identity in their families and child-rearing practices relative to their cisgender peers.

Children of trans and non-binary parents have varying and complex feelings connected to their parents' gender identities and expression. For instance, trans and non-binary parents must often carefully navigate conversations with their children during transition, as they may challenge their children's gender role beliefs along with the role their parent's identity plays in their own lives (Haines et al., 2014). School-age children may also experience bullying by classmates and even teachers or choose not to disclose their parent's gender identity to avoid bullying and harassment.

Little research specific to trans- and non-binary-headed families has been conducted, as they are often grouped with other LGBQ-headed families. The paucity of investigation allows for the perpetuation of negative stereotypes of trans and non-binary individuals and contributes to their erasure and marginalization (Pfeffer & Jones, 2020). In addition, there appears to be little research on different types of families headed by trans parents, including trans parents of color, as well as non-binary parents specifically.

1.2   Trans-Racial and Multi-Racial Families

By some estimates, nearly seven percent of the US population identifies as multi-racial, a segment of the population that is growing rapidly (Parker et al., 2015). Past research has demonstrated that multiracial individuals are less likely than single-race individuals to have a partner who identifies with just one race, and the number of multi-racial babies born since 1970 has increased tenfold (Parker et al., 2015).

Approximately 20 percent of LGBTQ couples reported being in an inter-racial or inter-ethnic relationship, compared to roughly 18 percent of married straight couples (Brainer et al., 2020; Gates, 2012; Kastanis & Wilson, 2014). Additionally, LGBTQ couples are more likely to create families in which the parents and children are of different races or ethnicities. For instance, LGBTQ couples adopt children trans-racially at higher rates relative to straight couples (Farr & Patterson, 2009). LGBTQ couples may be more likely to use child-centered approaches to adoption (where connections to previous caregivers/guardians may be part of post-adoption family life; Appell, 2010) than are non-LGBTQ couples, who are more likely to use a parent-centered approach (where adoptive parents may be considered "the only" parents in the familial picture; Appell, 2010). The likelihood of using child-centered approaches is supported by the data that on average, same-sex couples are more likely to adopt and foster children compared to their heterosexual counterparts (Bewkes et al., 2018).

Despite the disproportionate rates of multi-racial LGBTQ families with children, they are often not represented in studies of multi-racial families or of LGBTQ families (Brainer et al., 2020). As with multi-racial families headed by heterosexual and cisgender parents, a primary concern for white LGBTQ parents of children of color is to support their children in their racial identity development by acknowledging and confronting racism, power and white privilege, living and building relationships in a multiracial community, and helping their children to develop the skills necessary to navigate the institutional racism they will encounter throughout their lives (Ausbrooks & Russell, 2011). Given the discrimination they already face (Bewkes et al., 2018; Brodzinsky & Donaldson, 2011) LGBTQ may be uniquely well-equipped for trans-racial parenting practices that specifically that address oppression and discrimination.

2 Family Formation

2.1 Family Structure

Traditional notions of family are organized around a gender-based power structure, which do not necessarily apply to LGBTQ households (Warner, 1993). Common conceptualizations of "family" position heterosexuality as "normal," "natural," and "seeing itself as society," (Warner, 1993, xxii). There are several heteronormative assumptions of families, such as having a binary structure (i.e. mother and father), being cisgender, having cohabitating members, being heterosexual in orientation, and having some degree of heredity or relatedness (Allen & Demo, 1995). Yet, the strategies for building LGBTQ families are diverse and can include fostering, adopting, pregnancy with known or anonymous donors, surrogacy, or co-parenting with partners from previous relationships (Allen & Demo, 1995). Given the unique, diverse, and often complex ways in which LGBTQ people in relationships bring children into their lives (Gates, 2015), parenthood is not always an assumed life-choice for many LGBTQ individuals.

Heteronormative perspectives of family structure have historically centered the experiences of cisgender men and women, heterosexuality, as well as nuclear families (e.g. Ingraham, 2005; Jagose, 1996). Yet over the last two decades, there has been a national trend in the United States of increased social acceptance and support of LGBTQ people (Flores, 2014). With certain legislative changes in marriage equality (National Conference of State Legislatures, NCSL, 2015), military nondiscrimination practices (U.S. Department of Defense, 2016), and trans-inclusive health care options (e.g. Free State Legal, 2014), select dimensions of queerness are encompassed in heteronormative hegemony (Allen & Mendez, 2018). Heteronormativity now encapsulates binary transgender individuals who are socially recognized as their gender, gays and lesbians, as well as married gays and lesbians and their children (Allen & Mendez, 2018). As such, heteronormativity can not only uphold the familial structures of cisgender, married men and women, and their children, but also some queer people whose gender presentation, sexuality, and/or family constellations reinforce cis- and hetero-sexist family experiences (Allen & Mendez, 2018). This expansion of heteronormative values has created a *homonormativity* of LGBTQ individuals whose experiences follow the norms set by cis-/hetero-communities (Fish & Russell, 2018).

To better understand the uniqueness of queer family structures outside a heteronormative lens, it has been suggested that the study of families should recognize and honor the role of intersectional complexity along a variety of social dimensions (e.g. McGuire et al., 2016; Berkowitz, 2009). A number of factors are implicated in understanding the formation and concept of families. Race, class, ability, ethnicity, religion, geographical location and other dimensions of social location play a role in understanding family structures (Allen & Mendez, 2018; Fish & Russell, 2018). Often, the definition and concept of the LGBTQ family has been based on the inclusion of an LGBTQ-identified parent or child, an inherently heteronormative focus (Fish & Russell, 2018). However, honoring the complexities of intersectionality would pull us to recognize the exponential multiplicity of identities within a family, how individuals and relationships navigate such identities, and the fluidity of these constructs over the course of a lifetime (Ruppel et al., 2018).

Parenting constellations within queer families can be complex and involve more than two partners or parents (Tasker & Lavender-Stott, 2020; Pallotta-Chiarolli et al., 2020). *Polyparenting* situations in queer families can include biological parents, legally recognized parents, stepparents, or social parents (Park, 2013; Sheff, 2014; Tasker & Lavender-Stott, 2020). *Polyfamilies*, in which partners are in a polyamorous situation, include partners of any sexual orientation and gender, who are in exclusive intimate sexual relationships with more than one partner, and who may choose to reside together or otherwise combine or share their resources (Pallotta-Chiarolli, 2010; Pallotta-Chiarolli et al., 2013; Sheff, 2013; Sheff, 2016). They can be in *polyfidelitous* families, where their sexual relationships are confined to the partnership and closed to outsiders, or involve *polycules* of chosen family members involved in polyamorous relationships (Creation, 2019) or *polyaffective* relationships marked by nonsexual, emotional intimacy.

The concepts of "family of choice" or "chosen family" are often associated with the community or network LGBTQ people build in response to rejection from their families of origin (Etengoff & Daiute, 2015; Mitchell, 2008). Given the wide spectrum of family formation options among LGBTQ parents, families of choice often include former and current romantic partners, co-parents from blended families, and poly families. However, chosen family can also include close friends and family members outside the nuclear family structure. Given the importance that family of choice often holds for LGBTQ people (Blair & Pukall, 2015), it is often necessary to understand how LGBTQ parents and children define and make meaning of family.

Conceptualizing queer families, and decentering the cisgender, heterosexual narrative means examining the complex intersections of identity among family members and moving away from traditional, rigid, and narrow parameters and boundaries. The fluidity of social constructs such as gender and sexuality reinforce the idea that queer families that cannot be singularly defined, as the attempt to define limits the concept of queerness itself. Changes in the social-political landscape, individual development over the lifespan, and the ever-changing expansiveness of cultural norms further underscore the need for nuance and flexibility when interacting with queer family structures and the relational dynamics within them.

2.2 Foster Parenting and Adoption

Many LGBTQ parents are open to foster parenting and adoption, despite the social and legal challenges they may face. Same-sex couples are seven times more likely to be raising foster or adopted children and are more likely to engage in a lengthy decision-making process before fostering or adopting, compared to their different-sex counterparts (Boyer, 2007; Goldberg & Conron, 2018). Riggs, (2020) identified several themes from the research on LGBTQ foster parents. These include silencing of foster parents' sexuality, pathologization of sexuality, the expectation to demonstrate "appropriate" gender role models, resistance to placement matching for LGBTQ children in care, and the expectation for LGBTQ foster parents to educate child protection staff. However, there is a dearth of research on bisexual and transgender foster parents, and on white gay and lesbian parents raising foster children of color (Riggs, 2020).

LGBTQ adoptive parents are more likely to have chosen adoption as their "first choice" compared to non-LGBTQ parents (Mallon, 2011). LGBTQ adoptive parents also differ from non-LGBTQ adoptive parents in their willingness to adopt children who have a different ethnic/racial background (Farr et al., 2020). Similar to the research on LGBTQ foster parents, the research on LGBTQ adoptive parents relies on predominantly white lesbian and gay participants (Farr et al. 2020).

Laws about adoption by LGBTQ people vary by state and nation (Farr et al., 2020). The 2015 Supreme Court ruling on the national recognition of marriage equality made it possible for all married couples to petition for joint adoption. However, many states have passed laws allowing child welfare agencies to exclude LGBTQ foster and adoptive parents based on the agencies' religious beliefs. The legal inconsistencies regarding adoption laws in various states and countries can cause great stress and uncertainty among LGBTQ families.

2.3 Assisted Reproductive Technology

Some LGBTQ persons pursue parenthood through a variety of medical interventions including insemination and surrogacy, which are examples of assisted reproduction technology (ART). While ART has been available to the public since the 1980s, many years LGBTQ persons have experienced discrimination trying to access sperm banks to insurance providers (Bos & Gartrell, 2020; Karpman et al., 2018). Scientific advancement has provided more options for ART, including implantation of one person's egg into another person's womb so both parents can

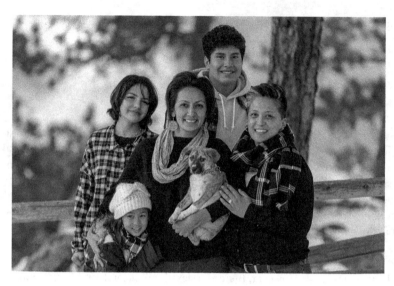

A caring and supportive family of LGBTQ parents, their children, and dog. Photo by Lou Felipe

contribute to reproduction (Bos & Gartrell, 2020). Thus, there are many options for people assigned female at birth to consider during family planning, including access to sperm donation (e.g. sperm bank, known donor), biological relationship to the child, and selection of person to carry the pregnancy to term. Access to these options often hinges on economic/class privilege: medical interventions are costly and not always covered by insurance. Another issue is that sperm banks do not often have donations from sperm donors of color, and when they do, these options are limited options compared to the availability and range of white donors. For example, with many more white donor options, it is easier for those seeking sperm from white donors to have the choice between anonymous donors and donors who are willing to be known by their offspring when the children conceived by the sperm reach adulthood. Karpman et al. (2018) conducted a qualitative study with 13 LBQ parents of color to examine how they arrived at the selection of a known donor, the characteristics that they prioritized in donor selection, and how their interactions with external institutions and histories of oppressive racialized family formation practices influenced their decision-making. Several participants shared that they utilized a known donor because sperm banks did not meet their needs politically or financially, and they often lacked adequate donor selection. There has been a move to encourage parents to choose willing-to-be-known donors for the sake of their children's right to know about their genetic history (Bos & Gartrell, 2020). However, many donors of color may opt to donate sperm anonymously, possibly as a reflection of cultural values. Of course, with the rise of genetic testing through services like 23&Me, donors who donated sperm anonymously may no longer be anonymous, which raises additional ethical issues.

Some men in same-sex relationships who wish to have children opt for surrogacy. This option requires a person with a uterus to carry the fetus to term. The most common type of surrogacy involves in-vitro fertilization of a donor-egg with sperm and then the implantation of the fertilized egg into the womb of the surrogate. Surrogacy can be done domestically, which is typically quite expensive. Domestic commercial surrogacy can, with an agency, cost around $150,000, making this option out of reach for many (Berkowitz, 2020). Research on men in same-sex relationships who create their offspring via surrogacy tend to utilize small convenience samples of white, wealthy cisgender men (Berkowitz, 2020). Some parents utilize transnational commercial surrogacy which employs women in the Global South to serve as surrogates for much less money (Nebeling Petersen, 2018). However, these arrangements can be exploitative and ethically problematic in a number of ways and many countries have outlawed commercial surrogacy entirely or limited it to married couples in different-sex marriages (Berkowitz, 2020).

While not all transgender parents seek assistive reproductive technology, they may face particular challenges when they do, particularly regarding discrimination and bias from service providers. Some transgender patients reported that their providers did not give them access to fertility information while they were discussing medical interventions such as hormone therapy (Hafford-Letchfield et al., 2019). Trans-masculine parents assigned female at birth may experience bias from providers if they choose to be gestational parents (Murphy, 2010). In addition, transgender parents may be misgendered on their children's birth certificates.

Non-gestational parents often experience invisibility and lack of recognition by people who do not view them as "real" parents. For example, Alexandre Costa et al. (2020) conducted a study with five Portuguese lesbian-identified families who conceived via donor insemination. They found that non-biological mothers had different experiences with their families of origin than did biological mothers. Biological mothers were questioned about why they wanted to have children, while non-biological mothers were questioned on how they could be a parent to a child to whom they were not related.

2.4   Children from Previous Relationships

Most frequently, LGBTQ parents have children in the context of previous different-sex romantic relationships (Goldberg et al., 2014). For some, the relationship and the family that form within the context of the relationship occurred before coming out. A sexual encounter with someone of a different sex may occur for the specific purpose of conception. For bi+ persons, the experience of being in a different-sex relationship can contribute to feelings of erasure and invisibility and this is can be compounded as a parent.

There are additional issues facing LGBTQ families with children from previous relationships. Some parents may realize a non-heterosexual sexual orientation and/ or a non-cisgender gender identity and come out to their partners and children. LGBTQ parents who enter into new relationships may experience rejection from their stepchildren rooted in discrimination. In a study of mostly white gay fathers and gay step-fathers, heterosexism both at the institutional level (e.g. religion, courts) and personal level were identified and put a strain on gay step-families (Jenkins, 2013).

3 Clinical Vignettes

3.1 Kanoa

Kanoa is a 32-year-old, queer, trans-masculine person (he/him pronouns) of Native Hawaiian descent. Kanoa and his partner Mona (who identifies as a bi-racial, Filipina and white, femme, pansexual, cisgender woman) are parents to two-year-old Jessie, the first grandchild on both sides of the family. Kanoa was the gestational parent and identifies as a "seahorse parent," a term used to describe trans men and/ or masculine-identifying gestational parents. Kanoa and Mona have been in a relationship for 10 years. They have been experiencing more conflict with each other since Jessie's birth. Mona worries about Kanoa's "moodiness" and impatience while parenting, and Kanoa feels that Mona does not often understand how much he is struggling emotionally.

A loving family embraces in a group hug. Photo Courtesy of August de Richelieu

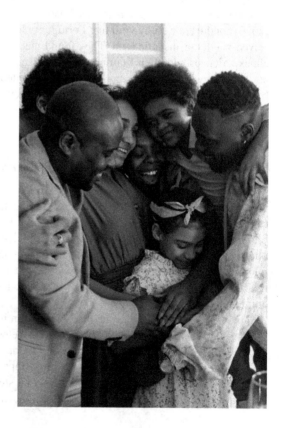

Kanoa has recently sought therapy to manage depressive symptoms and problems in his relationship with Mona. He reports feeling fatigued, lethargic, and irritable. He acknowledges he gets impatient with both Jessie and Mona and often feels ashamed about his inability to be present and calm with his family. Kanoa has thoughts that he is not a good father due to his impatience with Jessie. Kanoa, a high school teacher, feels generally supported in his work environment, although he does not currently find his work fulfilling. While his family of origin is not geographically close, Kanoa feels very emotionally connected to them. Mona's family is marginally supportive, although they display some discomfort and bias regarding Kanoa's status as Jessie's gestational parent. Kanoa, Mona, and Jessie live in a large urban area in the Pacific Northwest, and they have access to both a visible LGBTQ community and to communities of color.

3.1.1 Clinical Considerations

There are a number of important assessment areas to consider for Kanoa's case. A primary clinical consideration is to understand what names and pronouns queer, trans, and non-binary people use, but also the words they use to describe their bodies, parenting titles, and in this case, their gestational experience.

How does Kanoa think about his role as a parent, and particularly as a transmasculine, sea-horse father? How was he treated by service providers during the gestational period, and how do others treat him now? A contextual evaluation of his relationship to societal stressors, discrimination, and bias, not just to his family system, would be important areas to assess. In addition, it is likely that Kanoa may not have access to others with parenting paths similar to his, and he may experience feelings of isolation or disconnection as a result.

Given Jessie's age, it would be helpful to understand more about Kanoa's experience with the post-partum period. Could his depressive symptoms have started after Jessie's birth? A consultation with a trans-affirming gynecologist, and possibly psychiatrist, could help provide Kanoa with important information about how his body responded to the birthing experience. In addition, clinicians should consider whether Kanoa has had medical interventions, such as hormone replacement therapy, before and/or after having Jessie.

3.2 Aparna

Aparna (she/her/hers) is a 48-year-old cisgender, bisexual woman of Indian and Pakistani descent. As a child, Aparna's parents divorced, and she and her younger siblings lived full time with their mother. Moving from a two-parent household to a single-parent household was financially difficult for Aparna's mother. Consequently, Aparna was expected to take on a great deal of caretaking for her younger brothers, and she typically was unable to attend many social events at school or join many after school activities. She did have a serious boyfriend throughout high school, Marcus, a warm and thoughtful young man, for whom Aparna felt a great deal of affection. Aparna's relationship with Marcus ended once they graduated high school.

In college, Aparna, again, did not have a lot of involvement in school activities because she lived at home with her mother and brothers and chose to focus on supporting her family and studies, rather than getting too heavily involved with extracurricular activities. However, as an ethnic studies major, Aparna invested herself deeply into her schoolwork and was inspired by learning about diversity, equity, and systems of power, privilege and oppression. While volunteering to register young voters, she met Ray, a multiracial (Black and Pacific Islander) law student aspiring to become a civil rights attorney. Passionate about politics and human rights, the two had an immediate spark. They dated for several years and married shortly after graduating college.

Aparna has been married to her husband, Ray, for 15 years. Five years into their marriage, the couple separated for 6 months. To strengthen their marriage, the couple agreed to enter therapy together. While Aparna deeply and genuinely loves Ray, she disclosed that she has felt unresolved around her attraction to women, which was manifesting in the irritability she had toward her husband. In addition, the two had wanted to have children, but the couple experienced three pregnancy losses, which was deeply painful to the two of them. Aparna asserted her desire to more fully recognize her bisexuality, and the couple together realized the emotional toll that the pregnancy losses had on them both. Ray expressed his support of Aparna's sexuality and was committed to exploring avenues for Aparna to feel more recognized in her queer identity. The two also decided that they both wanted to pursue bringing children into their lives.

After years of navigating challenges with infertility, Aparna and Ray decided to become foster parents. Eventually, Aparna and Ray brought two children into their home: Jonathan and Brenda, who were 4 and 2, respectively, when they entered foster care. Jonathan and Brenda were siblings who witnessed a great deal of violence and experienced profound neglect with their biological parents. They were eventually removed from their home of origin and place into foster care. Aparna and Ray took them into their home, which was both challenging, yet fulfilling, for the couple. Eventually, Jonathan's and Brenda's birth parents lost their parental rights after 2 years of opportunity to engage and comply with court mandates to remain in their children's lives. However, they were inconsistent in their involvement with their children and eventually lost their legal rights as parents. Aparna and Ray, having been consistent and involved foster parents to the two children, then adopted Jonathan and Brenda.

3.2.1 Clinical Considerations

As a bisexual cisgender woman married to a heterosexual cisgender man, Aparna may not be fully seen or affirmed in her bisexual identity. She has clearly stated to her husband a need to assert and embrace her sexual orientation—a process that can be strengthened through thoughtful negotiations with her husband. There are added stressors in that the couple experienced infertility for a number of years, which is fraught with loss and grief for them both but has pronounced and unique psychological impacts for a cisgender woman desiring pregnancy. Consequently, Aparna is confronted not only with the feelings of invisibility as a bisexual person, but the invisibility of the emotional pain connected with infertility and stigma associated with pregnancy loss. Additionally, one of the "benefits" of being in a relationship with a cisgender man—the ability to biologically have children without outside assistance—was not actualized. This can deepen and complicate the level of loss and pain that Aparna experiences, who may feel inadequate or unfulfilled as both a bisexual person and as a woman. Further, issues of sexuality and procreation may have deep cultural implications as a woman of Indian and Pakistani heritage.

Upon fostering, then adopting, their children, Aparna and her partner will need to navigate a number of complicated relationships. For one, like many foster-to-adopt parents, there may be a great deal of contact with the children's family of origin. Such contact can have complicated and conflicting emotions about wanting to respect the biological family, as well as feelings of anger or contempt for the family members who maltreated the children. Further, Jonathan and Brenda will have intensive, complicated, and chronic needs that Aparna and Ray will need to support. The complexities of their children's trauma histories and emotional/behavioral needs may further tax the family.

A therapist working with Aparna will be faced with issues of sexuality, gender, partnership, parenthood, and adoption. Aparna's experiences as an individual and within a family system should be appreciated and assessed intersectionally, as none of these experiences occur in isolated contexts. Therapists are uniquely positioned to prompt reflections on intersectionality to better recognize the layers of stressors that one may experience, and to support improved relationship dynamics between and among different members of a family.

4 Conclusion

LGBTQ parenting communities are formed and maintained in a range of ways. While LGBTQ families display many forms of resilience, their experiences may vary based on encounters with various forms of interpersonal and systemic oppression. The intersectional experiences of LGBTQ families may greatly impact not only their daily lived experiences and stressors, but their values and coping strategies as well. Clinicians working with LGBTQ families will want to acknowledge and address their strengths, each unique family's needs, and the different forms of bias and discrimination LGBTQ parents may encounter.

References

Alexandre Costa, P., Tasker, F., Anne Carneiro, F., Pereira, H., & Leal, I. (2020). Reactions from family of origin to the disclosure of lesbian motherhood via donor insemination. *Journal of Lesbian Studies, 24*(1), 1–11.

Allen, K. R., & Demo, D. H. (1995). The families of lesbians and gay men: A new frontier in family research. *Journal of Marriage and Family, 57*(1), 111–127.

Allen, S. H., & Mendez, S. N. (2018). Hegemonic heternormativity: Toward a new era of queer family theory. *Journal of Family Theory & Review, 10*(1), 70–86. https://doi.org/10.1111/jftr.12241.

American Psychological Association (2021). APA Task Force on Psychological Practice with Sexual Minority Persons. *Guidelines for Psychological Practice with Sexual Minority Persons.* Retrieved from https://www.apa.org/about/policy/psychological-practice-sexual-minority-persons.pdf.

Appell, A. (2010). Reflections on the movement toward a more child-centered adoption. *Western New England Law Review, 32*(1), 1–32.

Ausbrooks, A. R., & Russell, A. (2011). Gay and lesbian family building: A strengths perspective of transracial adoption. *Journal of GLBT Family Studies, 7*(3), 201–216. https://doi-org.neumann.idm.oclc.org/10.1080/1550428X.2011.564936.

Bartlet, E., Bowling, J., Dodge, B., & Bostwick, W. (2017). Bisexual identity in the context of parenthood: An exploratory qualitative study of self-identified bisexual parents in the United States. *Journal of Bisexuality, 17*(4), 378–399.

Berkowitz, D. (2009). Theorizing lesbian and gay parenting: Past, present, and future scholarship. *Journal of Family Theory & Review, 1*(3), 117–132. https://doi.org/10.1111/j.1756-2589.2009.00017.x.

Berkowitz, D. (2020). Gay men and surrogacy. In A. E. Goldberg & K. R. Allen (Eds.), *LGBTQ-parent families.* New York: Springer. https://doi.org/10.1007/978-3-030-35610-1_8.

Bewkes, F.J. Mirza, S.A., Rooney, C., Durso, L.E., Kroll, J., & Wong, E. (2018). *Welcoming all families: Discrimination against LGBTQ foster and adoptive parents hurts children.* https://www.americanprogress.org/issues/lgbtq-rights/reports/2018/11/20/461199/welcoming-all-families/

Blair, K. L., & Pukall, C. F. (2015). Family matters, but sometimes chosen family matters more: Perceived social network influence in the dating decisions of same- and mixed-sex couples. *Canadian Journal of Human Sexuality, 24*(3), 257–270. https://doi.org/10.3138/cjhs.243-A3.

Bos, H., & Gartrell, N. (2020). Lesbian-mother families formed through donor insemination. In A. E. Goldberg & K. R. Allen (Eds.), *LGBTQ-parent families.* New York: Springer.

Boyer, C. A. (2007). The impact of adoption issues on gay and lesbian adoptive parents. In R. A. Javier, A. I. Baden, F. A. Biafora, & A. Camacho-Gingerich (Eds.), *The handbook of adoption* (pp. 228–241). Thousand Oaks, CA: Sage.

Brainer, A., Moore, M. R., & Banerjee, P. (2020). Race and ethnicity in the lives of LGBTQ parents and their children: Perspectives from and beyond North America. In A. Goldberg & K. Allen (Eds.), *LGBTQ-parent families.* New York: Springer.

Brodzinsky, D.M., & Donaldson, E.B., (2011). *Expanding resources for children III: Research-based best practice in adoption by gays and lesbians.* https://www.adoptioninstitute.org/wp-content/uploads/2013/12/2011_10_Expanding_Resources_BestPractices.pdf

Clark, K. A., Mays, V. M., & Cochran, S. D. (2017). Extreme violence and the invisibility of women who murder: The intersectionality of gender, race, ethnicity, sexual orientation, and gender identity equals silence. *Violence and Gender, 4*(4), 117–120. https://doi.org/10.1089/vio.2017.0036.

Collins, P. H. (1990). *Black feminist thought: Knowledge, consciousness, and the politics of empowerment.* Boston: Hyman.

Creation, K. (2019). *This heart holds many: My life as the nonbinary millennial child of a polyamorous family.* Portland, OR: Thorntree Press.

Crenshaw, K. (1991). Mapping the margins: Intersectionality, identity politics, and violence against women of color. *Stanford Law Review, 43*(6), 1241–1299. https://doi.org/10.2307/1229039.

Dierckx, M., Mortelmans, D., Motmans, J., & T'Sjoen, G. (2017). Resilience in families in transition: What happens when a parent is transgender? *Family Relations: An Interdisciplinary Journal of Applied Family Studies, 66*(3), 399–411. https://doi-org.neumann.idm.oclc.org/10.1111/fare.12282.

Estrellado, J. E. & Moore, A. A. (in press). Creating a queer feminist family model: Intersections of race and gender identity. In Doty, K. & Lowik, A.J. (Eds). The liminal chrysalis: Imagining reproductive and parenting futures beyond the binary. Demeter Press.

Etengoff, C., & Daiute, C. (2015). Online coming-out communications between gay men and their religious family allies: A family of choice and origin perspective. *Journal of GLBT Family Studies, 11*(3), 278–304. https://doi.org/10.1080/1550428X.2014.964442.

Farr, R. H., & Patterson, C. J. (2009). Transracial adoption by lesbian, gay, and heterosexual couples: Who completes transracial adoptions and with what results? *Adoption Quarterly, 12*(3–4), 187–204. https://doi.org/10.1080/10926750903313328.

Farr, R. H., Simon, K. A., & Bruun, S. T. (2017). LGBTQ relationships: Families of origin, same-sex couples, and parenting. In *Family dynamics and romantic relationships in a changing society* (pp. 110–136). Hershey: IGI Global.

Farr, R. H., Vázquez, C. P., & Patterson, C. J. (2020). LGBTQ adoptive parents and their children. In A. Goldberg & K. Allen (Eds.), *LGBTQ-parent families.* New York: Springer.

Fattoracci, E. S. M., Revels-Macalinao, M., & Huynh, Q.-L. (2020). Greater than the sum of racism and heterosexism: Intersectional microaggressions toward racial/ethnic and sexual minority group members. *Cultural Diversity and Ethnic Minority Psychology.* https://doi.org/10.1037/cdp0000329.

Fedewa, A. L., Black, W. W., & Ahn, S. (2015). Children and adolescents with same-gender parents: A meta-analytic approach in assessing outcomes. *Journal of GLBT Family Studies, 11*(1), 1–34. https://doi.org/10.1080/1550428X.2013.869486.

Fish, J. N., & Russell, S. T. (2018). Queering methodologies to understand queer families. *Family Relations, 67*(1), 12–25. https://doi.org/10.1111/fare.12297.

Flores, A. R. (2014). *National trends in public opinion on LGBT rights in the United States.* Los Angeles, CA: Williams Institute, UCLA School of Law.

Flores, A. R., Herman, J. L., Gates, G. J., & Brown, T. N. T. (2016). *How many adults identify as transgender in the United States?* Los Angeles, CA: The Williams Institute.

Free State Legal. (2014). *Maryland to provide nondiscriminatory health coverage to transgender state employees.* Retrieved from http://freestatelegal.org/victory-maryland-toprovide-nondiscriminatory-health-coverage-fortransgender-employees/US.

Gates, G. J. (2012). *Same-sex couples in census 2010: Race and ethnicity.* The Williams Institute. Retrieved from https://escholarship.org/uc/item/66521994

Gates, G. J. (2013). *LGBT parenting in the United States.* The Williams Institute. Retrieved from https://escholarship.org/uc/item/9xs6g8xx

Gates, G. J. (2015). Marriage and family: LGBT individuals and same-sex couples. *The Future of Children, 25*(2), 67–87. https://doi.org/10.1353/foc.2015.0013.

Goldberg, A. E., Gartrell, N. K., & Gates, G. (2014). *Research report on LGB-parent families.* Retrieved from https://williamsinstitute.law.ucla.edu/publications/report-lgb-parent-families/

Goldberg, A. E., & Sweeney, K. K. (2019). LGBTQ parent families. In B. H. Fiese, M. Celano, K. Deater-Deckard, E. N. Jouriles, & M. A. Whisman (Eds.), *APA handbook of contemporary family psychology: Foundations, methods, and contemporary issues across the lifespan* (Vol. 1, pp. 743–760). Washington, DC: American Psychological Association.

Goldberg, S. K., & Conron, K. J. (2018). *How many same-sex couples in the U.S. are raising children?* The Williams Institute. Retrieved from https://williamsinstitute.law.ucla.edu/research/parenting/how-many-same-sex-parents-in-us/

Hafford-Letchfield, T., Cocker, C., Rutter, D., Tinarwo, M., McCormack, K., & Manning, R. (2019). What do we know about transgender parenting?: Findings from a systematic review. *Health & Social Care in the Community.* https://doi.org/10.1111/hsc.12759.

Haines, B. A., Ajayi, A. A., & Boyd, H. (2014). Making trans parents visible: Intersectionality of trans and parenting identities. *Feminism & Psychology, 24*(2), 238–247. https://doi-org.neumann.idm.oclc.org/10.1177/0959353514526219.

Ingraham, C. (2005). *Thinking straight: The power, the promise, and the paradox of heterosexuality.* New York, NY: Routledge.

Jagose, A. (1996). *Queer theory: An introduction.* New York, NY: New York University Press.

Jenkins, D. A. (2013). Boundary ambiguity in gay stepfamilies: Perspectives of gay biological fathers and their same-sex partners. *Journal of Divorce & Remarriage, 54*(4), 329–348. https://doi.org/10.1080/10502556.2013.780501.

Jeong, Y. M., Veldhuis, C. B., Aranda, F., & Hughes, T. L. (2016). Racial/ethnic differences in unmet needs for mental health and substance use treatment in a community-based sample of sexual minority women. *Journal of Clinical Nursing, 25*(23–24), 3557–3569. https://doi.org/10.1111/jocn.13477.

Karpman, H. E., Ruppel, E. H., & Torres, M. (2018). "It wasn't feasible for us": Queer women of color navigating family formation. *Family Relations, 67*(1), 118–131. https://doi.org/10.1111/fare.12303.

Kastanis, A., & Wilson, B. (2014). *Race/ethnicity, gender, and socioeconomic wellbeing of individuals in same- sex couples.* Los Angeles, CA: The Williams Institute, UCLA School of Law.

Lorde, A. (1984). *Sister outsider.* Trumansburg, NY: Crossing Press.

Mallon, G. P. (2011). The home study assessment process for gay, lesbian, bisexual, and transgender prospective foster and adoptive families. *Journal of GLBT Family Studies, 7,* 9–29. https://doi.org/10.1080/1550428X.2011.537229.

Mays, V. M., Juster, R. P., Williamson, T. J., Seeman, T. E., & Cochran, S. D. (2018). Chronic physiologic effects of stress among lesbian, gay, and bisexual adults: results from the national health and nutrition examination survey. *Psychosomatic Medicine, 80*(6), 551–563.

McGuire, J. K., Kuvalanka, K. A., Catalpa, J. M., & Toomey, R. B. (2016). Transfamily theory: How the presence of trans* family members informs gender development in families. *Journal of Family Theory & Review, 8*(1), 60–73.

Mitchell, V. (2008). Choosing family: Meaning and membership in the lesbian family of choice. *Journal of Lesbian Studies, 12*(2–3), 301–313. https://doi.org/10.1080/10894160802161497.

Murphy, T. F. (2010). The ethics of helping transgender men and women have children. *Perspectives in Biology and Medicine, 53*(1), 46–60. https://doi.org/10.1353/pbm.0.0138.

National Conference of State Legislatures. (2015). *Same-sex marriage laws.* Retrieved from https://www.ncsl.org/research/human-services/same-sex-marriage-laws.aspx

Nebeling Petersen, M. (2018). Becoming gay fathers through transnational commercial surrogacy. *Journal of Family Issues, 39*(3), 693–719. https://doi.org/10.1177/0192513X16676859.

Paceley, M. S., Fish, J. N., Conrad, A., & Schuetz, N. (2019). Diverse community contexts and community resources for sexual and gender minority youth: A mixed-methods study. *Journal of Community & Applied Social Psychology.* https://doi.org/10.1002/casp.2417.

Pallotta-Chiarolli, M. (2010). *Border sexualities, border families in schools.* Lanham, MD: Rowman & Littlefield Publishers.

Pallotta-Chiarolli, M., Haydon, P., & Hunter, A. (2013). "These are our children": Polyamorous parenting. In A. Goldberg & K. Allen (Eds.), *LGBT-parent families.* New York, NY: Springer.

Pallotta-Chiarolli, M., Sheff, E., & Mountford, R. (2020). Polyamorous parenting in contemporary research: Developments and future directions. In A. Goldberg & K. Allen (Eds.), *LGBTQ-parent families*. New York: Springer.

Park, S. M. (2013). *Mothering queerly, queering motherhood: Resistingmonomaternalism in adoptive, lesbian, blended, and polygamous families*. Albany, NY: SUNY Press.

Parker, K., Horowitz, J. M., Morin, R., & Lopez, M. H. (2015). *Multiracial in America: Proud, diverse and growing in numbers*. Retrieved from https://www.pewsocialtrends.org/2015/06/11/multiracial-in-america/#the-size-of-the-multiracial-population

Patterson, C. J. (2017). Parents' sexual orientation and children's development. *Child Development Perspectives, 11*(1), 45–49. https://doi.org/10.1111/cdep.12207.

Pfeffer, C. A., & Jones, K. B. (2020). Transgender-parent families. In A. Goldberg & K. Allen (Eds.), *LGBTQ-parent families* (pp. 199–214). Cham: Springer.

Riggs, D. W. (2020). LGBTQ foster parents. In A. Goldberg & K. Allen (Eds.), *LGBTQ-parent families*. New York: Springer.

Ruppel, E., Karpman, H., & Terres, M. (2018). "It wasn't feasible for us": Queer women of color navigating family formation. *Family Relations, 67*, 117–130.

Sheff, E. (2013). Solo polyamory, singleish, single, and poly. *Psychology Today*. Retrieved from https://www.psychologytoday.com/blog/the-polyamorists-next-door/201310/solo-polyamory-singleish-single-poly

Sheff, E. (2016). *When someone you love is polyamorous: Understanding poly people and relationships*. Portland: Thorntree Press.

Sheff, E. A. (2014). Seven forms of non-monogamy. *Psychology Today* [Online]. Retrieved from http://www.psychologytoday.com/blog/the-polyamorists-next-door/201407/seven-forms-non-monogamy

Stotzer, R.L., Herman, J.L., & Hasenbush, A. (2014). *Transgender parenting: A review of existing research*. Retrieved from https://escholarship.org/uc/item/3rp0v7qv

Tasker, F., & Lavender-Stott, E. S. (2020). LGBTQ parenting post-heterosexual relationship dissolution. In A. Goldberg & K. Allen (Eds.), *LGBTQ-parent families*. New York: Springer.

Tornello, S. L. (2020). Division of labor among transgender and gender non-binary parents: Association with individual, couple, and children's behavioral outcomes. *Frontiers in Psychology, 11*. https://doi-org.neumann.idm.oclc.org/10.3389/fpsyg.2020.00015.

U.S. Department of Defense. (2016). *Secretary of Defense Ash Carter announces policy for transgender service members* [Press release]. Retrieved from https://www.defense.gov/News/News-Releases/News-Release-View/Article/821675/secretary-of-defense-ash-carter-announces-policy-for-transgender-service-members

van Gelderen, L., Bos, H. M. W., Gartrell, N., Hermanns, J., & Perrin, E. C. (2012). Quality of life of adolescents raised from birth by lesbian mothers: The US National Longitudinal Family Study. *Journal of Developmental and Behavioral Pediatrics, 33*(1), 17–23. https://doi.org/10.1097/DBP.0b013e31823b62af.

Warner, M. (1993). *Fear of a queer planet*. Minneapolis: University of Minnesota Press.

"My Wings May Be Broken, But I'm Still Flying": Queer Youth Negotiating Expansive Identities, Structural Dispossession, and Acts of Resistance

María Elena Torre and Shéár Avory

1 "My Wings May Be Broken, But I'm Still Flying": Queer Youth Negotiating Expansive Identities, Structural Dispossession, and Acts of Resistance

Over the past few decades, there has been an increase in literature focusing on experiences of lesbian, gay, bisexual, transgender, queer, intersex, asexual, and gender expansive (LGBTQIA+ GE) youth. Since the late 1990s, GLSEN (formerly known as the Gay, Lesbian, Straight Education Network) has produced annual reports focusing on the experiences of LGBTQ+GE students in K-12 schools—highlighting experiences such as bullying, homophobic an transphobic languages by peers and teachers, and issues related to retention, absences, and dropouts (see Kosciw et al., 2020). Studies have found that LGBTQIA+GE youth are significantly more likely to have express suicidality (i.e., ideations or attempts), in comparison to their cisgender and heterosexual counterparts (Marshal et al., 2011; Perez-Brumer et al., 2017; Toomey et al., 2018). Previous studies have also reported that LGBTQIA+GE youth report significantly greater symptoms of mental health issues, such as depression, posttraumatic stress disorder (PTSD), and anxiety (Burns et al., 2015; Lucassen et al., 2017) and that LGBTQ youth were at risk for substance use and abuse, such as alcohol, tobacco, marijuana, illicit drugs, and prescription drugs (Zaza et al., 2016). Previous literature has found that LGBTQ+GE youth (especially LGBTQ+GE youth of color) are more likely than their heterosexual and cisgender counterparts to be overrepresented in both the criminal punishment system and child welfare system (Nadal, 2020) and are significantly more likely to experience homelessness (Choi et al., 2015; Waguespack & Ryan, 2019) (Fig. 1).

M. E. Torre (✉) · S. Avory
The Public Science Project, Critical Social Psychology Program, The Graduate Center of the City, University of New York, New York, NY, USA
e-mail: mtorre@gc.cuny.edu

K. L. Nadal and M. R. Scharrón-del Río (ed.), *Queer Psychology*,
https://doi.org/10.1007/978-3-030-74146-4_12

217

Fig. 1 A young person
expressing themselves
through makeup and
artistry. Photo Courtesy of
Jameson Mallari Atent

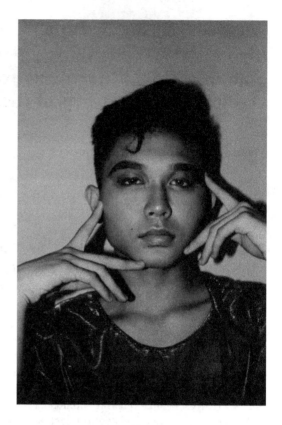

In spite of this growth in literature, there is very little scholarship on the experiences of LGBTQ+GE children under 12 years old—as majority of studies on queer and trans youth focus on LGBTQ+GE adolescents (Mackenzie & Talbott, 2018). Yet, previous scholars have described how LGBTQ+GE adults begin to recognize their gender identities and sexualities from their childhood years (Savin-Williams & Cohen, 2004; Vance et al., 2014), as well as the multiple ways that positive and negative childhood and adolescent experiences (e.g., in families, cultural groups and communities, and schools, etc.) influence sexual orientation and gender identity development (Adames & Chavez, 2022; Puzio & Forbes, 2022). Further, GLSEN and Harris Interactive (2012) found that about one-tenth of their elementary school student sample did not adhere to traditional gender role norms, which resulted in increased bullying and decreased feelings of safety at school.

Taken together, the current literature on LGBTQ +GE adolescents and children is generally helpful in identifying some of the disparities encountered by LGBTQ+GE youth; however, one major critique to this academic literature is that scholars have generally positioned LGBTQIA+ GE youth as they were merely objects of study. In fact, to date, the limited national studies of LGBTQGE experiences that exist have been produced primarily by adults, focused on experiences of health, "risk," and discrimination, and include few young people under 18. The experiences of LGBTQ+GE youth, (as individual and as collectively) have been typically described from above—from a "God's eye" perspective (Harding, 1991) of scholarly expertise, from an academic community whose history introduced and diagnosed pathology, exclusion, and soul-crushing harm in the guise of "treatment". In doing so, scholars have failed to truly understand actual youth perspectives and instead have relied on a narrative that was created for them, instead of by them.

1.1 What's Your Issue? (WYI)

In a radical departure from this convention, this chapter will offer a discussion of LGBTQIA+GE youth experiences—anchored in findings from *What's Your Issue?* (WYI)—a national participatory action research project conducted by queer and trans youth (a majority of whom were youth of color) that featured a survey taken by 6073 youth, aged 14–24, from every state in the nation, as well as Puerto Rico and Guam. The WYI research collective was brought together by the Public Science Project (PSP) at the Graduate Center of the City University of New York, that works in solidarity with communities interested in using social science to interrupt injustice and create freedom spaces. A radically diverse, intergenerational, research collective from across the U.S., we rooted ourselves in the legacies of ACTUP and indigenous and disability movements that insisted on the rights of people and communities to name the terms and conditions of research essential to their survival. As such, we were (and continue to be) committed to the principal and practice of "no research about us without us."

We share the experiences, dreams, and desires that these young people entrusted to us as a contribution to informing action, education, policy and aiming to shift and further research with the purpose of supporting gender and sexuality justice. We write as two members of the larger research collective—both whom are queer and view each other as colleagues. The second author (Shéar) is a Black Indigenous trans femme who not so long ago completed two decades, and the first author (María) is a white woman from a Spanish immigrant family who has nearly completed five. Our relationship was borne of love and solidarity, grown over 6 years, across different experiences and changing relationships to power and vulnerability, through shared commitments, and, at times, stark disagreements.

Our desire with this writing is twofold: first and foremost we wish to bring LGBTQIA+ & GE youth lives to center as narrators of their own experiences, and second we hope to demonstrate the power of critical participatory action research (CPAR) as a justice approach for research *with* communities that is committed to dignity, respect, self-determination, and solidarity (Torre et al., 2012). With *What's Your Issue?* we share possibilities for reimagining research relationships, wherein those historically "studied" become architects of the work, no longer passive and "in need," but active contributors, building the necessary knowledge, visions, and tools for more just futures (Fine et al., 2018; Torre et al., 2018). In this way, every aspect of *WYI*—from creating the survey to analyzing and interpreting the data, to deciding the important findings—was led by young people who identify as LGBTQ+GE and who have had very different experiences shaped by race, ethnicity, gender, class, dis/ability, family and community relationships, and experiences with housing, schools, police, and the medical community. We share the findings of the research as simultaneously a traditional and nontraditional way of discussing the state of queer youth in the U.S. on their own terms. This chapter shares the "issues"—ideas, experiences, and a set of priorities for us to join them in taking action.

1.2   Language and Ethical Commitments

While we understand gender and sexuality as distinct identities, we recognize that in popular usage, words to describe gender and sexuality often overlap. Indeed, as queer youth have reminded us time and time again, language at best is dynamic and shifting as individuals, communities, and movements develop and grow, and at worst limiting and insufficient, filled with binaries that betray our realities. Our intention to be inclusive as possible, so in the spirit of the WYI research collective, we use "LGBTQIA+GE" and "queer" interchangeably to represent youth who identify as lesbian, gay, bisexual, transgender, queer, intersex, asexual, and gender expansive. Honoring our commitment to self-determination, in instances where we reflect on experiences and ideas of specific

The WYI collective made two non-negotiable ethical commitments to those who took the WYI survey. The first was one of action—to share what we learned far and wide, with those who took the survey, with youth organizers, policy makers, advocates, families of LGBTQIA&GE youth, academics, and beyond, with the intent of igniting change. The second was to never engage in "damage-centered" research or representation, whose exclusive focus on individual suffering has often obscured structural causes and led to myopic portrayals of queer youth as depressed, suicidal, and "at risk." As a collective, we committed to an ongoing analysis of both oppressive systems and the experiences of individual lives, recognizing the ways structures and practices are ever-present in shaping our opportunities and daily experiences, emotions, and feelings. As you read, we ask you, in the spirit of action, to think about how to incorporate what you learn into *your work, relationships, organizing, policy-making, and educational efforts.* We also encourage you to visit www.whatsyourissue.org to learn more about our methodology and to watch videos produced by WYI youth researchers on identities, activism, housing precarity, dignity schools, all at the intersections of gender, sexual, racial, and disability justice.

1.3   Perspectives of LGBTQ+GE Youth

The data from our participants was analyzed a WYI collective—which consisted of researchers from the Public Science Project and 40 LGBTQGE young people from 10 different communities across the country (i.e., Seattle, Los Angeles, Tucson, Detroit, St. Louis, Jackson, New Orleans, Jersey City, New York, and Boston). What follows are a reflection of our analyses—a palette of the experiences, struggles, and yearnings shared with us. A national look at the lives of LGBTQIA+GE youth reveals that they are:

- blazing new pathways for expressing gender, sexuality, and race/ethnicity—insisting on recognition of their complexity, fluidity, intersectionality and multiplicity and unapologetically rejecting the binaries and categories of generations who came before,
- contending with disproportionately high rates of discrimination, harassment and moral exclusion—particularly youth of color and trans and gender expansive youth—and multiple forms of structural dispossession, including housing insecurity, aggressive policing, and alienation from/harassment in schools, and
- leading vibrant lives committed to civic engagement, activism, community organizing and solidarity even as they endure high rates of dispossession and discrimination.

Across our analysis we were committed to representing the youth in their fullness—refusing to isolate one feature of their experience from others. As you read, we encourage you to do the same, to hold both the challenges and struggles LGBTQIA+GE youth shared with us, as well as their critical ideas, creativity, joy, and humor—and to remember as one survey-taker described, "My wings may be broken, but I'm still flying #transforlife".

1.4   Blazing New Expansive Identities: Representation, Recognition and Justice

The WYI survey invited young people to express their full humanities—their dreams, desires, and struggles. Trusting us with their hopes and sense of possibility, as well as their histories of betrayal and alienation from public institutions, intimates, peers, and strangers, we begin with a montage of youth in their own words. The WYI survey opened with the question, "What 5 words or phrases would you use to describe yourself?" The responses below, with the size of the words reflecting how frequently they were used, force us to recognize the gorgeous multiplicity of queer youth lives.

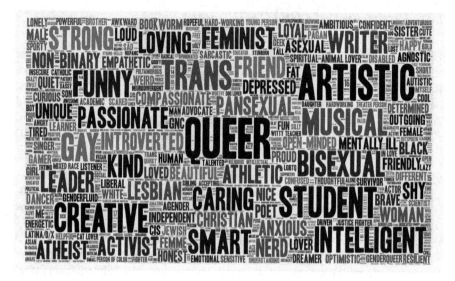

The 10 most repeated words were: queer (1028), artistic (808), student (597), trans (547), creative (526), gay (498), musical (442), funny (432), intelligent (413), bisexual (403), smart (363).

From the East Coast to the West; from urban, suburban, and rural communities; from across racial/ethnic and gender lines; large numbers of youth are rejecting binaries, and embracing complexity, critiquing hegemony, and engaging intersectional solidarities. Whether responding to seemingly "straight" forward questions about identity or sharing ideas about what banner would represent them, it is clear across our data that conventional identity labels, "boxes," and categories do not do justice to multilayered lives of contemporary LGBTQGE youth. To demonstrate this, Jai' Celestial Shavers, a youth organizer from BreakOUT! New Orleans stated: "LGBTQ young people insist on a range of identities. We don't 'fit' into boxes; we don't believe in those boxes. They don't work for us. They do not represent the range of our racial, gender or sexual lives." Further, a queer Black female participant shared "#honorthecomplexities."

The WYI collective was painfully aware of cost of denying their queer peers the ability to use their own language to describe their identities before being asked to check demographic boxes—even if survey takers were encouraged to checking off as many listed options as desired. Having felt the repeated sting of not being seen, not being recognized, we felt obligated to provide an intentional space for self-determination in each of our demographic questions. Our intention was to communicate that we valued and respected the specific ways that *participants themselves* identified. This simple move later allowed us insight into the vast and diverse ways LGBTQGE youth define themselves in relation to gender, race/ethnicity, and sexuality.

1.4.1 Gender

More than half (57%) of the youth identified as trans or gender expansive, with 42% identifying as cisgender, meaning they identify with a gender that "matches" the sex they were assigned at birth. When given the opportunity to describe their gender in their own words, dominant categories of "female" and "male" faded as exclusive categories, often replaced or joined with more specific terms. Terms like trans, non-binary, genderfluid, and agender were each used by more than 400 young people in the survey. Forty-three percent of youth used more than one term to describe their gender, writing in more than 100 different terms, 60 of which were used by at least 5 other survey takers. Examples included: Genderfluid; Genderqueer; Femme; GNC; Transmasculine; Demigirl; Androgynous/Androgyne; Gender neutral/neutrois; Bigender; Genderflux; No gender/No labels; Genderless; and Trans femme (to name a few). Regarding pronouns, one-third of the participants used "they" as one of their pronouns and others offered write-in responses like, "All of them!", "No preference", or "My name". A few participants used the open-ended pronoun question to share additional aspects fundamental to their identities, often with witty, serious, or critique-filled responses such as "he, his, clarinet" and "he, his, Palestine."

Youth noted that adults in their lives have more and less comfort with the proliferation of new words, identities, and expressions. When youth were asked to share their "proudest or happiest moment", many wrote about having pronouns and names respected, moments when they were "being seen" and recognized as who they are. Many participants specifically spoke about the joy in having their true gender recognized. For instance, a Queer, Gender Non-Binary, Latinx, Guatemalan shared: "My happiest moment was deconstructing gender with a group of middle schoolers in a program I did about a year ago. I told them how I didn't feel like a girl or a boy and a lot of them got it. I felt super hopeful about our future!" Similarly, a Pansexual, Agender, Mixed Native American and White participant disclosed: "My happiest moment was when I was 18 and discovered the 'agender' label for my identity and was accepted by my online friends." Finally, a participant who identifies as a Heteroflexible, Transgender male, Chinese American shared:

> [When] I got my name legally changed. I was 18 years old and a senior in high school. With my little sister, we went to the courthouse in the early morning. We had to wait through several other cases until mine came. Then it was my turn. The judge approved my name change and I went downstairs to get my certificate of change. I was so happy I finally would be recognized by the name I identify with.

While these examples demonstrate that recognizing youths' gender affirming pronouns and names is a matter of justice; it is crucial to note that such affirmation is also a predictive factor for positive mental health (Olson-Kennedy et al., 2018) (Fig. 2).

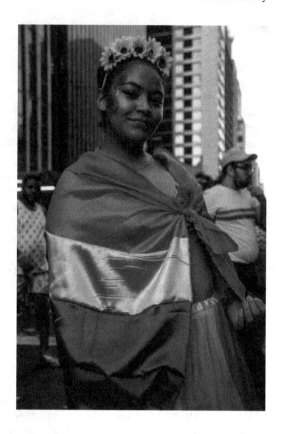

1.4.2   Race and Ethnicity

Like with the other demographic categories, the survey asked youth to identify their
own ethnicity and race before asking them to select from pre-existing options. The
127 racial and ethnic identities youth specified ranged from broader racial/ethnic
categories historically found on the US Census (such as White, Hispanic/Latino,
Black or African American, Asian or Asian American, Native Hawaiian, Pacific
Islander, Native American or Alaska Native, Arab, etc.) to identities that are often
grouped into larger categories or not present on large scale national surveys (e.g.,
Filipino, Jamaican, and Chamorro). Youth again responded at times with a sense of
humor about their own group while others offered social commentary, with many
blending the two. These commentaries offered critiques of dominant views and
marginalization of their racial/ethnic groups, of legacies of colonialism and the
trans-Atlantic slave trade, such as: "Biracial; Black American, no cultural connection to Africa (thanks, colonialism)"; "Latin@/Indigenous; Fuck borders"; "I am
South East Asian and people tend to think lowly of my people"; and "African-
American in political situations but Black when I interact with others like me". In
some cases, participants identified their privileged identities: "White privileged
with a mixed race background" and "White as marshmallow fluff". In others cases,

participants described what it means to belong to multiple racial/ethnic groups at the same time; examples include: "Black and Puerto Rican mother/fully Korean father, I was never Black enough and never Korean enough" and"Mixed Black; slavery-who knows?"

1.4.3 Sexual Orientation

Similar patterns emerged as youth described of their sexual orientation in their own words, with traditional terms failing to capture the complexity of new identities. Terms such as "gay" and "lesbian" were used by only a little more than a third (35%) of youth, with more young people using "queer" (47%) and/or multiple terms to describe their sexual orientation. Sixty percent of youth selected or wrote-in 2 or more sexual orientation terms, with the most frequent being: bisexual (used by 1062 youth), queer (1060), pansexual (904), gay (823), asexual (631), lesbian (555), and demisexual (216). Youth descriptions were serious, careful, and often very specific. At the same time, many were tender and filled with humor, such as "Any with a heart, I don't care about the parts", "¯_(ツ)_/¯", "Ladies ladies ladies" and "nebulous and changing". In addition, a survey-takers offered a corrective to our narrow construction of sexuality, with 446 youth adding something specifically about romantic attraction in their sexual orientation.

1.4.4 Naming Ourselves and Our Issues on Our Own Terms

Adding to the beautiful and complex mosaic of how queer youth name themselves, we close this section with responses to the question: "If you were designing a sign or banner about you, what would it say?" With sharp clarity, youth rejected the singularity of simple nouns and passive categories. Identity for contemporary LGBTQ+GE youth appears less about description or assimilation, and more about proclamation and recognition. Rather than squeezing into a "box," there is an active piercing of boundaries and contesting of binaries with LGBTQGE youth reimagining intersectional selves, on their own terms, and as an act of justice. Like with self-descriptions, youth banners rejected binaries, embraced complexity, and critiqued dominant perspectives, and expressed intersectional solidarities.

Marked with the wisdom of lived experience, participants' self-descriptors can be read as signposts of desire, social commitments, and resistance. For example, a Demisexual, Genderfluid, African American and Native American participant shared "Don't put people into boxes. Humans are way too complex to be judged solely based on race, gender, or sexuality." A Pansexual, Female to male transgender, Femme male, Genderfluid, South East Asian, Lao participant wrote: "Yellow pansexual trans boy magic." A Queer, Pansexual, Questioning Polyamory, Cisgendered female, White, Muslim participant shared: "This queer Shi'a Muslim woman supports demilitarization of police because #BlackLivesMatter." A participant who identified as "Dykeness, Cisgender, Mexican to the core, Maya/Aztec" described herself as "Woman, Queer, Immigrant, Mexican … how much more pow-erful can I get in this country?" The WYI banners speak to a strong, unapologetic insistence on being recognized in full vibrant complexity, even as most survey-tak-ers endured harassment, betrayal, and/or microaggressions on the streets, in school, in the media, by government, and even sometimes at home.

1.5 Contending with Discrimination, Harassment, and Structural Dispossession

While youth demand recognition on their own terms, and join others' struggles for human justice, the disproportionately high rates of structural dispossession, wit-nessed in part through persistent discrimination, harassment, and moral exclusion, particularly youth of color and trans and gender expansive youth, is staggering. Hostile treatment from public institutions in the form of aggressive and violent policing, alienation from and harassment in schools and in healthcare settings, has been consistently documented (Chmielewski et al., 2016; Cohen, 2010; Kosciw et al., 2020; Stoudt et al., 2011), as have negative experiences queer youth have faced at the hands of the families, places of worship, and neighborhood communi-ties (Nadal, 2020). These experiences too often leave LGBTQ+GE youth in a pre-carious place in terms of life's basic necessities, with high rates of housing insecurity, inconsistent schooling and health care, and negative encounters with the criminal (in)justice system (Kosciw et al., 2020; Nadal, 2020; Waguespack & Ryan, 2019). WYI issue suggests precarity experiences are exponentially higher for queer youth of color and gender expansive youth (Frost et al., 2017). Since much of the research on LGBTQIA+GE youth focuses on the consequences of the structural injustice they face, we will only briefly review the ways the WYI youth experiences mirror these deeply troubling trends, pausing only to lift the experiences of queer youth of color and gender expansive youth to highlight the dynamics of the intersecting oppressions white supremacy, gender discrimination, and heteronormativity.

1.5.1 Discriminatory and Aggressive Policing

Queer youth experiences with policing reflect the racialized experiences of youth nationally, wherein youth of color are disproportionately targeted. (Chmielewski et al., 2016; Cohen, 2010; Nadal, 2020; Stoudt et al., 2011). WYI shared similar experiences—whether they lived in cities, towns or rural areas. In fact, nearly twice as many LGBTQIA+GE youth of color (32%) reported negative contact with police (being stopped, frisked, or arrested), as compared to their white LGBTQIA+GE peers (17%). In addition to negative physical contact, WYI Youth reported high levels of feeling disrespected by the police, with trans and gender expansive youth (46%) more likely to report feeling disrespected than their cis peers (33%). Given these experiences it is perhaps not surprising that only 5% of the WYI Youth overall report that they "turn to the police for help or support" when they have a problem.

1.5.2 Unequal Schooling

Over half (58%) of all WYI youth in middle or high school reported negative experiences with schooling ('*teachers don't respect young people like me', frequently feel like dropping out, experienced being suspended from school, and/or stopped attending school*). When looked at closely, stark patterns of racial and gender disparity surface, with students of color and trans students reporting more negative experiences that white and cis students, aligning with previous literature on LGBTQ+GE students in middle school and high school (Kosciw et al., 2020). Moreover, queer youth experiences with school suspension display similar patterns of disparities produced by racial discrimination as we see in experiences with police, where regardless of gender, youth of color report more negative experiences. It is hard not to see the imprint of entrenched racism and white supremacy when public institutions such as schooling and policing, that when LGBTQGE young people are engaged by their disciplinary arms, racial disparities spike.

1.5.3 Housing Precarity

Confirming national studies that have documented the disproportionately high rates of experiences of housing insecurity and homelessness among LGBTQGE youth (Choi et al., 2015; Waguespack & Ryan, 2019), 40% of WYI youth reported experiences of homelessness. Racism and gender discrimination intensify housing precarity, with trans and gender expansive youth (46%) and youth of color (46%) reporting substantially more housing insecurity than their cis (32%) and white (36%) peers. Youth struggling with housing insecurity, relied on creativity and community, finding shelter in a variety of ways, often shuffling between multiple situations: from nights in their family home to couches and floors of friends, to extended family to foster care, group homes, shelters, and residential treatment programs. Creating resources where there are none, youth wrote about finding shelter in alternative spaces like subways and buses, abandoned buildings, military barracks, community-based organizations, and sanctuary spaces. Older youth reported more housing insecurity than their younger peers, with 45% of 18 and over reporting housing insecurity as compared to 34% of youth aged 14 to 17. This disparity underscores that for too many queer youth, particularly youth of color and trans and gender expansive youth, some things don't "get better."

 The significant rates of housing insecurity, alienation in schools, negative experiences with police, and social discrimination experienced by LGBTQGE youth is unsurprisingly associated with a wide range of negative consequences that impact well-being (physically and psychologically) as well as one's material stability. Unsurprisingly, the youth that reported experiences of destabilized housing also reported an avalanche of negative outcomes, witnessing or experiencing violence (84%); experiencing physical health issues: (82%); negative school experiences (70%); not having enough to eat (61%); being stopped, frisked, or arrested by the police (34%); and losing a job (23%).

These patterns provide an important reminder of the intersectional relationships between different forms of structural violence. LGBTQ+GE youth who shared stories of navigating these intersections, spoke not only of pain and betrayal, but also of desire and incredible, relentless commitments to lives of meaning, recognition and participation. For instance, a participant who identifies as two-spirit, same-gender loving, indigenous, and Mexican shared:

> My housing situation was not stable after being kicked out by my parents twice and constantly having to ask friends and partner at that time to let me stay at their place. I then lost my part-time job right after that. Months after that I got a full-time job and was able to save enough money to get my own apartment and not have to worry burdening people with favors or worried about where I would be staying the following night.

The stories of survivance are as much a testament to humans' capacity to grow and thrive despite remarkable obstacles, as they are a commentary on the many ways that oppressive systems harm and burden people of historically marginalized groups (Fig. 3).

1.6 Civic Engagement, Activism, Community Organizing and Solidarity

While social and psychological toll of persistent oppression, of intersecting dynamics of "cis"tematic heterosexism, transphobia, racism, capitalism, disability discrimination, undeniably and unequally shapes the lived experiences of LGBTQIA+GE youth, these experiences do not tell the totality of queer youth lives. As one WYI research collective member often reminded us: "We are more than a collection of our struggles." In fact, one of the most remarkable lessons LGBTQIA+GE taught us through their responses was that pain and struggle often lives side by side to fierce resistance all within the same body. We do not wish to brush aside the soul crushing associations between economic, housing, or food insecurities and psychological distress that was present in our data (Frost et al., 2017). However, time and time again, we witnessed the pain and consequences of these inequities not only share space with, but often fuel desire, imagination, resourcefulness, and commitments to self, each other, and a more just world.

To demonstrate this, we share the experiences of Kat, a youth organizer in Detroit who shares:

> I have been in the system since I was 13; I ran away from family violence at home, lived on the streets, in shelters, juvenile facilities, and then went back into sleeping in a vacant apartment in an abandoned building. Then I met Lance from Detroit Represent! who offered me a place to stay, and I learned the importance of activism and giving back. So now, as an activist and an organizer, I work on campaigns for housing, against domestic violence and for the human rights of young people living on the streets of Detroit.

Fig. 3 Two young people striking a pose during a Pride celebration. Photo Courtesy of Ronê Ferreria

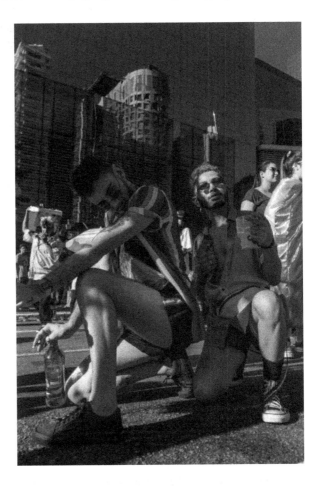

Kat's experiences illustrate that just as the tremendous discrimination and inequality hold material, social, and psychological consequences, these experiences of injustice can also inspire lives of activism and willful resistance.

Moreover, analyses of our the WYI data of youth engaged in activism demonstrated a buffering impact of activism on mental and physical health and suicidal ideation. The more discrimination youth reported, the more activism they engaged. The relationship between discrimination is stronger for trans and gender expansive youth and youth of color and relatively weaker for cis and white youth (Fine et al., 2018). For example, a Fluid, Two-Spirit, Quiche, Guatemalan stated: "I don't just carry ancestral Trauma, I carry ancestral two- spirit Knowledge. #decolonize systems from the root." Similarly, a Queer/Pansexual, Non-binary/Trans/Gender Variant, Hispanic/Latin@, Colombian participant described: "I have survived, and I can survive a lot more."

Just as LGBTQIA+GE unapologetically demand recognition they work for justice with equal passion. Youth reported high levels of activism across geographic regions, with a full half of youth engaging 5 or more forms of activism in the last 12 months. They are on the streets and online engaging in both in-person activities

(92% report talking with family and friends, 59% attended meetings or demonstrations, 49% engaged in outreach, 39% attended or facilitated a training, 24% worked with neighborhood members) and more individual activities (88% engaged activism through social media, 80% signed a petition, 28% contacted a public official). Activism is not necessarily the result of participating in organized activist settings, as interestingly only 30% of the youth reported being involved in a community based or youth leadership organizations. Areas or "issues" in which youth were most active included LGBTQ justice (61%), feminism and gender justice (51%), anti-racist organizing (35%), disability rights (18%), health and wellness (17%), environmental justice (16%), immigration justice (13%), economic justice (13%). Committed to multiple issues of justice struggles, 58% of youth reported being involved in 2 or more areas, and 20% were involved in 4 or more.

While queer youth engage deliberate and disruptive actions to demand change, many also engage in what we've come to call "intimate" activisms—the *care work of building relationships and community* (Luttrell, 2013). Even as many have been so deeply wounded by prejudice and discrimination by institutions and policies, and/or by strangers and people who love or have loved them, queer youth take up the political work of care and community, marked by a tremendous generosity, and sense of social, community, and family responsibility. Nearly a quarter of youth missed one or more days of school to "take care of family responsibilities" and 83% said they have helped a friend struggling with depression. Youth reported being as committed to "making a difference in someone else's life" (94%) as to pursuing a "personal goal" (97%). These intimate activisms, often as hidden even as they are bold, are relational everyday enactments of interruption, care and solidarity. These activisms are delicate challenges to family, friends, teachers, and strangers who vocalize discriminatory attitudes, so that they and "others" might be not only be seen but recognized with justice. For instance, a pansexual, queer, Filipino and Iranian participants asserted:

> Fighting the good fight and believing what's right. This doesn't necessarily mean being out in the streets (but good for you if you are); it could be asserting yourself and correcting others when they make offensive or problematic comments. It's about recognizing one's own microaggressions and unjust prejudices and working to correct them.

Similarly, a Queer, Fluid, Bi-racial participant advocated:

> To me there is Big Activism and little activism. Big activism is protesting in the streets, is going to rallies and creating petitions, it is driving people to polls to make sure they can vote because you know that they aren't the people that those in positions of power want voting. Big Activism is actions that you take publicly on a larger scale than yourself. Little activism is just as important and I only call it little because of the way it seems smaller in proportion, not because of its relative importance.:ittle activism is all of the things you do every day to make the lives of those discriminated against better, it could be asking for preferred pronouns, setting up a safe space in your office, it could be tweeting about #BlackLivesMatter or making sure that people #StayWoke. It is a hundred little things that begins the death of a thousand cuts for the status quo.

In these ways, it is clear that these LGBTQ+GE are committed to advocating for justice.

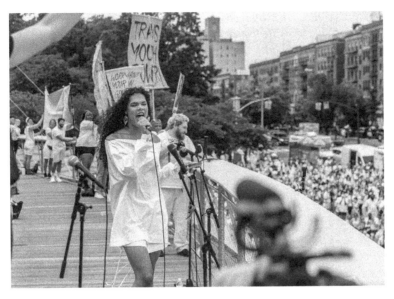

Fig. 4 Author shéár avory speaks at the second historic trans youth liberation march in New York City in June 2021. Photo by: shéár avory

1.7 Empathy, Care and Connection

Alongside, and sometimes through, youth resistance, activism, humor (e.g., "Want a tissue for that cis-sue?"), joy, and persistence, LGBTQ+GE youth also showcase enormous amounts of empathy and connection. Across open-ended sections of the survey or where youth could select what was important or concerning to them, youth expressed concern for one another. Linking their own experiences to those of others. They wanted to know how other youth were feeling, surviving, hoping, planning, organizing, and (perhaps most importantly) loving and building. The connections between justice for themselves and justice for others in the activism sections was palpable in their banners, their hopes and dreams, and the ways they cared for each other (Fig. 4).

2 Reflections on Growing up Queer in America: My Life as a Case Study by Shéár Avory

2.1 Embracing Complexity & Demanding Recognition

Life is as nuanced and complex as the galaxies in the sky, if I were to write an "I Poem" it would go something like this.
  I am currently 22.

I identify as a Black and Indigenous non binary trans femme.

Some call me the nightlife femme fatal; my friends call me the coffee haus queen.

I am a national social justice advocate and have been advocating for social justice since I was in the second grade, according to my mom

(My elementary school got a salad bar after my letter to the superintendent).

My activism is committed to racial, gender, economic, environmental and disability justice, with a particular focus on the empowerment of young people.

I am a California native living in New York

I am a survivor of conversion therapy and suicidality.

I am a proud ungraduated student of 13 public schools, whose path counters all the norms.

My path has been unique, but it has been my own.

I am a former foster youth that emancipated into homelessness at the age of 17 and experienced homelessness from the ages of 17–21 in Los Angeles and New York.

I didn't know that this would be my path, but it has been, and as I've grown, I've learned that this path, my path, is not only unique, but shared—it's one well worn by trans women and nonbinary femmes, especially those of color.

I am a trans femme who wishes the medical community had real conversations with young people about fertility options.

I have come to accept that healing is a lifelong, nonlinear journey … but that the sun always rises.

New York has been a beacon of hope for the LGBTQ community—youth like me—all gravitate here, still

I came to New York around the same age that Marsha was dancing on the piers, so I carry that spirit, that energy, that history, present within me

I know my ancestors are with me, guiding me.

Hope has been my driving force, even as I carry the scars of intergenerational trauma, discrimination, and abuse, I rise in the lowest of the lows and find myself always searching for hope—even as a very young person, being punished I would stare out the window and dream about my future.

My younger self would be proud.

My future self is looking forward to meeting me.

2.2   Navigating Structural Dispossession and Precarity

From age 5 to 10, my father forced me to undergo conversion therapy. At age 10, I was placed in foster care. I never finished high school because I was traumatically bullied in elementary, middle, and high school. Two weeks after my 18th birthday, I left Los Angeles for New York City. I wasn't able to find stable housing and was eventually thrown out of a youth shelter, along with two other Black trans women. We were actively pushing back against transphobia (especially the lack of life necessities and resources that we were experiencing) in the shelter. That was the catalyst that began a cycle of chronic homelessness that eventually lead to incarceration.

At this point I felt like my only other option was to get into a domestic partnership, hoping this might open other avenues for finding shelter. My partner at the time thought we could apply for a couples shelter and that they could take care of me. As typically happens, we then entered a revolving door of eligibility and ineligibility, and we eventually were back on the streets. We ended up going to rural Pennsylvania to stay with relatives. Unfortunately, family violence brought the police to where we were staying, and we encountered a whole new level of terror—winding up in jail in Trump country with confederate flags everywhere.

I was placed in a men's facility and experienced relentless transphobia. As an 18-year-old, I was lectured by a police captain about chromosomes, X and Y. It was petrifying just being in his office. I was in constant fear of being beaten and raped. I was only allowed out of my cell for an hour a day, and people called me all kinds of names. It was so violent. Even though I had all my identity documents updated to reflect my name and gender, none of it protected me from the abuse. I experienced firsthand the unfortunate reality of the "cradle to prison pipeline" endured by trans people, particularly trans women and femmes of color.

As an activist, my response is always to fight, to speak to the manager, or to file a complaint. However, for the first time in my life, I didn't fight for my rights. I couldn't. I was so afraid, I honestly thought I was going to be killed.

I share this difficult reflection to acknowledge that the work of movements is always to protect and empower people. I know in my heart that I would very likely still be incarcerated if I didn't have the privilege—that everyone should have—of being so connected to community. It was my connection to grassroots activists that saved my life. My first phone call was to my Mom, who then called a lawyer I had met while interning at the Lambda Legal Defense Fund when I was in New York. I had never told anyone I was homeless when I worked there, as there's a lot of shame when you're a young person and don't have a place to live.

This chain of support was then bolstered by activists in LA, Philly and New York—an action that still seems so miraculous. But it was really people in the community who came together to help, bringing whatever they could. And luckily, I was able to get out.

2.3   Engaging Activism and Community

I'm a real time activist. No matter what I experience I always return to activism. It's been part of my survival! It's where I find hope. When I reflect, it's clear that activism has been a response to real time experiences that I am living through, and I know must change. How better to inform community and movement responses to injustice, or build policy to shift disparity then from the direct experiences and leadership of people who are living through those experiences as they're happening?

My entire life has been filled with conflict and I alongside too many young people like me—trans youth, youth of color, poor and working-class youth, have experienced far too many grotesque experiences. These lived experiences have fueled my passion and coupled with the learning I have done in community, have completely informed my activism.

To conclude, my story is one of the devastating realities that trans femmes of color too often face when they don't have a safe and secure place to grow as a young person. Yet, it is also a story of community at its best when we rally around each other. My hope is that other queer and trans folks will not have to go through the types of obstacles that I did. However, if they do, I hope they will have a community that can help them to get the resources they need, so that they can survive and eventually thrive.

3   Conclusion: A National Agenda by and for Queer Youth

LGBTQIA+GE youth demand big changes and small—structural transformations and radical shifts in their intimate relationships. They are generous, empathic, activist and still, given the tremendous burden of enduring ever increasing institutional and interpersonal violence, many are hurting. The harms queer youth experience can be addressed with the right social and political will. Youth who attended schools with LGBTQIA+GE affirming policies, inclusive curriculum, out teachers and/or adults, access to LGBTQIA+GE supportive mental health services, Gender and Sexuality Alliances and teachers who are supportive to LGBTQIA+GE students, reported fewer negative school experiences. Changing the culture of schools to affirm queer youth lives matters. And this is only the beginning.

We leave you with a final piece of data—"our issues" (or a national agenda, if you will) synthesized from our analysis of all the qualitative from the 6000+ youth that took the *What's Your Issue?* survey. LGBTQ+GE youth want an end to structural oppression—namely racism, poverty, sexism, homophobia, transphobia, ageism, and ableism. They want financial security—schools where LGBTQ+GE youth can thrive and economic opportunities. They want loving relationships, which consists of accepting families, healthy partnerships, and caring communities. They want freedom—the freedom to live as they are; safety and security; and accessibility and inclusion. Finally, they want health and happiness, which includes accessible health care, stable mental health, and physical health.

We close indebted to all the youth who took our survey and offering their thoughts, ideas, experiences, and desires with the hope of creating a more robust, holistic national portrait of their lives—one that details the structural injustices they are subjected to and pays equal attention to the creativity, complexity, joy and gifts they have to offer. It is on us, now, to challenge dominant narrow constructions of gender and sexuality; embrace complexity and solidarities; dismantle discriminatory policies and practices, and build anti-racist, LGBTQIA+GE affirming institutions and communities were queer youth can not only grow, but flourish.

References

Adames, H. Y., & Chavez, D. (2022). Reclaiming all of me: The racial queer identity framework. In K. L. Nadal & M. Scharron-del Río (Eds.), *Queer psychology: Intersectional perspectives* (pp. 59–80). New York: Springer.

Burns, M. N., Ryan, D. T., Garofalo, R., Newcomb, M. E., & Mustanski, B. (2015). Mental health disorders in young urban sexual minority men. *The Journal of adolescent health : official publication of the Society for Adolescent Medicine, 56*(1), 52–58.

Chmielewski, J. F., Belmonte, K. M., Fine, M., & Stoudt, B. G. (2016). Intersectional inquiries with LGBTQ and gender nonconforming youth of color: Participatory research on discipline disparities at the race/sexuality/gender nexus. In R. J. Skiba, K. Mediratta, & M. K. Rausch (Eds.), *Inequality in school discipline* (pp. 171–188). New York: Palgrave Macmillan.

Choi, S. K., Wilson, B. D. M., Shelton, J., & Gates, G. (2015). *Serving our youth 2015: The needs and experiences of lesbian, gay, bisexual, transgender, and questioning youth experiencing homelessness*. Los Angeles: The Williams Institute with True Colors Fund.

Cohen, C. J. (2010). *Democracy remixed: Black youth and the future of American politics*. New York: Oxford University Press.

Fine, M., Torre, M. E., Frost, D., Cabana, A., & Avory, S. (2018). Refusing to check the box: Participatory inqueery at the radical rim. In K. Gallagher (Ed.), *The methodological dilemma revisited: Creative, critical and collaborative approaches to qualitative research for a new era* (pp. 11–31). London: Routledge.

Frost, D. M., Fine, M., Torre, M. E., & Cabana, A. (2017, August). *Precarity and Activism in the Face of Economic Hardship: Results from a National Participatory Action Survey of LGBTQ & GNC Youth*. Paper presented at the European Conference on Developmental Psychology. Utrecht, The Netherlands.

GLSEN and Harris Interactive. (2012). *Playgrounds and prejudice: Elementary school climate in the United States, a survey of students and teachers*. New York: GLSEN. Retrieved from https://www.glsen.org/sites/default/files/2020-04/Playgrounds_Prejudice.pdf.

Harding, S. (1991). *Whose science? Whose knowledge?: Thinking from women's lives*. Ithaca: Cornell University Press.

Kosciw, J. G., Clark, C. M., Truong, N. L., & Zongrone, A. D. (2020). *The 2019 National School Climate Survey: The experiences of lesbian, gay, bisexual, transgender, and queer youth in our nation's schools*. New York: GLSEN.

Lucassen, M. F. G., Stasiak, K., Samra, R., Frampton, C. M. A., & Merry, S. N. (2017). Sexual minority youth and depressive symptoms or depressive disorder: A systematic review and meta-analysis of population-based studies. *Australian & New Zealand Journal of Psychiatry (51)*8, 774–787.

Luttrell, W. (2013). Children's counter-narratives of care: Towards educational justice. *Children and Society, 27*, 195–308.

Mackenzie, S., & Talbott, A. (2018). Gender justice/gender through the eyes of children: A Photovoice project with elementary school gender expansive and LGBTQ-parented children and their allies. *Sex Education, 18*(6), 655–671.

Marshal, M. P., Dietz, L. J., Friedman, M. S., Stall, R., Smith, H. A., McGinley, J., & Brent, D. A. (2011). Suicidality and depression disparities between sexual minority and heterosexual youth: A meta-analytic review. *Journal of Adolescent Health, 49*, 115–123.

Nadal, K. L. (2020). *Queering law and order: LGBTQ communities and the criminal justice system*. Lanham, MD: Rowman & Little.

Olson-Kennedy, J., Okonta, V., Clark, L. F., & Belzer, M. (2018). Physiologic response to gender-affirming hormones among transgender youth. *Journal of Adolescent Health, 62*(4), 397–401.

Perez-Brumer, A., Day, J. K., Russell, S. T., & Hatzenbuehler, M. L. (2017). Prevalence and correlates of suicidal ideation among transgender youth in California: Findings from a representative, population-based sample of high school students. *Journal of the American Academy of Child & Adolescent Psychiatry, 56*, 739–746.

Puzio, A., & Forbes, A. (2022). Gender identity as a social developmental process. In K. L. Nadal & M. Scharron-del Río (Eds.), *Queer psychology: Intersectional perspectives* (pp. 33–58). New York: Springer.

Savin-Williams, R. C., & Cohen, K. M. (2004). Homoerotic development during childhood and adolescence. *Child and Adolescent Psychiatric Clinics of North America, 13*(3), 529–549. https://doi.org/10.1016/j.chc.2004.02.005.

Stoudt, B. G., Fine, M., & Fox, M. (2011). Growing up policed in the age of aggressive policing policies. *New York Law School Law Review, 56*, 1331.

Toomey, R. B., Syvertsen, A. K., & Shramko, M. (2018). Transgender adolescent suicide behavior. *Pediatrics, 142*, 1–8.

Torre, M., Fine, M., Stoudt, B., & Fox, M. (2012). Critical participatory action research as public science. In P. Camic & H. Cooper (Eds.), *The handbook of qualitative research in psychology: Expanding perspectives in methodology and design* (2nd ed.). Washington, DC: American Psychological Association.

Torre, M. E., Fine, M., Cabana, A., Frost, D., Avory, S., Fowler-Chapman, T., & The What's Your Issue? Youth Research Collective. (2018). Radical wills (and won'ts): Critical participatory inqueery. In S. Talburt (Ed.), *Youth sexualities: Public feelings and contemporary cultural politics* (Vol. 2, pp. 169–191). Westport, CT: Praeger.

Vance, S. R., Ehrensaft, D., & Rosenthal, S. M. (2014). Psychological and medical care of gender nonconforming youth. *Pediatrics, 134*(6), 1184–1192.

Waguespack, D., & Ryan, B. (2019). State index on youth homelessness. True Colors and the National Law Center on Homelessness and Poverty.

Zaza, S., Kann, L., & Barrios, L. C. (2016). Lesbian, gay, and bisexual adolescents: Population estimate and prevalence of health behaviors. *Journal of the American Medical Association, 316*(22), 2355–2356.

Issues for LGBTQ Elderly

Christian D. Chan and Nicole Silverio

1 Issues for LGBTQ Elderly

Research focused on lesbian, gay, bisexual, transgender, and queer (LGBTQ) older adults has expanded over the past decade with significant attention to later stages of the lifespan. Witnessing this growing area in psychological research and practice, the field of gerontology has similarly expanded to meet the needs of policy and practice as an interdisciplinary enterprise (see Espinoza, 2016; Hash & Rogers, 2017; Porter & Krinsky, 2014; South, 2017). The significance of these advances has played an important role for two main purposes. The first impetus involves the combination of health professions (e.g., counseling, psychology, nursing) and disciplines (e.g., sociology, law, anthropology) attempting to meet the needs of older adults and to shift the discourse around gerontology and older adults within their respective professional communities (Adams, 2016; Linscott & Krinsky, 2016). The second motivation emboldens researchers to focus on this stage in the lifespan to illuminate opportunities for how older adults generally view themselves in light of their personal journeys and coinciding generational changes across time periods (Arthur, 2015). Both factors operate as a response to the growing stereotyping, bias, and negative responses toward older adults. Within LGBTQ communities, the plethora of social identities has not rendered the overall group immune to such issues of marginalization. In fact, LGBTQ elders frequently face a myriad of stressors that involve active and implicit forms of exclusion, harm, and violence, which tend to

---

The original version of this chapter was revised. The correction to this chapter is available at https://doi.org/10.1007/978-3-030-74146-4_18

C. D. Chan (✉) · N. Silverio
Department of Counseling and Educational Development, The University of North Carolina at Greensboro, Greensboro, NC, USA
e-mail: cdchan@uncg.edu; njsilver@uncg.edu

© The Author(s), under exclusive license to Springer Nature Switzerland AG 2021, Corrected Publication 2022
K. L. Nadal and M. R. Scharrón-del Río (ed.), *Queer Psychology*, https://doi.org/10.1007/978-3-030-74146-4_13

237

accumulate over the lifespan (Porter & Krinsky, 2014). Within an already marginalized group of identities, LGBTQ elders have been subject to horizontal aggression, namely involving ageism, and face backlash for negative societal responses to the aging process (Porter & Krinsky, 2014; Woody, 2014). Considering this stage in lifespan development, LGBTQ elders have likely endured multiple instances of trauma that overlap with incidents of oppression and violence (Woody, 2015) (Fig. 1).

Although research attempting to address the plight of LGBTQ older adults have several areas to cover with marginalization and health disparities, the platform to expand this area within psychology and other disciplines continues to receive extensive attention and motivates researchers and practitioners alike to shift affirmative practices in a profoundly meaningful way. Notably, the experiences of LGBTQ elders are not solely problem-centered, as researchers have elucidated significant findings that detail experiences of survival, cultural capital, community cultural wealth, and resistance in response to oppression (Chacaby & Plummer, 2016; Chaney & Whitman, 2020; Hash & Rogers, 2017). Conceptualizing this framework of practice for older LGBTQ elders, this population can benefit from honoring responses to both oppression and resilience. As this chapter unearths the complexity of these social and psychological experiences, several areas allude to meaningful affirmative and culturally responsive practices that can embrace a section for gerontology, older adults, and elders across LGBTQ communities. Under the premise of intersectionality, it will be important for psychology researchers and practitioners to continue exploring both areas of oppression and resilience for LGBTQ elders instead of relegating the population to one single set of experiences (Porter et al., 2016; Van Sluytman & Torres, 2014). Augmenting the goals of expanding culturally responsive and affirmative practices in psychology for LGBTQ elders, we attend to three main goals in the chapter: (a) an overview of contemporary research involving LGBTQ elders, aging, and gerontology; (b) theoretical underpinnings of intersectionality to reflect LGBTQ elders with other dimensions of culture and forces of oppression; and (c) considerations for practice and research areas with LGBTQ elders. For the purpose of the chapter, the use of LGBTQ is inclusive and involves populations minoritized across gender identity, gender expression, sexual identity,

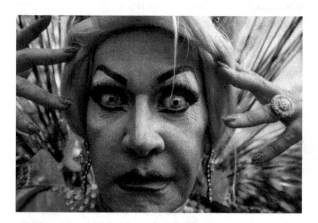

Fig. 1 A drag queen serving fierce looks in an LGBTQ Pride Parade. Photo by Tarek Mahammed

and affectional identity (Griffith et al., 2017). The use of elders and older adults is interchangeable due to differing illustrations across disciplines and their nomenclature in research and practice.

1.1 Minority Stress

Research on older adults features a plethora of issues that exacerbate psychosocial factors precipitating minority stress (see Correro & Nielson, 2020; Kim & Fredriksen-Goldsen, 2017). The Williams Institute, one of the largest community advocacy organizations focused on LGBTQ communities, took a unique interest in illuminating several issues among LGBTQ older adults (Choi & Meyer, 2016). In particular, researchers have taken note that LGBTQ older adults are generally at the margins in the broader landscape of behavioral health, mental health, and physical health research, which has essentially illuminated a constellation of health disparities (Foglia & Fredriksen-Goldsen, 2014; Goldhammer et al., 2019). Indeed, the chronic stress endured by LGBTQ older adults throughout the lifespan culminates in a predisposed risk for mental health issues, medical conditions, and disproportionate health disparities (Hash & Rogers, 2017). Compromised immune systems and medical issues have become an even larger focus for gerontological practitioners during the pandemic of COVID-19, given that the conditions of minority stress elicit a decrease in healthcare usage, access, and help-seeking (Jen et al., 2020; Meyer & Choi, 2020).

Researchers have taken a notable interest in identifying the needs of LGBTQ older adults from the standpoint of minority stress due to convergent forms of racism, genderism, heterosexism, and ageism (Arthur, 2015; Bettis et al., 2020; Choi & Meyer, 2016; Correro & Nielson, 2020; Woody, 2014, 2015). These overlapping forms of oppression do not preclude other structural inequities linked to classism and ableism, which likely exacerbate a number of preexisting conditions and access to care. Minority stress was initially conceptualized as a taxonomy of stressors, including events, people, and incidents, that predispose historically marginalized individuals to suicidal ideation, higher mortality rates, poorer physical health outcomes, and increased rates of mental health disorders (see Meyer, 1995, 2003). Meyer (2010, 2020) has advanced this model to illustrate how multiple marginalized identities may conflate the incidence of these risks for physical and mental health disorders. Additionally, Meyer (2020) has revamped this model to support resilience as an integral factor in ameliorating the risks of minority stress. Originally conceptualized in response to the experiences of LGBTQ communities, key components in classifying the definitions of minority stress are referred to as proximal stressors and distal stressors (Meyer, 1995). Distal stressors are defined as objective events that occur in the lives of historically marginalized communities, yet they are considered external to the individual (Douglass & Conlin, 2020; Meyer, 2003). For LGBTQ older adults, a distal stressor could be witnessing a verbal attack on another LGBTQ older adult in their housing environment. Conversely, proximal stressors are characterized as subjective events and reflect internalization of a stressor, such as a discrimination event (Correro & Nielson, 2020; Meyer, 2003). For instance, LGBTQ older adults could face the proximal stressor of negotiating fears of coming out in the workplace and internalized shame for being inauthentic to self.

There are significant connotations related to LGBTQ older adults that distinguish their experiences in the broad landscape of minority stress research. Namely, LGBTQ older adults face numerous events linked to past historical events and concurrent events of discrimination (Hash & Rogers, 2017). The chronic daily incidence of these events over a lifetime can potentially heighten rejection sensitivity and internalized stigma, which ultimately affect outcomes of mental health (Correro & Nielson, 2020; Meyer, 2020). Additionally, the subjective nature of proximal stressors for LGBTQ older adults can draw from a single or combination of discrimination events in one's life, which means that the internalized response could emerge from a past experience, current experience, or combination of both. Different from the broad grouping of LGBTQ communities, minority stress affects the help-seeking and healthcare access of LGBTQ older adults (Choi & Meyer, 2016; Correro & Nielson, 2020). For many LGBTQ older adults, they may already face experiences of social isolation that heighten their hesitation to utilize medical and mental health care or lack the access needed to secure an affirmative provider (Bettis et al., 2020; Porter & Krinsky, 2014; Serafin et al., 2013). In the scope of minority stress, LGBTQ older adults may face accelerated negative outcomes of aging and disorders consistent with this stage of the lifespan, such as dementia (Correro & Nielson, 2020; Fredriksen-Goldsen et al., 2018; Yarns et al., 2016).

1.2 Social Determinants of Health

Combined with factors related to minority stress, a myriad of social determinants contribute to LGBTQ older adults' access to care. In the frame of health equity, this issue is especially prominent for psychologists, mental health practitioners, counselors, and related healthcare professionals to examine as a public health issue (Espinoza, 2016; Yarns et al., 2016), given the way how multiple inequities can overlap at a single point in time and throughout the lifespan (Bowleg, 2017; Chan & Henesy, 2018). For this reason, specific regions already marred by mental health care shortages relate to the likelihood for whether older adults can access care, feel safe to do so, and find an affirmative provider (Bettis et al., 2020; Lecompte et al., 2020; Porter et al., 2016). Indeed, a number of these issues are pervasively affecting social conditions and psychosocial factors that exacerbate underlying medical conditions and mental health issues (Correro & Nielson, 2020; Yarns et al., 2016).

1.2.1   Physical Health and Mortality

Due to the relationship between psychosocial factors and underlying medical conditions, researchers have typically found that stressful events and their corresponding responses result in lower outcomes of wellness (Correro & Nielson, 2020; Meyer, 2020). The accumulation of these experiences leads researchers to links between health inequities and predisposing discrimination events. Numerous healthcare disciplines have identified concerns in their research about the overrepresentation of physical illness, underlying medical conditions, chronic illness, and obesity among LGBTQ older adults (Choi & Meyer, 2016; Kim et al., 2017). Of important note, physical and chronic illnesses are highest in older transgender adults, which warrants specific attention for practitioners and researchers (Fredriksen-Goldsen et al., 2013; Yarns et al., 2016). Healthcare workers and researchers have also distinctively found that sexual health concerns cannot be precluded, given that many LGBTQ older adults continue to remain sexually active throughout the lifespan (Brennan-Ing et al., 2020; Hillman, 2017; Schubert & Pope, 2020). Regarding promotion of sexual health, discrimination experiences and stereotypes may also challenge access to care and engagement in services for LGBTQ older adults living with HIV (Johnson Shen et al., 2019). Similar to indications of minority stress, LGBTQ older adults may be responding with their own historical trauma (Hash & Rogers, 2017) or internalize stigma about their sexual health in relation to heterosexism, genderism, and ageism (Brennan-Ing et al., 2020). For LGBTQ older adults, the constellation of stressors, medical issues, and mental health disorders increases the risk of mortality through physical health risks (Kim et al., 2017) and suicidal ideation (Brennan-Ing et al., 2014). Correro and Nielson (2020) elaborated further with examples of the physical effects and health disparities emanating from minority stress, such as hypertension, high blood pressure, cardiovascular issues, and diabetes. Kim et al. (2017), in particular, observed that health risks are exacerbated for older LGBT people of Color, specifically older LGBT Black and Latino populations. Results from the Choi et al. (2018) study also indicated that LGB Latino older adults reported more food insecurity, diabetes, and lack of health insurance.

At worst, LGBTQ older adults refrain from seeking care due to negative healthcare experiences or brace themselves for everyday discrimination in their healthcare experiences (Correro & Nielson, 2020; Foglia & Fredriksen-Goldsen, 2014). The culmination of discrimination experiences and overall lack of affirmative providers generally results in lower rates of help-seeking (Burton et al., 2020), and culturally responsive encounters can buffer the problematic experiences associated with negative healthcare encounters (Flynn et al., 2020; Porter & Krinsky, 2014). Instigated by these experiences, only a sample of practitioners are trained to work with older adults (Hash & Rogers, 2017) or covered by Medicare to provide mental health services (Fullen, 2018). LGBTQ older adults may not have the means for transportation to access medical or mental healthcare (Bettis et al., 2020), which is further complicated when they are living alone (Choi et al., 2018; Choi & Meyer, 2016). Burton et al. (2020) specifically suggested that the patient or client relationship is ultimately a crucial factor for LGBTQ older adults to access care. In light of the Burton et al. (2020) findings, trusting relationships and therapeutic alliances for mental health providers are consistently established as the most effective intervention in culturally responsive practices (Sue et al., 2019).

1.2.2 Mental Health and Substance Use

Numerous researchers have referenced the public health crisis related to mental health of LGBTQ older adults (e.g., Chaney & Whitman, 2020; Fredriksen-Goldsen et al., 2015; Yarns et al., 2016). McCann & Brown (2019), in particular, noted the global crisis indicating that LGBTQ older adults' combination of mental health and discrimination concerns is not isolated to a single country. Correro and Nielson (2020) also documented the ramifications of minority stress and its cumulative effect on cognitive decline among LGBTQ older adults, which can potentially elicit more risks for dementia. Chronic incidents of discrimination, social isolation, and addressing societal expectations can lead LGBTQ older adults to serious psychological consequences (King & Richardson, 2017). According to Choi and Meyer (2016), LGBTQ older adults reported higher rates of mood disorders (e.g., anxiety, depression) and suicidal ideation in comparison to their heterosexual and cisgender counterparts. Notably, transgender, non-binary, and gender nonconforming older adults face higher rates in comparison to cisgender LGB community members (Hoy-Ellis & Fredriksen-Goldsen, 2017; Yarns et al., 2016), and bisexual individuals reported more incidents of psychological distress than gay and lesbian individuals (Choi et al., 2018). These studies further elaborate how LGBTQ older adults are uniquely situated at their stage of the lifespan not only with one single event of oppression, but rather, the overlapping psychosocial effects from oppression (Woody, 2014, 2015; Yarns et al., 2016). As a unique concern for LGBTQ older adults in comparison to LGBTQ individuals at other lifespan stages, LGBTQ older adults may be susceptible to heightened internalized stigma from longer histories of trauma, have fewer means to access mental health care, and face social isolation (Bettis et al., 2020; Choi & Meyer, 2016). Although LGBTQ individuals are similarly susceptible to the health disparities related to minority stress, practitioners must consider that decreased access to social networks can result in a lower likelihood of participating in mental health care (King & Richardson, 2017).

With the overview of risks, minority stressors, and potential social isolation experiences, multiple LGBTQ older adults may resort to substance use as a coping mechanism. Combined with managing psychologically distressing events, inadequate means to potential social networks for older LGBTQ adults could result in illicit substance use conflated with the lack of care and barriers to help-seeking. One primary risk pervasive to LGBTQ older adults is the potential social isolation, given a disconnection from friends and family, grief, and death of loved ones (Arthur, 2015; Burton et al., 2020; Goldhammer et al., 2019). Notably, Choi et al. (2018) noted that older LGB adults in California showed higher rates of smoking. Substance use research reflects these disparities as a major concern, given that many LGBTQ older adults access healthcare far less than their counterparts across cohorts of adults (e.g., emerging adults, midlife; Choi & Meyer, 2016). Talley et al. (2016) have raised attention to the comorbidity of substance use, underlying medical conditions, and mental health distress among LGBTQ older adults, where a lifetime of substance use coping mechanisms exacerbate the stress placed on preexisting medical conditions. Talley et al. (2016) also posited that chronic substance use to cope with psychological distress from discrimination can result in medical conditions and physical health issues later in life.

1.2.3 Housing, Eviction, and Financial Issues

Another significant area related to social determinants of health is food insecurity, financial issues, and housing for LGBTQ older adults. The housing issue layers into several social determinants of health, given that LGBTQ older adults may be living with caregivers, by themselves, or in nursing homes. Specifically in nursing homes, LGBTQ older adults may directly experience bigotry, incivility, and discrimination from other residents in nursing homes or nursing home workers (Hafford-Letchfield et al., 2018). A study by Putney et al. (2018) indicated that LGBTQ older adults' fears about nursing homes and assisted living are primarily enacted through potential abuse, mistreatment, and identity concealment. Related to the Putney et al. (2018) study, Serafin et al. (2013) reinforced this claim by bringing more attention to LGBT elders and how they conceal their identities upon transitioning into nursing homes.

Unfortunately, LGBTQ older adults living among themselves or with caregivers are not immune to these deleterious effects. Choi and Meyer (2016) reported an increasing prevalence of LGBTQ older adults facing eviction from current housing, higher payments for housing and rent, or denial of housing applications. Although specific to California, the Choi et al. (2018) report indicated that LGB older adults, especially Latinos, were more likely to be food insecure. The accumulation of housing issues and food insecurity precipitate alarming concerns for LGBTQ older adults, as many transition into less income-earning and career opportunities later in life (Chaney & Whitman, 2020; Putney et al., 2018). Putney et al. (2020), in particular, identified that inclusive housing options for LGBTQ older adults are paramount to buffer the effects of isolation. As practitioners consider the implications of oppression specific to LGBTQ older adults, they could explore responses to potential discriminatory events and the cultural context associated with these housing environments (Goldhammer et al., 2019; Serafin et al., 2013). Additionally, practitioners could identify policies that protect or inhibit LGBTQ older adults in their housing conditions (Espinoza, 2016; McCann & Brown, 2019). As findings from the Putney et al. (2018) revealed, LGBTQ older adults are searching for housing with affirmative cultures and policies that embrace their identities.

1.3   Life Transitions, Trauma, and Surviving Multiple Eras

Within gerontological scholarly spaces, researchers and policymakers are focusing on LGBTQ older adults due to late adulthood transitions and distinct historical events that precipitate stress and resilience (Hash & Rogers, 2017; McCann & Brown, 2019). Practitioners should consider that the landscape has perpetually shifted for LGBTQ older adults, considering that they likely endured shifts in healthcare and mental health practices (Goldhammer et al., 2019). For some LGBTQ older adults, their sexual identity, gender identity, and gender expression was criminalized, despite the activism formed by previous generations of LGBTQ communities (Choi & Meyer, 2016; King & Richardson, 2017). Being gay, for instance, was considered a disorder in the DSM until 1973, and there are still major issues with the diagnosis of gender dysphoria (Hash & Rogers, 2017). Conflated with medical criminalization and ostracization, legislation in the United States and globally was rampant with sodomy laws that sustained long-term systemic harm for LGBTQ communities (Choi & Meyer, 2016). For some LGBTQ older adults, the timing of the HIV/AIDS pandemic left them with profound experiences of loss while simultaneously carrying homophobic and transphobic stigma over decades (de Vries & Herdt, 2012; Serafin et al., 2013).

Additionally, a rising number of recent research studies have revealed elder abuse and neglect among LGBTQ older adults to be a pervasive problem at this stage in the lifespan (see Bloemen et al., 2019; McCann & Brown, 2019; Robson et al., 2018). Given this alarming finding, mental health issues and traumatic stress can manifest in response to incidents of abuse (Westwood, 2019). Due to risk factors and discriminatory experiences, such as social isolation, LGBTQ older adults may underreport incidents of abuse or, in more dire circumstances, conceal their sexual identity and gender identity as a coping mechanism. There is an overwhelming fear of transitioning into healthcare settings, assisted living, or nursing homes as a result of abuse incidents instigated against LGBTQ older adults (Serafin et al., 2013; Witten, 2012). For LGBTQ older adults, practitioners and researchers can draw from a wider taxonomy in their conceptualization of abuse. Abuse can include interpersonal violence from caregivers, intimate partners, family members, healthcare providers, and other individuals within their living environments (Westwood 2019). Abuse can also be classified into elder abuse and neglect with LGBTQ older adults excluded from adequate care (Serafin et al., 2013; Westwood, 2019). Additionally, abuse can stem from systemic and epistemic violence through discrimination, explicit violence, and microaggressions (Choi & Meyer, 2016).

1.4   Caregivers and Social Isolation

For LGBTQ older adults, caregivers and social isolation have emerged as a significant priority for intervention, given that successful outcomes of health and wellness are tied to social networks. Researchers (e.g., Fredriksen-Goldsen et al., 2013, 2017; McCann & Brown, 2019; Putney et al., 2018; Yarns et al., 2016) have pinned social isolation as a pervasive issue for LGBTQ older adults, given that numerous LGBTQ older adults who self-disclose their identities or relocate may lose contact with critical networks. In turn, transitions among family and social networks alter LGBTQ older adults' access to medical and mental health care. Isolation has also made LGBTQ older adults susceptible to increased mental health risks, psychological distress, and suicidal ideation (Goldhammer et al., 2019). The plight of isolation for LGBTQ older adults can manifest in feelings of loneliness, which compound with mental health disorders and symptoms (Yarns et al., 2016). The fear of isolation can incite an impending doom related to cognitive and physical decline and societal expectations on the aging process (Choi & Meyer, 2016; Zelle & Arms, 2015).

For LGBTQ older adults, families and kinship may be crucial factors in ameliorating the effects of oppression because these connections instill coping mechanisms and access to preventive care (Choi & Meyer, 2016; Yarns et al., 2016). LGBTQ older adults may be more apt to engage in counseling and mental health services with a stronger network of social connections. Similarly, social dimensions are characteristic of a holistic profile of wellness for LGBTQ older adults (Chaney & Whitman, 2020). Putney et al. (2020) highlighted these social bonds are interpersonal and contextual factors contributing to the overall safety and health of the population (Fig. 2).

2   Intersectionality and Its Connection to LGBTQ Older Adults

Intersectionality has become a radical force across numerous disciplines, especially psychology and counseling, for its intuitive applications to practice, policy, and social justice (see Bowleg, 2012; Bowleg & Bauer, 2016; Chan & Erby, 2018; Grzanka et al., 2017; Singh et al., 2020; Warner et al., 2016). Notably, intersectionality plays a consistent role in examining multiple overlapping forms of oppression and how they conflate into larger systems of health inequities (Bowleg, 2017; Chan & Erby, 2018; Chan & Henesy, 2018; Hankivsky et al., 2014). Using the lens of intersectionality can serve as a catalyst for affirmative practices, specifically for LGBTQ older adults (Adams, 2016; Arthur, 2015), and raises the salience of policies and structural conditions affecting multiply marginalized communities (Crenshaw, 1989; Grzanka, 2020). Although intersectionality has been sourced to the work of Crenshaw (1989) and Collins (1986), intersectionality should be considered in the broader scheme of its intellectual forerunners (e.g., Anzaldúa, 1987; Combahee River Collective, 1995; Davis, 1983; Hooks, 1984; Lorde, 1984; Moraga & Anzaldúa, 1983). These intellectual forerunners drew from personal narratives that critically examined the clashes among their identities, the forces of oppression that culminated in these cultural clashes, and the opportunities to integrate these

Fig. 2 Dr. Debra Joy
Perez and Billy
Fields share a
moment at the 2015
LGBTQ Scholars of Color
National Conference in
New York City. Photo
Courtesy of Riya Ortiz/
Red Papillon Photography

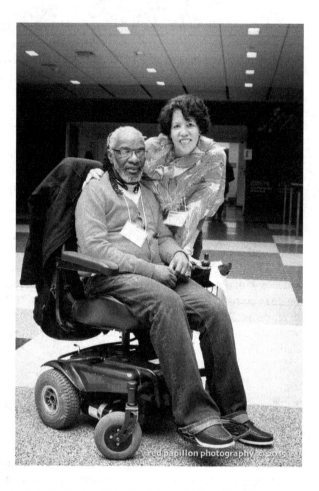

intersections (Chan & Howard, 2020; Moradi & Grzanka, 2017). Otherwise, inter-sectionality will be essentially reduced to a commodity of multiple identities or diverse identities without its premise in dismantling problematic power structures, a social justice ethos, and deconstruction of race (Chan & Henesy, 2018; Collins, 2015; Moradi & Grzanka, 2017). Too often, the approach is co-opted and erased from the genealogy of women of Color, queer women of Color, and Black feminism (Moradi & Grzanka, 2017), which first centered the movement in response to endemic racism within white feminist spaces (Collins, 2019; Crenshaw, 1989).

To effectively use intersectionality as an approach, scholars and practitioners must use several principles that continue to dismantle the inequities affecting LGBTQ older adults (Bowleg, 2017; Warner et al., 2016). Intersectionality is con-tingent on six themes from Collins and Bilge (2020) that demonstrate the depth of its framework: (a) power, (b) social context, (c) social inequality, (d) relationality, (e) complexity, and (f) social justice. Relationality and complexity work in tandem as these two principles characterize how individuals consist of multiple identities and carry unique experiences shaping each of their identities (Collins & Bilge,

2020). For LGBTQ older adults, using these two principles can reaffirm their experiences, capital, and integration of identities as protective factors and sources of resilience (Arthur, 2015; Woody, 2014, 2015). In the Woody (2014) study, aging African American lesbian and gay participants specifically reported that surviving multiple forms of oppression over several generations contributed to their resilience. Several scholars based in intersectionality have posited that intersectionality must draw from an analysis of power (Bowleg & Bauer, 2016; Collins, 2015) and structural oppression (Bowleg, 2017; Grzanka, 2020). Intersectionality represents a promising framework to elucidate the experiences of LGBTQ older adults, especially LGBTQ older adults of Color (Arthur, 2015; Bloemen et al., 2019). For instance, practitioners should consider structural forces, such as white supremacy, and how they foundationally undergird heterosexism, genderism, and ageism. Practitioners can contextualize how these forces impact LGBTQ older adults' experiences over time and in the current state of society.

Although LGBTQ older adults are explicitly connected to heterosexism, genderism, and ageism, researchers and practitioners must unveil other intersecting forms of oppression, such as racism, classism, and ableism (Hash & Rogers, 2017; Johnson Shen et al., 2019). A plethora of researchers have commented that LGBTQ older adults of Color and racism must be further explored in the larger scope of gerontological research (Goldhammer et al., 2019; King & Richardson, 2017). Additionally, multiple researchers have noted the disparities associated with HIV exclusions in LGBTQ older adults, which illustrates an increased need to examine ableism within this population. Other than merely realizing multiple forms of oppression, researchers and practitioners must clearly foreground their practices of intersectionality in a social justice agenda (Collins, 2019). Using this mindset will reflect systematic changes that unsettle inequities and propels communities toward action (Bowleg, 2017; Hankivsky et al., 2014). This issue is especially relevant for policymakers who are unaware of the litany of injustices and health disparities facing LGBTQ older adults today (Espinoza, 2016; Hash & Rogers, 2017). Aside from empowering LGBTQ older adults with affirmative practices, practitioners should reflect their conversations on the possibilities for changing the cultural contexts affecting LGBTQ older adult clients.

3   Case Example

In this hypothetical case example, Mona is a lesbian 68-year-old Asian older cisgender woman with Indonesian and Chinese heritage and has accumulated a sizable amount of income due to financial planning within the last few years. Mona has recently retired from a successful position with her last company after a long-term leadership position in business. Mona uses the pronouns she, her, and hers. She has been living together with her partner who is also a lesbian cisgender woman, but with a white racial identity and a career in education. Her partner is still employed as a student affairs practitioner. They have been living in an urban city and have been married for several years with strong levels of marital, relational, and sexual satisfaction.

Upon retiring, Mona has changed her most recent medical provider to ensure that she is able to receive insurance coverage for the medical services. While visiting a new provider several times over the past few months, Mona has noticed that staff have foregone any discussions about her sexual health and generally meet with her for only 5 min. Mona has speculated that staff at the new provider have seemingly rushed her appointments and physically avoid her. At one point, she mentioned living with her partner to which the staff quickly shifted the topic of conversation. One day, the provider perpetuated a stereotype about Asian older adults and their usage of healthcare. The combination of these experiences has left Mona conflicted about continuing with this provider, although this provider is covered under her insurance and closest in location to her house. Mona tried to broach these issues among her friends and family, particularly white individuals in her social network, where many have dismissed the experiences or tried to explain the rationale behind their actions. Some friends, including her partner, suggested that the experiences may have been likely a result of heterosexist microaggressions. She has been working with a counselor for her own wellness over the past 2 years and bring these new life transitions to the counseling sessions (Fig. 3).

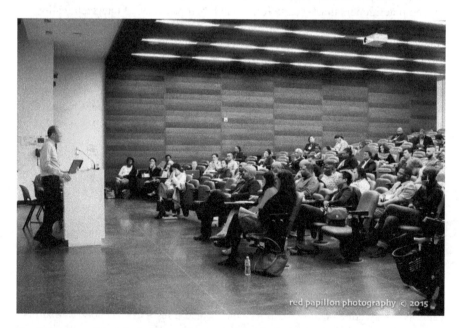

Fig. 3 Dr. Barry Chung lecturing on his experiences as a gay Asian American before an captive audience. Photo Courtesy of Riya Ortiz/Red Papillon Photography

4   Considerations for Reflecting Intersectionality in Practice

Within clinical practice, psychologists, counselors, and mental health practitioners are tasked with a responsibility to examine the accumulating effects sustained by health inequities and overlapping forms of oppression. There are three main areas related to intersectionality that are applicable to the case example. Given the potential health inequities and social determinants of health affecting LGBTQ older adults, practitioners can consider that a combination of factors might have been present in this case example. With LGBTQ older adults, they may face a variety of barriers in accessing healthcare, which may limit choices to access an affirmative provider. As demonstrated in the story, Mona has had several successes over her lifetime, including financial security, housing, and social connection. However, a life transition altered the pressures of finding another provider and shaped her choices for a healthcare provider. Social conditions and contextual factors influence the ability to seek certain providers, where specific providers may not institute the same affirmative approach. Although Mona's past experiences with discrimination were not extensively discussed, practitioners must be attuned to the ways that life transitions may place a client at the nexus of multiple forms of marginalization (Arthur, 2015; Correro & Nielson, 2020). The contextual factors in this scenario alluded to the prominent issue that agencies, healthcare, and society are contending with gaps in training affirmative and culturally responsive practitioners (Hash & Rogers, 2017; McCann & Brown, 2019). Many training programs across healthcare disciplines are suffering from the omission of cultural aspects in the lives of clients, consumers, and patients (Lecompte et al., 2020), which render practitioners less likely to detect interpersonal and structural forms of marginalization (Choi & Meyer, 2016).

Although intersectionality highlights the constellation of oppression events that Mona could have encountered previously and currently, it behooves practitioners to address the strengths and resilience sustained over her lifetime (Chacaby & Plummer, 2016; Meyer, 2015). Given intersectionality's focus on relationality and complexity, Mona's experiences can map profound experiences of discrimination and resilience reflecting her multiple identities. Exclusively perceiving LGBTQ older adults in a deficit perspective can also be harmful (Arthur, 2015). However, this perspective does not mean that practitioners should diminish the cascading effects of oppression. Practitioners can incorporate Mona's successes and responses to oppression as factors that ameliorate the psychological consequences with racism, heterosexism, and genderism throughout her life and specific to this incident (Choi & Meyer, 2016; Woody, 2014; Yarns et al., 2016).

The story of Mona is only a sample of the diverse spectrum of experiences among LGBTQ older adults. Researchers and practitioners must dedicate more efforts to tackling the epidemic and crises facing LGBTQ older adults of Color (Foglia & Fredriksen-Goldsen, 2014; Fredriksen-Goldsen et al., 2013, 2017; Kim et al., 2017; Van Sluytman & Torres, 2014), given the disproportionate amount of racism and white supremacy taking place over decades. In this scenario, Mona simultaneously experienced heterosexism and racism, which often manifested as a combination of implicit and explicit acts (e.g., avoidance, stereotypes, discomfort around sexuality). One element that should be highlighted was how individuals within Mona's social network, particularly white individuals, perpetuated horizontal oppression (i.e., oppression within oppressed communities). By dismissing Mona's experiences with her healthcare providers, the accumulation of these experiences may contribute to Mona's likelihood of seeking help from future healthcare providers in the future (Flynn et al., 2020). Individuals in her own community overlooked the racism and racial microaggressions that could have played a distinct role in this incident. An apparent dynamic surfaced between Mona and her partner who also disregarded the racialized experience and focused primarily on the heterosexist act. Intersectionality provides a way to make sense of exclusionary practices and marginalization that takes place within historically marginalized communities (Chan & Erby, 2018).

5 Conclusion

Although researchers, psychologists, counselors, and mental health professionals are taking an interest in LGBTQ older adults and elders, the multitude of research studies in the past decade have demonstrated a more urgent need to increase research, practice, and policy supporting the population (Espinoza, 2016; Hash & Rogers, 2017). LGBTQ older adults may have overlap with youth and emerging adults, but in the context of lifespan development, practitioners and researchers must consider the historical events that precede stress and resilience experiences. Using intersectionality can be an effective approach to conceptualize the myriad forms of oppression and draw on multiple dimensions for cultural capital, knowledge, and wealth (Singh, 2019). For many LGBTQ older adults, their experiences with resilience and survival are likely contingent on integrating multiple dimensions of their social identities, becoming conscious about inequitable conditions, and affirming the intersections of their identities.

References

Adams, M. (2016). An intersectional approach to services and care for LGBT elders. *Generations, 40*(2), 94–100.

Anzaldúa, G. (1987). *Borderlands/la Frontera*. San Francisco: Aunt Lute Books.

Arthur, D. P. (2015). Social work practice with LGBT elders at end of life: Developing practice evaluation and clinical skills through a cultural perspective. *Journal of Social Work in End-of-Life & Palliative Care, 11*(2), 178–201. https://doi.org/10.1080/15524256.2015.1074141.

Bettis, J., Kakkar, S., & Chan, C. D. (2020). Taking access to the community: An ecological systems framework for in-home counseling with older adults. *Adultspan Journal, 19*(1), 54–64. https://doi.org/10.1002/adsp.12087.

Bloemen, E. M., Rosen, T., LoFaso, V. M., Lasky, A., Church, S., Hall, P., Weber, T., & Clark, S. (2019). Lesbian, gay, bisexual, and transgender older adults' experiences with elder abuse and neglect. *Journal of the American Geriatrics Society, 67*(11), 2338–2345. https://doi.org/10.1111/jgs.16101.

Bowleg, L. (2012). The problem with the phrase women and minorities: Intersectionality—an important theoretical framework for public health. *American Journal of Public Health, 102*(7), 1267–1273. https://doi.org/10.2105/AJPH.2012.300750.

Bowleg, L. (2017). Towards a critical health equity research stance: Why epistemology and methodology matter more than qualitative methods. *Health Education & Behavior, 44*(5), 677–684. https://doi.org/10.1177/1090198117728760.

Bowleg, L., & Bauer, G. (2016). Invited reflection: Quantifying intersectionality. *Psychology of Women Quarterly, 40*(3), 337–341. https://doi.org/10.1177/0361684316654282.

Brennan-Ing, M., Seidel, L., Larson, B., & Karpiak, S. E. (2014). Social care networks and older LGBT adults: Challenges for the future. *Journal of Homosexuality, 61*(1), 21–52. https://doi.org/10.1080/00918369.2013.835235.

Brennan-Ing, M., Kaufman, J. E., Larson, B., Gamarel, K. E., Seidel, L., & Karpiak, S. E. (2020). Sexual health among lesbian, gay, bisexual, and heterosexual older adults: An exploratory analysis. *Clinical Gerontologist*, 1–13. https://doi.org/10.1080/07317115.2020.1846103.

Burton, C. W., Lee, J.-A., Waalen, A., & Gibbs, L. M. (2020). "Things are different now but": Older LGBT adults' experiences and unmet needs in health care. *Journal of Transcultural Nursing, 31*(5), 492–501. https://doi.org/10.1177/1043659619895099.

Chacaby, M.-N., & Plummer, M. L. (2016). *A two-spirit journey: The autobiography of a lesbian Ojibwa-Cree elder*. Winnipeg, Manitoba: University of Manitoba Press.

Chan, C. D., & Erby, A. N. (2018). A critical analysis and applied intersectionality framework with intercultural queer couples. *Journal of Homosexuality, 65*(9), 1249–1274. https://doi.org/10.1080/00918369.2017.1411691.

Chan, C. D., & Henesy, R. K. (2018). Navigating intersectional approaches, methods, and interdisciplinarity to health equity in LGBTQ+ communities. *Journal of LGBT Issues in Counseling, 12*(4), 230–247. https://doi.org/10.1080/15538605.2018.1526157.

Chan, C. D., & Howard, L. C. (2020). When queerness meets intersectional thinking: Revolutionizing parallels, histories, and contestations. *Journal of Homosexuality, 67*(3), 346–366. https://doi.org/10.1080/00918369.2018.1530882.

Chaney, M. P., & Whitman, J. S. (2020). Affirmative wellness counseling with older LGBTQ+ adults. *Journal of Mental Health Counseling, 42*(4), 303–322. https://doi.org/10.17744/mehc.42.4.02.

Choi, S. K., Kittle, K., & Meyer, I. H. (2018). *Aging LGB adults in California: Findings from the 2015–2016 California health interview survey*. The Williams Institute. Retrieved from https://williamsinstitute.law.ucla.edu/wp-content/uploads/Aging-LGB-CA-Aug-2018.pdf

Choi, S. K., & Meyer, I. H. (2016). *LGBT aging: A review of the research findings, needs, and policy implications*. The Williams Institute. Retrieved from http://williamsinstitute.law.ucla.edu/wp-content/uploads/LGBT-Aging-A-Review.pdf

Collins, P. H. (1986). Learning from the outsider within: The sociological significance of black feminist thought. *Social Problems, 33*(6), S14–S32. https://doi.org/10.2307/800672.

Collins, P. H. (2015). Intersectionality's definitional dilemmas. *Annual Review of Sociology, 41*(1), 1–20. https://doi.org/10.1146/annurev-soc-073014-112142.

Collins, P. H. (2019). *Intersectionality as critical social theory*. Durham and London: Duke University Press.

Collins, P. H., & Bilge, S. (2020). *Intersectionality* (2nd ed.). Cambridge, UK: Polity Press.

Combahee River Collective. (1995). Combahee River Collective statement. In B. Guy-Sheftall (Ed.), *Words of fire: An anthology of African American feminist thought* (pp. 232–240). New York: New Press. (Originally published in 1977).

Correro, A. N., & Nielson, K. A. (2020). A review of minority stress as a risk factor for cognitive decline in lesbian, gay, bisexual, and transgender (LGBT) elders. *Journal of Gay & Lesbian Mental Health, 24*(1), 2–19. https://doi.org/10.1080/19359705.2019.1644570.

Crenshaw, K. (1989). Demarginalizing the intersection of race and sex: A black feminist critique of antidiscrimination doctrine, feminist theory and antiracist politics. *University of Chicago Legal Forum, 1989*(1), 139–167. https://chicagounbound.uchicago.edu/cgi/viewcontent.cgi?art icle=1052&context=uclf.

Davis, A. Y. (1983). *Women, race & class.* New York: Vintage Books.

de Vries, B., & Herdt, G. (2012). Aging in the gay community. In T. M. Witten & A. E. Eyler (Eds.), *Gay, lesbian, bisexual & transgender aging: Challenges in research, practice, and policy* (pp. 84–129). Baltimore: The Johns Hopkins University Press.

Douglass, R. P., & Conlin, S. E. (2020). Minority stress among LGB people: Investigating relations among distal and proximal stressors. *Current Psychology, 2020.* https://doi.org/10.1007/s12144-020-00885-z.

Flynn, P. M., Betancourt, H., Emerson, N. D., Nunez, E. I., & Nance, C. M. (2020). Health professional cultural competence reduces the psychological and behavioral impact of negative healthcare encounters. *Cultural Diversity and Ethnic Minority Psychology, 26*(3), 271–279. https://doi.org/10.1037/cdp0000295.

Foglia, M. B., & Fredriksen-Goldsen, K. I. (2014). Health disparities among LGBT older adults and the role of nonconscious bias. *Hastings Center Report, 44*(S4), S40–S44. https://doi.org/10.1002/hast.369.

Fredriksen-Goldsen, K. I., Emlet, C. A., Kim, H. J., Muraco, A., Erosheva, E. A., Goldsen, J., & Hoy-Ellis, C. P. (2013). The physical and mental health of lesbian, gay male, and bisexual (LGB) older adults: The role of key health indicators and risk and protective factors. *The Gerontologist, 53*, 664–675. https://doi.org/10.1093/geront/gns123.

Fredriksen-Goldsen, K. I., Jen, S., Bryan, A. E. B., & Goldsen, J. (2018). Cognitive impairment, alzheimer's disease, and other dementias in the lives of lesbian, gay, bisexual and transgender (LGBT) older adults and their caregivers: Needs and competencies.(report). *Journal of Applied Gerontology, 37*(5), 545–569. https://doi.org/10.1177/0733464816672047.

Fredriksen-Goldsen, K. I., Kim, H. J., Bryan, A. E., Shiu, C., & Emlet, C. A. (2017). The cascading effects of marginalization and pathways of resilience in attaining good health among LGBT older adults. *The Gerontologist, 57*(1), S72–S83. https://doi.org/10.1093/geront/gnw170.

Fredriksen-Goldsen, K. I., Kim, H. J., Shiu, C., Goldsen, J., & Emlet, C. A. (2015). Successful aging among LGBT older adults: Physical and mental health-related quality of life by age group. *The Gerontologist, 55*, 154–168. https://doi.org/10.1093/geront/gnu081.

Fullen, M. C. (2018). Ageism and the counseling profession: Causes, consequences, and methods for counteraction. *The Professional Counselor, 8*(2), 104–114. https://doi.org/10.15241/mcf.8.2.104.

Goldhammer, H., Krinsky, L., & Keuroghlian, A. S. (2019). Meeting the behavioral health needs of LGBT older adults. *Journal of the American Geriatrics Society, 67*(8), 1565–1570. https://doi.org/10.1111/jgs.15974.

Griffith, C., Akers, W., Dispenza, F., Luke, M., Farmer, L. B., Watson, J. C., . . . Goodrich, K. M. (2017). Standards of care for research with participants who identify as LGBTQ. *Journal of LGBT Issues in Counseling, 11*(4), 212–229. https://doi.org/10.1080/15538605.201 7.1380549.

Grzanka, P. R. (2020). From buzzword to critical psychology: An invitation to take intersectionality seriously. *Women & Therapy, 43*(3), 244–261. https://doi.org/10.1080/02703149.202 0.1729473.

Grzanka, P. R., Santos, C. E., & Moradi, B. (2017). Intersectionality research in counseling psychology. *Journal of Counseling Psychology, 64*(5), 453–457. https://doi.org/10.1037/cou0000237.

Hafford-Letchfield, T., Simpson, P., Willis, P. B., & Almack, K. (2018). Developing inclusive residential care for older lesbian, gay, bisexual and trans (LGBT) people: An evaluation of the *Care Home Challenge* action research project. *Health & Social Care in the Community, 26*(2), e312–e320. https://doi.org/10.1111/hsc.12521.

Hankivsky, O., Grace, D., Hunting, G., Giesbrecht, M., Fridkin, A., Rudrum, S., Ferlatte, O., & Clark, N. (2014). An intersectionality-based policy analysis framework: Critical reflections on a methodology for advancing equity. *International Journal for Equity in Health, 13*(1), 50–78. https://doi.org/10.1186/s12939-014-0119-x.

Hash, K. M., & Rogers, A. (2017). Introduction to LGBT aging. *Annual Review of Gerontology & Geriatrics, 37*(1), 1–12. https://doi.org/10.1891/0198-8794.37.1.

Hillman, J. (2017). The sexuality and sexual health of LGBT elders. *Annual Review of Gerontology and Geriatrics, 37*(1), 13–26. https://doi.org/10.1891/0198-8794.37.13.

Hooks, B. (1984). *Feminist theory: From margin to center.* Boston: South End Press.

Hoy-Ellis, C. P., & Fredriksen-Goldsen, K. I. (2017). Depression among transgender older adults: General and minority stress. *American Journal of Community Psychology, 59*(3–4), 295–305. https://doi.org/10.1002/ajcp.12138.

Jen, S., Stewart, D., & Woody, I. (2020). Serving LGBTQ/SGL elders during the novel corona virus (COVID-19) pandemic: Striving for justice, recognizing resilience. *Journal of Gerontological Social Work, 63*(6–7), 607–610. https://doi.org/10.1080/01634372.2020.1793255.

Johnson Shen, M., Freeman, R., Karpiak, S., Brennan-Ing, M., Seidel, L., & Siegler, E. L. (2019). The intersectionality of stigmas among key populations of older adults affected by HIV: A thematic analysis. *Clinical Gerontologist, 42*(2), 137–149. https://doi.org/10.1080/07317115.2018.1456500.

Kim, H., Jen, S., & Fredriksen-Goldsen, K. I. (2017). Race/Ethnicity and health-related quality of life among LGBT older adults. *The Gerontologist, 57*(1), S30–S39. https://doi.org/1093/geront/gnw172.

Kim, H.-J., Jen, S., & Fredriksen-Goldsen, K. I. (2017). Race/ethnicity and health-related quality of life among LGBT older adults. *The Gerontologist, 57*(Suppl 1), 39. https://doi.org/10.1093/geront/gnw172.

King, S. D., & Richardson, V. E. (2017). Mental health for older LGBT adults. *Annual Review of Gerontology & Geriatrics, 37*(1), 59–75. https://doi.org/10.1891/0198-8794.37.59.

Lecompte, M., Ducharme, J., Beauchamp, J., & Couture, M. (2020). Inclusive practices toward LGBT older adults in healthcare and social services: A scoping review of quantitative and qualitative evidence. *Clinical Gerontologist*, 1–12. https://doi.org/10.1080/07317115.2020.1862946.

Linscott, B., & Krinsky, L. (2016). Engaging underserved populations: Outreach to LGBT elders of color. *Generations, 40*(2), 34–37.

Lorde, A. (1984). *Sister outsider: Essays and speeches.* Trumansburg, NY: Crossing Press.

McCann, E., & Brown, M. J. (2019). The mental health needs and concerns of older people who identify as LGBTQ: A narrative review of the international evidence. *Journal of Advanced Nursing, 75*(12), 3390–3403. https://doi.org/10.1111/jan.14193.

Meyer, I. H. (1995). Minority stress and mental health in gay men. *Journal of Health and Social Behavior, 36*(1), 38–56. https://doi.org/10.2307/2137286.

Meyer, I. H. (2003). Prejudice, social stress, and mental health in lesbian, gay, and bisexual populations: Conceptual issues and research evidence. *Psychological Bulletin, 129*(5), 674–697. https://doi.org/10.1037/0033-2909.129.5.674.

Meyer, I. H. (2010). Identity, stress, and resilience in lesbians, gay men, and bisexuals of color. *The Counseling Psychologist, 38*(3), 442–454. https://doi.org/10.1177/0011000009351601.

Meyer, I. H. (2015). Resilience in the study of minority stress and health of sexual and gender minorities. *Psychology of Sexual Orientation and Gender Diversity, 2*(3), 209–213. https://doi.org/10.1037/sgd0000132.

Meyer, I. H. (2020). Rejection sensitivity and minority stress: A challenge for clinicians and interventionists. *Archives of Sexual Behavior, 49*(7), 2287–2289. https://doi.org/10.1007/s10508-019-01597-7.

Meyer, I. H. & Choi, S. K. (2020). *Vulnerabilities to COVID-19 among older LGBT adults in California*. The Williams Institute. Retrieved from https://williamsinstitute.law.ucla.edu/publications/older-lgbt-covid-ca

Moradi, B., & Grzanka, P. R. (2017). Using intersectionality responsibly: Toward critical epistemology, structural analysis, and social justice activism. *Journal of Counseling Psychology, 64*(5), 500–513. https://doi.org/10.1037/cou0000203.

Moraga, C., & Anzaldúa, G. (Eds.). (1983). *This bridge called my back: Writings by radical women of color* (2nd ed.). New York: Kitchen Table/Women of Color Press.

Porter, K. E., & Krinsky, L. (2014). Do LGBT aging trainings effectuate positive change in mainstream elder service providers? *Journal of Homosexuality, 61*(1), 197–216.

Porter, K. E., Brennan-Ing, M., Chang, S. C., dickey, l. m., Singh, A. A., Bower, K. L., & Witten, T. M. (2016). Providing competent and affirming services for transgender and gender nonconforming older adults. *Clinical Gerontologist, 39*(5), 366–388. https://doi.org/10.1080/07317115.2016.1203383.

Putney, J. M., Hebert, N., Snyder, M., Linscott, R. O., & Cahill, S. (2020). The housing needs of sexual and gender minority older adults: Implications for policy and practice. *Journal of Homosexuality*, 1–18. https://doi.org/10.1080/00918369.2020.1804261.

Putney, J. M., Keary, S., Hebert, N., Krinsky, L., & Halmo, R. (2018). "Fear runs deep:" The anticipated needs of LGBT older adults in long-term care. *Journal of Gerontological Social Work, 61*(8), 887–907. https://doi.org/10.1080/01634372.2018.1508109.

Robson, C., Gutman, G., Marchbank, J., & Kelsey, B. (2018). Raising awareness and addressing elder abuse in the LGBT community: An intergenerational arts project. *Language and Literacy, 20*(3), 46–66. https://doi.org/10.20360/langandlit29408.

Schubert, A., & Pope, M. (2020). Sexuality beyond young adulthood: Affordances and barriers to sexual expression in the nursing home. *Journal of Counseling Sexology & Sexual Wellness: Research, Practice, and Education, 2*(1), 35–47. https://doi.org/10.34296/02011022.

Serafin, J., Smith, G. B., & Keltz, T. (2013). Lesbian, gay, bisexual, and transgender (LGBT) elders in nursing homes: It's time to clean out the closet. *Geriatric Nursing, 34*(1), 81–83. https://doi.org/10.1016/S0197-4572(12)90405-X.

Singh, A. A. (2019). *The racial healing handbook: Practical activities to help you challenge privilege, confront systemic racism, and engage in collective healing*. Oakland, CA: New Harbinger Publications.

Singh, A. A., Appling, B., & Trepal, H. (2020). Using the multicultural and social justice counseling competencies to decolonize counseling practice: The important roles of theory, power, and action. *Journal of Counseling & Development, 98*(3), 261–271. https://doi.org/10.1002/jcad.12321.

South, K. T. (2017). The impact of public policy on LGBT aging. *Annual Review of Gerontology & Geriatrics, 37*, 161–174. https://doi.org/10.1891/0198-8794.37.161.

Sue, D. W., Sue, D., Neville, H. A., & Smith, L. (2019). *Counseling the culturally diverse: Theory and practice* (8th ed.). Hoboken, NJ: Wiley.

Talley, A. E., Gilbert, P. A., Mitchell, J., Goldbach, J., Marshall, B. D. L., & Kaysen, D. (2016). Addressing gaps on risk and resilience factors for alcohol use outcomes in sexual and gender minority populations. *Drug and Alcohol Review, 35*(4), 484–493. https://doi.org/10.1111/dar.12387.

Van Sluytman, L. G., & Torres, D. (2014). Hidden or uninvited? A content analysis of elder LGBT of color literature in gerontology. *Journal of Gerontological Social Work, 57*(2–4), 130–160. https://doi.org/10.1080/01634372.2013.877551.

Warner, L., Settles, I., & Shields, S. (2016). Invited reflection: Intersectionality as an epistemological challenge to psychology. *Psychology of Women Quarterly, 40*(2), 171–176. https://doi.org/10.1177/0361684316641384.

Westwood, S. (2019). Abuse and older lesbian, gay bisexual, and trans (LGBT) people: A commentary and research agenda. *Journal of Elder Abuse & Neglect, 31*(2), 97–114. https://doi.org/10.1080/08946566.2018.1543624.

Witten, T. M. (2012). The aging of sexual and gender minority persons: An overview. In T. M. Witten & A. E. Eyler (Eds.), *Gay, lesbian, bisexual & transgender aging: Challenges in research, practice, and policy* (pp. 1–58). Baltimore, MD: The Johns Hopkins University Press.

Woody, I. (2014). Aging out: A qualitative exploration of ageism and heterosexism among aging African American lesbians and gay men. *Journal of Homosexuality, 61*(1), 145–165.

Woody, I. (2015). Lift every voice: Voices of African-American lesbian elders. *Journal of Lesbian Studies, 19*(1), 50–58. https://doi.org/10.1080/10894160.2015.972755.

Yarns, B. C., Abrams, J. M., Meeks, T. W., & Sewell, D. D. (2016). The mental health of older LGBT adults. *Current Psychiatry Reports, 18*(6), 1–11. https://doi.org/10.1007/s11920-016-0697-y.

Zelle, A., & Arms, T. (2015). Psychosocial effects of health disparities of lesbian, gay, bisexual, and transgender older adults. *Journal of Psychosocial Nursing and Mental Health Services, 53*(7), 25–30. https://doi.org/10.3928/02793695-20150623-04.

Queer Vocational and Workplace Considerations

Sarah N. Baquet, Vincent M. Marasco, and Jehan A. Hill

1 Queer Vocational and Workplace Considerations

To understand the career experiences of queer-identified persons, it is necessary to examine the significance of cultural contexts and systemic influences, as well as the policies and political realities that shape the world of work within the United States. This chapter aims to address the career and workplace considerations of queer individuals by highlighting (1) intersectional and queer theory, (2) emergent career issues including political and social issues and, (3) career development theory considerations. Authors conclude with the theoretical case application of August, a mid-career non-binary queer person who is seeking career counseling. The authors recognize the increasing inclusivity of lesbian, gay, bisexual, transgender, gender expansive, queer, intersex, asexual, and pansexual (LGBTGEQIAP+) communities. The word queer has been reclaimed from its original derogatory origins and is now widely used to describe individuals who identify within the broader LGBTGEQIAP+ communities. Therefore, 'queer' will be used throughout this chapter in reference to any individuals who identify within these distinct communities (Fig. 1).

S. N. Baquet (✉)
Department of School Psychology, Counseling, and Leadership, Brooklyn College-City University of New York, Brooklyn, NY, USA
e-mail: Sarah.Baquet@brooklyn.cuny.edu

V. M. Marasco
School of Education and Counseling, Purdue University Northwest, Hammond, IN, USA
e-mail: vmarasco@pnw.edu

J. A. Hill
Department of Counseling and Higher Education, Northern Illinois University, DeKalb, IL, USA
e-mail: jhill2@niu.edu

© The Author(s), under exclusive license to Springer Nature Switzerland AG 2021
K. L. Nadal and M. R. Scharrón-del Río (ed.), *Queer Psychology*,
https://doi.org/10.1007/978-3-030-74146-4_14

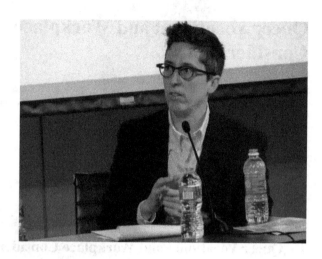

Fig. 1 Graphic Artist Alison Bechdel discusses her work at the Queers & Comics Conference in 2015. Photo Courtesy of Center for LGBTQ Studies

2 Queer Theory and Intersectionality Framework

To understand the workplace experiences and career development of queer individuals, it is necessary to engage with Queer and Intersectional Theory. More specifically, embodying Queer Theory through an intersectional framework when working with the queer population is essential to dismantle the systemic heterosexist and gendered ideologies of the workplace. Scholars have noted that Queer theory alone does not adequately integrate intersectional concepts when discussing systemic social justice concerns (Cor et al., 2018). However, with an intersectional lens, practitioners are better equipped in addressing the complex nature of additional social inequities layered within the dominant ideologies of the workplace. In the following section, the authors briefly outline the integration of an intersectional framework with the major tenants of queer theory.

Both intersectionality and queer theory strive to dismantle and challenge social structures. By integrating intersectional thought and key queer theory tenants, practitioners can initiate and validate the critical exploration of the limitations, lived experiences, and career adaptability of queer individuals. Queer theory is a postmodern philosophy that guides focus to deconstruct binary constructs such as female/male or gay/straight. It is useful to confront restrictive social constructs within workplace settings such as gender performance and sexual identity classifications (Goodrich et al., 2016; Plummer, 2005). Queer theory predicates that inherent in cultural systems like the workplace, power is used to shape meaningful institutional practices based on sex and gender, which therefore must be scrutinized and dismantled (Carroll & Gilroy, 2001; Manalansan, 2015). In clinical work, queer theory has informed affirmative practices which are used to actively promote the well-being of various sexual and gender identities and expressions. Affirming practices are essential given the unique "affectional and developmental experiences" of queer individuals (Ginicola et al., 2017, p. ix), and the compounding effects of stress on minority individuals (Meyer, 2014).

The integration of an intersectional framework, which originated from Black feminist scholarship and shifted the moral priorities of feminist inclusivity (Knapp, 2005), requires examination of the process by which individuals negotiate the fluidity, variability, and interactive processes that occur between and within their social identities, social groupings, institutions, and social practices (Bowleg, 2008; Collins & Bilge, 2016). This is critical in providing affirmative career counseling as an individual's social identities not only deeply impact one's lived experiences, but their beliefs about and understanding of gender and sexuality (Choo & Ferree, 2010). Key connecting elements that emerged as scholars engaged in queer- intersectional frameworks are the acknowledgment of identity intersections creating both oppression and opportunity; identities manifest social groupings, invisibility, subordination, and hierarchies; and the importance of equity, social action, and social justice paradigms (Collins & Bilge, 2016). Both Queer and intersectional frameworks are important in the identification of emergent queer issues in the workplace.

3   Emergent Career Issues

Title VII of the Civil Rights Act XE "Civil Rights Act" (1964) was a founding legislative action which codifies equal workplace protections and opportunity of all individuals living within the United States, regardless of race, class, religion, sex, or community of origin. This advocacy-based legal protection theoretically shielded employees of all backgrounds from discriminatory workplace decision-making within the federal government, public and private sectors, employment agencies and labor organizations; and is enforced by the Equal Employment Opportunity Commission (Dorton, 2020). However, queer individuals have not explicitly been protected in the workplace, creating a civil rights gap within the original 1964 legislative law. The Equality Act (2019) would ensure full federal non-discrimination protections, adding both *sexual orientation and gender identity* to the protected classes within the existing laws. In June 2020, The United States Supreme Court ruled in Bostock v. Clayton County XE "Bostock v. Clayton County" (2020) that gender identity and sexual orientation are included under the definition of "sex" as defined in Title VII, a landmark case for queer workplace rights. This ruling does not address states with at-will employment legislation.

Although a promising forward movement for the rights of queer persons in workplace settings, homophobic and heterosexist policies and decision-making procedures continue to exist in areas such as housing, employment, and healthcare (Buddel, 2011; Dorton, 2020). Workplace policies have been noted as "empty promises" as they often do not offer enough applicable protections (Lloren & Parini, 2017, p. 299). Rather, individual states, municipalities, and businesses have had to establish and implement protective policies to offer protections (American Civil Liberties Union [ACLU] 2020). This demonstrates the continued importance of workplace protections and anti-discrimination advocacy while also highlighting the critical significance of understanding the impact of dominant systemic ideologies on career experiences for queer-identified persons.

3.1 Dominant Workplace Ideologies

Advances in creating social equity have recently gained momentum politically; however, dominant social ideologies continue to impact the career experiences of queer individuals. Connections between capitalism, social class structure, and scripts of the dominant culture within the U.S. have been noted in the literature, highlighting problematic, meritocratic belief systems that further marginalize queer and oppressed populations (Smith, 2005). As continued employment and career development is a precursor to social class mobility, these systemic ideologies keep queer-identified persons in a cycle of poverty and fuel classism (Burnes & Singh, 2016). Social class structures highlight the need for additional career considerations connected to the lack of access to various forms of capital queer individuals experience throughout their career lives.

Further, sexist and genderist belief systems can be seen when examining the historical institution of work in the U.S. and holds continued prominence within professional contexts. Heteronormativity, or the presumption of heterosexuality, permeates every facet of career experience. The systemically sexist, gendered, heteronormative belief systems present within the U.S. workforce creates fear surrounding the queer identity, stigmatizes any non-heterosexual form of behavior (i.e., homophobia), creates privilege surrounding the heterosexual identity, and leads to deeply engrained workplace discrimination (Buddel, 2011). Much of the literature on queer individual experience in the workplace is often conducted through the dominant lens, using racially and culturally homogenous participant samples; and therefore, fails to capture the unique intersections (i.e., race, sexual/gender identity, age, ability) on workplace discrimination experiences (Cheng et al., 2017) (Fig. 2).

3.2 Discrimination in the Workplace

Discrimination in the workplace is a common experience for queer-identified persons, and research has demonstrated that many queer individuals anticipate discrimination as a part of their career and employment (Parnell et al., 2012). Scholars have examined types of discrimination experienced and found queer individuals experience verbal stigmatization and intrusive questions; exclusion from work teams, projects, and social opportunities; and moral and physical harassment (DeSouza et al., 2017; Lloren & Parini, 2017). Those who experience discrimination often face both covert discrimination (disguised or subtle prejudice) and overt discrimination (open expression of prejudice) simultaneously throughout their career lifespan. Covert discrimination (i.e., daily microaggressions) can lead to a

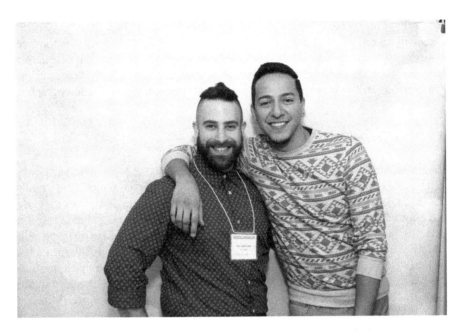

Fig. 2 Two friends attending an LGBTQ community event. Photo courtesy of Center for LGBTQ Studies

greater level of internalized self-doubt compared to experiences of overt workplace racism, though both contribute to workplace trauma. These experiences saturate the career cycle of individuals with oppressed and marginalized identities, and includes job selection (Abrams et al., 2016), access to fair wages (Devaraj et al., 2018), and the emotional stress when encountering adversity in the work environment (Miner & Costa, 2018).

3.2.1 Sexism and Genderism

Sexism typically refers to prejudices and discrimination based upon the biological sex of an individual. Genderism, like sexism, is discrimination based on gender identity and expression, and recognizes the many forms of gender variance and expression. Sexism has been conflated with genderism, making it challenging to ignore Western societies historical marginalization and oppression of the female gender (Dahl, 2015) and gender minorities. This historical perspective has shaped societal expectations and communication with genders deemed lower (e.g. female, transgender) by the constructed Western social scale which greatly influences one's vocational identity and journey. Observing hostile sexism in the workplace also negatively impacts performance, self-esteem, and career goals for women, while empowering male counterparts (Bradley-Geist et al., 2015). This discrepancy underlines the impact that sexism and genderism have on career aspirations. Within the work setting, perspectives of gender minorities are often not represented. This is especially true for transgender individuals whose voices go unheard in workplace contributing to exclusivity and isolation in the professional environment (Alexandra Beauregard et al., 2018). The absences of genderqueer and female voices in the career setting creates problematic dynamics, further marginalizing this demographic.

3.2.2 Heterosexism

Heterosexism represents an ideology within the U.S. that grants privilege and power to heterosexuals while systemically marginalizing queer communities (Chesir-Teran, 2003). Heterosexism is rampant in the education system, impacting the early stages of career development of queer youth (Chesir-Teran, 2003), continuing as a part of young adulthood during career selection (Douglass et al., 2017), and ultimately impacting job satisfaction (Miner & Costa, 2018). Heterosexism in the workplace contributes to lower job satisfaction and complex psychological impacts for queer individuals. Heterosexist workplace environments Heterosexist workplace have also been shown to increase levels of fear and anger of employees (Miner & Costa, 2018). Systemic heterosexism creates experiences of invisibility and perpetuates discrimination based on sexual identity both within and outside career identity formation. Sexual minorities encounter both external and internal stress from societal expectations (Meyer, 2010, 2014; Sutter & Perrin, 2016). Meyer, (2010, 2014) described this phenomenon as minority stress and specifically attributed it to the experiences that queer individuals face. Queer individuals experience added stress in the workplace from feelings of obligation to disclose their sexual orientation; a conflicting stress from feeling pressure to hide a part of their identity; and stress from internalizing messages of negativity and oppression (Meyer, 2010, 2014; Sutter & Perrin, 2016), referred to as internalized homophobia. Examples of heterosexism include an employer's presumptions of heterosexuality and refusal to integrate a partner into work-life due to the view of marriage as a heteronormative institution (Buddel, 2011). These discriminatory experiences and internalization of negative messages is compounded when the individual faces multiple, marginal social status such as race.

3.2.3 Racism

Racism is deeply embedded in Western society, and this pervasive structure of oppressive power is intended to benefit those of the dominant culture while creating systemic barriers for ethnic and racial minorities (Delgado & Stefancic, 2012). Racism is prevalent through all aspects of a person of color's (POC) career journey, starting with the school system and leading into the workforce. Educational institutions are situated within the dominant White cultural lens, and perspectives outside of this worldview are dismissed and their relevance questioned within the classroom (Delgado Bernal, 2002; Delgado & Stefancic, 2012; Haskins & Singh, 2015). When setting career goals as adolescents, the anticipation of racial discrimination during their career journey impacts students of color when examining their career self-efficacy and decision-making process (Conkel-Ziebell et al., 2019). Once a POC enters the workforce, their skin color impacts their ability to advance their income. A study conducted by Devaraj et al., (2018), suggested that "darker skin tone is negatively related to income" (p. 15). Highlighting the inequitable access to fair wages based on phenotype and social constructs of race, and the preferences for certain lighter skin tones over darker tones. For queer POC, common vernacular associated with coming out and understanding diversity are rooted in White, dominant systems reinforcing the idea of conformity to Western standards. Companies which seek to promote inclusivity within the workplace often utilize diversity frameworks situated in White normativity translating to a corporate approach to multiculturism (Ward, 2008) which further marginalizes queer POC in the work setting.

3.2.4   Ageism

Roughly 48 million Americans aged 65 year or older reside in the United States (United States Census Bureau, 2018). This number is projected to grow with the number of older Americans expected to be one in five by 2030 (Rural Health Information Hub, n.d.). Unfortunately, negative stereotypes associated with aging, known as ageism, are also on the rise (Myers & Shannonhouse, 2012; Ng et al., 2015). Ageism, especially rampant in societies which emphasize youth-centered social structures, influences job satisfaction (Macdonald & Levy, 2016) and work engagement (Bayl & Griffin, 2014). In addition to the on-the-job implications, ageism also impacts an applicant's opportunity to secure new job placement. Abrams et al., (2016) found that when reviewing job applicants, younger appearing profiles are shown higher preference than older appearing applicants. Despite many positive career characteristics associated with ageing, ageism can impact older adults' vocational experiences based on the bias's society holds regarding aging. Furthermore, queer identifying older adults have experienced years of oppressive work environments and policies pathologizing sexual identity. This discrimination leads to fear based protective factors which could include engaging in a heterosexual relationship in order to be perceived as passing to advance within the workplace (Burlew & Wise, 2017). For queer older adults, systemic oppression related to past and present discrimination has impacted the work environment and career advancement.

3.2.5   Ableism

Ableism refers to the invalidation of a person's ability level and permeates society, impacting the lives of individuals with physical, cognitive and psychiatric disability (Smart, 2012). Dominant ableist beliefs marginalize and oppress people with disabilities (PWD), creating systemic barriers "which in turn compromises their opportunities to convert it into economic, cultural, social and emotional capital" (Loja et al., 2013, p. 200). Many of these compromised opportunities impact PWD throughout their career cycle, where ableism influences recruitment, hiring, career advancement and socialization (Bonaccio et al., 2020). For example, individuals who are d/Deaf or Hard-of-Hearing (HH) encounter the pressures to adhere to standards of the dominant culture in order to experience professional success. While facing the pressure to assimilate to the dominant culture, they are concurrently encountering adversity such as needing to be the sole voice of d/Deaf or HH community in the workplace (Howells, 2018). Queer PWD encounter multiple oppressive factors, including the process of coming out regarding their sexual identity and disclosing their disability (Miller et al., 2019). These intersecting identities highlight how ingrained heteronormativity and ableism is in the workplace, creating systemic barriers throughout the career cycle, impacting career placement and advancement for individuals with disabilities.

4 Affirming Career Development Framework

Career development theories examine pathways toward enhancing professional growth and job satisfaction, as well as a person's overall career trajectory. Career development occurs across the lifespan and is not static as individuals continue to explore interests and opportunities. Acknowledgment of career theory is helpful in conceptualizing client issues in career counseling. As outlined in the above sections, for Queer identifying individuals, the career journey is influenced by oppressive institutional and societal heterosexism (Meyer, 2010, 2014; Sutter & Perrin, 2016). Queer people deal with multiple obstacles including but not limited to isolation, rejection, and workplace identity challenges, often leading to an impaired sense of self (Grossman & D'Augelli, 2007; Maree, 2014). The uniqueness associated with the career development of the queer community and their intersecting identities should be understood by mental health professionals in order to provide affirming career counseling services (Roland & Burlew, 2017). Due to the importance of a queer affirming and intersectional paradigm, the authors highlight the integration of two major career theories which can be uniquely positioned within a queer affirming and intersectional lens, to serve clients who hold marginalized identity statuses within the workplace; Super's Lifespan Life Space Model and Savickas's Career Constructionist Theory.

4.1 Lifespan Life Space and Career Construction

When utilizing Super's Lifespan Life Space model, counselors can focus on career maturity which balances the idea of choice, ability level, and interests (Super, 1955). Savickas's Career Constructionist theory explores career adaptability, which refers to barrier's individuals encounter within themselves, society, and the work environment that influences the construction of their career story (1997). Authors explore career development considerations that occur from adolescence to older adulthood through the lens of Super (1980, 1990) approach and Savickas's developmental tasks of career adaptability (1997, 2005).

4.1.1   Early

Adolescents and early adulthood signify a critical time in career and sexual identity development. According to Super (1980), 1990), adolescents begin to understand how their values impact career goals and crystallize their vocational plans. Once they reach their mid-twenties, many begin to implement their vocational goals. Expanding upon Super's developmental model, the career construction theory (Savickas, 2005) has similar tasks in adolescents and early adulthood. During this period, individuals explore career options, searching for occupations based upon access to resources and knowledge. For queer folks, the adversity experienced from external and internal stressors takes precedent, impacting vocational processes (Belz, 1993). Progress through these developmental career tasks may be affected due to the experiences associated with having an oppressed identity (Schmidt & Nilsson, 2006). When engaging in career explorations, counselors need to take into consideration the client holistically. Career planning is a unique part of the vast identity development occurring during this stage in an individual lifespan (Norman et al., 2017).

4.1.2   Middle

As adolescents and early adults transition into careers, they begin middle adulthood. At this time, the integration of sexual identity as part of self-concept is helpful to all aspects of well-being, including career aspirations (Schmidt & Nilsson, 2006). During this stage, which Super (1990) suggests ranges from 25 to 45, individuals establish themselves in a career in which they will remain over many years. Savickas, (2005) describes a cycle for adults in middle or later years where individuals select a job, reach a point where they no longer find opportunities for advancement, and then begin to disengage from the occupation. Depending on the place in life, many may select a new position or begin the stages of entering retirement. Career constructionist theory recognizes the power the dominant cultural holds on the career journey, Savickas, (2005) described it as the following: "individuals mentally structure the story of their own work life using the social structure provided by society's grand narrative of a career" (p. 49), implying the pressure associated with societal expectations to achieve certain career goals regardless of adversity. For counselors working with queer individuals during this stage in their career journey, Dispenza & Pulliam, (2017) suggest recognizing the uniqueness of each client, becoming aware of multicultural competencies (Ratts et al., 2016), and approaching the client from a place of affirmation and empathy.

4.1.3 Later Life

Once an individual reaches the age of 45, Super (1990) suggests people reach a stage of maintaining the level of career advancement that they have achieved. Once they begin to reach the age of retirement, they also may begin the process disengaging from certain work-related activities. As discussed previously, Savickas, (2005) also utilized the term disengagement to describe this transition to retirement. For queer clients, it imperative for counselors to be cognizant of stigmatization, legal discrimination, and prejudices that the older population has encountered. Their career selection was impacted by safety concerns, and potentially needing to keep a part of their identity invisible to maintain employment (Burlew & Wise, 2017). Further, due to the implications of stigma and discrimination on career success and social class, many queer individuals may not experience the same sense of financial security needed for career disengagement and retirement (Burnes & Singh, 2016). Career constructionist theory connects with this reality encountered by queer older adults, who may have felt pressure to structure their career story around narratives dictated by dominate society regarding who is worthy to work. Career counselors should be aware of historical injustices encountered by clients and help them process adversity and make meaning of their lived experiences. Counselors should be prepared to discuss resources and social support with their clients, while also exploring career or retirement satisfaction (Burlew & Wise, 2017) (Fig. 3).

5 Case of August

In this section, the authors explore how career counselors can utilize affirmative career counseling practice through the examination of August, a fictional client based on real-life client interaction and experience. The authors outline the considerations for the counseling process and demonstrate specific interventions under a career constructivist framework for providing August with affirming, comprehensive, and effective career counseling services.

Our case study client, who goes by the name August, is a 39-year-old Multi-Ethnic Person of Color (POC) with a Bachelor of Arts degree in Business Marketing, and recently completed their Master of Science in Advertising. August does not identify within a gender binary system, shares they are gender fluid, bisexual, and uses they/their/them pronouns. August resides in an urban community in a large metropolitan area with their partner Sam. August discloses that although once close with their immediate family unit, they now have little-to-no contact due intolerance and homophobic discourse in their family. August is originally from a rural town and moved to the city almost 20 years ago to pursue a career in Business Marketing

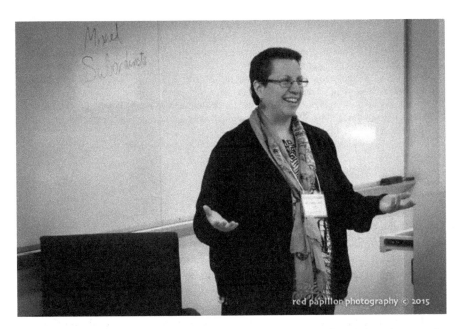

Fig. 3 Dr. Marie Miville (a Latina lesbian counseling psychology professor) shares her expertise at an conference. Photo Courtesy of Riya Ortiz/Red Papillon Photography

while seeking acceptance and understanding from new communities. August is seeking career counseling services specifically to explore her growing dissatisfaction with their current role as the Digital Communications Support Coordinator for a large pharmaceutical company. They disclose that they often feel drained, unmotivated, and angry after a workday, unable to decompress even on days off. August shares that they have not felt as if they can connect with anyone in the workplace, which is important for their career satisfaction, and discloses that they have started to feel this disconnection within their social and supportive communities outside of work. August is considering leaving the company for new opportunities. However, this is a major decision that will greatly impact August's long-term career goals, as they have been with the same company for 15 years and feels they have been ready for a leadership position for some time now. August has discussed their professional relationships with coworkers and describes few individuals that identify as allies who "still don't get it sometimes," and recounts an instance in which an offensive advertisement was developed by a former coworker. Additionally, with their recent completion of a master's degree in marketing, August is eligible for a new opening of Marketing Director. This position would significantly increase their visibility, salary, and leadership power within the company. These variables are particularly important in their consideration, as August shares they have often felt overlooked for previous promotions; one of the driving forces behind their motivation for completing their master's degree. They share with you,

"I often feel overlooked within my department in the company and have never been considered for promotions that I worked hard for. Sometimes it feels like I have to work twice as hard as my counterparts to receive any recognition at all. I know I look, dress, speak, and carry myself different than many of my professional peers. Sometimes I wonder if the comments I hear are reportable to human resources. I had one manager in my early career tell me I did not have what it takes to lead a team because I am intimidating, and people cannot relate to me. Something he stated was essential within the Business Marketing field. I also feel let down, I thought marketing would be much more accepting for someone like me, but I haven't always felt that way".

5.1 Case Discussion

The infusion of affirmative practices, intersectional queer theory, and career counseling begins at the outset of the therapeutic alliance, and includes practices such as using gender inclusive intake forms, creating a professional environment conducive to safety and acceptance, discussing client and counselor identities (e.g., personal pronouns, stage of queer- and racial-identity development), honest discussions of power and privilege, and an initial identification of relevant treatment goals informed by client values and strengths. August is a queer-identified bisexual, multi-ethnic individual with an advanced degree who experiences different levels of privilege and marginalization. For example, privilege due to an advanced degree, potential marginalization via erasure of their bisexual identity, and has experiences of discrimination based on their multi-ethnic identity. Work with August must also include awareness of their developmental stage and where they are at in their coming out processes. August is entering a point in their career where they feel discouraged regarding advancement in their current position. August's mid-life career reassessment and reported feelings of anger are a result of layered contextual and cultural variables within the workplace setting (i.e., imposter syndrome; feeling othered; isolation; lack of collegial support; overlooked for earned promotion). Many of these professional interactions are driven by systemic racism and heterosexism within the workplace and are perpetrated by individuals in leadership roles. Thus, rendering the client invisible for advancement and promotion. The contextual dimensions and existing information provided underscore the professional frustration and dissatisfaction reported by August. The structuring of their career narrative is heavily influenced by societal biases associated with their intersecting identities causing them to explore other career opportunities rather than feeling secure within their current occupation. August's discussion of potential professional allies encapsulates the often-isolating experiences of queer persons in their workplaces.

Collaboration with August is useful to identify and define their presenting problem(s) and treatment goal(s), while relying on August's expertise in their own lives is critical. Allowing collaboration to guide goal setting in treatment increases cultural sensitivity, particularly how counselor positionality informs assumptions regarding goal setting. The counselor can then work to avoid integrating personal bias about presenting concerns. Potential goals in the case of August may focus on building and reconstructing their career narrative; developing coping skills to address negative outcomes of stress; development of communication and relationship skills to use with allied coworkers; and, making a decision whether to stay or leave their current company and accepting the decision. Additionally, affirmative counselors should include interventions which focus on resilience and building sources or communities of support outside of career environments.

5.2 Constructing and re-Authoring Career Narratives

As therapeutic rapport strengthens, August and the counselor can begin to focus on the *Career Construction Interview* (CCI), which will begin to outline August's *career life story* (Savickas, 2005). Central counselor characteristics needed include honesty, congruence, compassion, truthfulness, and mutual respect, which the counselor can communicate by utilizing person centered interventions such as self-disclosure, validation, active listening, and reflection of feeling (Maree, 2013). An affirming counselor guides the career life story process by encouraging August to narrate both career experiences and development, while articulating the subjective meaning-making of their life experiences.

Important considerations through CCI would include the counselor encouraging August to explore autobiographical accounts of how their intersecting identities have informed their interpersonal relationships, self-concept, significant work transitions, role models, and accounts of career decision-making. Once August and the counselor determine they have discussed a saturated account of August's career narrative, counseling transitions into exploring themes in understanding their verbal and behavioral content of career interviews. With themes processed, August and the counselor are able to re-author (also known as re-storying) their career and life story. This technique emphasizes that August is the expert in their own life, creates opportunity to discover new meaning, find healing with their current feelings of anger and disconnection, and re-establish their career identity. Additional interventions the counselor can explore with August while empowering their career decisions and affirming their experiences within a disaffirming workplace include externalization and deconstruction. Externalization can help August reframe their current workplace issues as external, meaning their problems are not inherently their own. Deconstruction, which is often helpful throughout theme identification, allows the counselor and August to break down larger issues (i.e., feelings of disconnection) to specific circumstances (i.e., receiving othering messages through a workplace ad) (Watson, 2013). This helps August clarify the key issues surrounding their decision making, externalize the problem(s), and reduce overgeneralization.

5.3 Case Conclusion

August's presenting career concerns are further compounded by a heterosexist work environment, where isolation and lack of support are impacting advancement in the company. This systemic barrier situated within their current workplace resulted in disengagement from a career that August has spent significant time cultivating experiences and skills in order to obtain a leadership position. Utilizing an affirmative career counseling approach, August and their counselor facilitated dialogue surrounding empowerment and addressed feelings associated with institutional and societal marginalization. Through career constructivist counseling, August was able to mentally restructure their own career story taking into account societal pressures based on dominant cultural expectations. This re-authoring of their story allowed August to engage in self-advocacy and inquire about workplace protections regarding discrimination in their current position. They also began to explore other pharmaceutical companies that promote inclusivity in the workplace and encourage transparency regarding promotion. August was able to understand their anger and disconnection which assisted their externalization of the specific workplace issues, ultimately leading to empowerment and enhanced self-concept. In order to address systemic oppressions, the counselor became involved in their counseling state organizations to advocate for legislative actions regarding discriminatory workplace practices.

References

Abrams, D., Swift, H. J., & Drury, L. (2016). Old and unemployable? How age-based stereotypes affect willingness to hire job candidates. *Journal of Social Issues, 72*(1), 105–121. https://doi-org.caldwell.idm.oclc.org/10.1111/josi.12158.

Alexandra Beauregard, T., Arevshatian, L., Booth, J. E., & Whittle, S. (2018). Listen carefully: Transgender voices in the workplace. *International Journal of Human Resource Management, 29*(5), 857–884. https://doi.org.caldwell.idm.oclc.org/10.1080/09585192.2016.1234503.

American Civil Liberties Union. (2020). *The rights of lesbian, gay, bisexual and transgender people*. American Civil Liberties Union. Retrieved from https://www.aclu.org/other/rights-lesbian-gay-bisexual-and-transgender-people

Bayl, S. P. H., & Griffin, B. (2014). Age discrimination in the workplace: Identifying as a late-career worker and its relationship with engagement and intended retirement age. *Journal of Applied Social Psychology, 44*(9), 588–599. https://doiorg.caldwell.idm.oclc.org/10.1111/jasp.1225.

Belz, J. R. (1993). Sexual orientation as a factor in career development. *The Career Development Quarterly, 41*(3), 197–200. https://doi.org/10.1002/j.2161-0045.1993.tb00370.x.

Bonaccio, S., Connelly, C. E., Gellatly, I. R., Jetha, A., & Martin Ginis, K. A. (2020). The participation of people with disabilities in the workplace across the employment cycle: Employer concerns and research evidence. *Journal of Business and Psychology, 35*, 135–158. https://doi.org/10.1007/s10869-018-9602-5.

Bostock v. Clayton County 590 US. (2020). Retrieved from https://www.oyez.org/cases/2019/17-1618

Bowleg, L. (2008). When black+lesbian+woman≠black lesbian Woman: The methodological challenges of qualitative and quantitative intersectionality research. *Sex Roles, 59*(3), 312–325. https://doi.org/10.1007/s11199-008-9400-z.

Bradley-Geist, J. C., Rivera, I., & Geringer, S. D. (2015). The collateral damage of ambient sexism: Observing sexism impacts bystander self-esteem and career aspirations. *Sex Roles, 73*, 29–42. https://doi.org/10.1007/s11199-015-0512-y.

Buddel, N. (2011). Queering the workplace. *Journal of Gay & Lesbian Social Services: The Quarterly Journal of Community & Clinical Practice, 23*(1), 131–146. https://doi.org/10.108 0/10538720.2010.530176.

Burlew, L. D., & Wise, S. (2017). Career development. In C. B. Roland & L. D. Burlew (Eds.), *Counseling LGBTQ adults throughout the life span*. Alexandria: American Counseling Association. Retrieved from http://www.counseling.org/knowledge-center/lgbtq-resources.

Burnes, T. R., & Singh, A. A. (2016). "Gay in the bank, queer in the streets": The intersection of LGBTQQ and social class identities. *Journal of LGBT Issues in Counseling, 10*(1), 55–71. https://doi.org/10.1080/15538605.2015.1138096.

Carroll, K., & Gilroy, P. J. (2001). Teaching "outside the box": Incorporating queer theory in counselor education. *Journal of Humanistic Counseling, Education & Development, 40*(1), 49–58.

Cheng, J., Klann, E. M., Zounlome, N. O. O., & Chung, Y. B. (2017). Promoting affirmative career development and work environment for LGBT individuals. In K. Maree (Ed.), *Psychology of career adaptability, employability and resilience* (pp. 265–282). Cham, Switzerland: Springer. https://doi.org/10.1007/978-3-319-66954-0_16.

Chesir-Teran, D. (2003). Conceptualizing and assessing heterosexism in high schools: A setting-level approach. *American Journal of Community Psychology, 31*(3), 267–279. http://dx.doi.org.caldwell.idm.oclc.org/10.1023/A:1023910820994.

Choo, H. Y., & Ferree, M. M. (2010). Practicing intersectionality in sociological research: A critical analysis of inclusions, interactions, and institutions in the study of inequalities. *Sociological Theory, 28*(2), 129–149.

Civil Rights Act of 1964, Pub. L. No. 88-352, 78 Stat. 241 (1964). Retrieved from https://www.dol.gov/agencies/oasam/centers-offices/civil-rights-center/statutes/title-vii-civil-rights-act-of-1964

Collins, P. H., & Bilge, S. (2016). Intersectionality. Cambridge: Polity.

Conkel-Ziebell, J. L., Gushue, G. V., & Turner, S. L. (2019). Anticipation of racism and sexism: Factors related to setting career goals for urban youth of color. *Journal of Counseling Psychology, 66*(5), 588–599. https://doi-org.caldwell.idm.oclc.org/10.1037/cou0000357.

Cor, D. N., Chan, C. D., & Pérez, J. C. (2018). Queering the curriculum: Queer intersectionality in counselor education. *Women and Language, 1*, 79.

Dahl, U. (2015). Sexism: A femme-inist perspective. *New Formations*, (86), 54–73. http://dx.doi.org.caldwell.idm.oclc.org/10.3898/NEWF.86.03.2015.

Delgado Bernal, D. (2002). Critical race theory, latCrit theory and critical race gendered epistemologies: Recognizing students of color as holders and creators of knowledge. *Qualitative Inquiry, 8*(1), 105–126.

Delgado, R., & Stefancic, J. (2012). *Critical race theory: An introduction* (2nd ed.). New York: New York University Press.

DeSouza, E. R., Wesselman, E. D., & Ipsas, D. (2017). Workplace discrimination against sexual minorities: Subtle and not-so-subtle. *Canadian Journal of Administrative Sciences/Revue Canadienne des Sciences de l'Administration, 34*(2), 121–132. https://doi.org/10.1002/cjas.1438.

Devaraj, S., Quigley, N. R., & Patel, P. C. (2018). The effects of skin tone, height, and gender on earnings. *PLoS One, 13*(1) http://dx.doi.org.caldwell.idm.oclc.org/10.1371/journal.pone.0190640.

Dispenza, F., & Pulliam, N. (2017). Career development. In C. B. Roland & L. D. Burlew (Eds.), *Counseling LGBTQ adults throughout the life span*. Alexandria: American Counseling Association. Retrieved from http://www.counseling.org/knowledge-center/lgbtq-resources.

Dorton, K. (2020). Who is going to protect the LGBTQ community from discrimination—Congress or the courts? *Campbell Law Review, 42*(2).

Douglass, R. P., Velez, B. L., Conlin, S. E., Duffy, R. D., & England, J. W. (2017). Examining the psychology of working theory: Decent work among sexual minorities. *Journal of Counseling Psychology, 64*(5), 550–559. https://doiorg.caldwell.idm.oclc.org/10.1037/cou0000212.

Equality Act, H.R.5, 116th Cong. (2019). Retrieved from https://www.congress.gov/bill/116th-congress/house-bill/5/text

Ginicola, M. M., Smith, C., & Filmore, J. M. (2017). Preface. In M. M. Ginicola, C. Smith, & J. M. Filmore (Eds.), *Affirmative counseling with LGBTQI+ people* (pp. ix–xiii). Alexandria, VA: ACA.

Goodrich, K. M., Luke, M., & Smith, A. J. (2016). Queer humanism: Toward epistemology of socially just, culturally responsive change. *Journal of Humanistic Psychology, 56*(6), 612–623. https://doi.org/10.1177/0022167816652534.

Grossman, A. H., & D'Augelli, A. R. (2007). Transgender youth and life-threatening behaviors. *Suicide & Life Threatening Behavior, 37*(5), 527–537.

Haskins, N. H., & Singh, A. (2015). Critical race theory and counselor education pedagogy: Creating equitable training. *Counselor Education and Supervision, 54*(4), 288–301. https://doi.org/10.1002/ceas.12027.

Howells, R. C.. (2018). *Can you hear me now?: Exploring the experiences of students who are d/deaf and hard of hearing in CACREP accredited counseling programs*. Doctoral Dissertation, Idaho State University.

Knapp, G-A. (2005). Race, Class, Gender: Reclaiming Baggage in Fast Travelling Theories. *European Journal of Women's Studies. 12*(3):249–265. https://doi.org/10.1177/1350506805054267.

Lloren, A., & Parini, L. (2017). How LGBT-supportive workplace policies shape the experience of lesbian, gay men, and bisexual employees. *Sexuality Research & Social Policy, 14*, 289–299. https://doi.org/10.1007/s13178-016-0253-x.

Loja, E., Costa, M. E., Hughes, B., & Menezes, I. (2013). Disability, embodiment and ableism: Stories of resistance. *Disability & Society, 28*(2), 190–203. https://doi.org/10.1080/09687599.2012.705057.

Macdonald, J. L., & Levy, S. R. (2016). Ageism in the workplace: The role of psychosocial factors in predicting job satisfaction, commitment, and engagement. *Journal of Social Issues, 72*(1), 169–190. https://doi-org.caldwell.idm.oclc.org/10.1111/josi.12161.

Manalansan, M. F. (2015). Queer theory. In R. A. Scott & M. C. Buchmann (Eds.), *Emerging trends in the social and behavioral sciences: An interdisciplinary, searchable, and linkable resource*. Hoboken, NJ: Wiley.

Maree, J. G. (2013). *Counselling for career construction: Connecting life themes to construct life portraits—Turning pain into hope*. Rotterdam, The Netherlands: Sense Publishers.

Maree, J. G. (2014). Career construction with a gay client: A case study. *British Journal of Guidance & Counselling, 42*(4), 436–449. https://doi-org.proxy.library.nyu.edu/10.1080/03069885.2014.886670.

Meyer, I. H. (2010). Identity, stress, and resilience in lesbians, gay men, and bisexuals of color. *The Counseling Psychologist, 38*(3), 442–454. https://doi.org/10.1177/0011000009351601.

Meyer, I. H. (2014). Minority stress and positive psychology: Convergences and divergences to understanding LGBT health. *Psychology of Sexual Orientation and Gender Diversity, 1*(4), 348–349. https://doi.org/10.1037/sgd0000070.

Miller, R. A., Wynn, R. D., & Webb, K. W. (2019). "This really interesting juggling act": How university students manage disability/queer identity disclosure and visibility. *Journal of Diversity in Higher Education, 12*(4), 307–318. https://doi.org/10.1037/dhe0000083.

Miner, K. N., & Costa, P. L. (2018). Ambient workplace heterosexism: Implications for sexual minority and heterosexual employees. *Stress & Health: Journal of the International Society for the Investigation of Stress, 34*(4), 563572. https://doiorg.caldwell.idm.oclc.org/10.1002/smi.2817.

Myers, J. E., & Shannonhouse, L. R. (2012). Combating ageism: Advocacy for older persons. In C. C. Lee (Ed.), *Multicultural issues in counseling: New approaches to diversity* (pp. 151–170). Alexandria, VA: American Counseling Association.

Ng, R., Allore, H. G., Trentalange, M., Monin, J. K., & Levy, B. R. (2015). Increasing negativity of age stereotypes across 200 years: Evidence from a database of 400 million words. *PLoS One, 10*(2), e0117086. https://doi.org/10.1371/journal.pone.0117086.

Norman, D., Hunter, Q., & O'Hara, M. (2017). Career development. In C. B. Roland & L. D. Burlew (Eds.), *Counseling LGBTQ adults throughout the life span.* Alexandria: American Counseling Association. Retrieved from http://www.counseling.org/knowledge-center/lgbtq-resources.

Parnell, M. K., Lease, S. H., & Green, M. L. (2012). Perceived career barriers for gay, lesbian, and bisexual individuals. *Journal of Career Development, 39*(3), 248–268. https://doi.org/10.1177/0894845310386730.

Plummer, K. (2005). Critical humanism and queer theory: Living with the tensions. In N. Denzin & Y. Lincoln (Eds.), *Handbook of qualitative research* (3rd ed., pp. 357–373). Thousand Oaks, CA: Sage.

Ratts, M. J., Singh, A. A., Nassar-McMillan, S., Butler, S. K., & McCullough, J. R. (2016). Multicultural and social justice counseling competencies: Guidelines for the counseling profession. *Journal of Multicultural Counseling and Development, 44*(1), 28–48. https://doi.org/10.1002/jmcd.12035.

Roland, C. B., & Burlew, L. D. (Eds.). (2017). *Counseling LGBTQ adults throughout the life span.* Retrieved from http://www.counseling.org/knowledge-center/lgbtq-resources

Rural Health Information Hub. (n.d.). *Demographic changes and aging population—RHIhub aging in place toolkit.* Retrieved from https://www.ruralhealthinfo.org/toolkits/aging/1/demographics

Savickas, M. L. (2005). The theory and practice of career construction. In S. D. Brown & R. W. Lent (Eds.), *Career development and counseling: Putting theory and research to work* (pp. 42–70). Hoboken, NJ: John Wiley & Sons.

Schmidt, C. K., & Nilsson, J. E. (2006). The effects of simultaneous developmental processes: Factors relating to the career development of lesbian, gay, and bisexual youth. *The Career Development Quarterly, 55*(1), 22–37. https://doi.org/10.1002/j.2161-0045.2006.tb00002.x.

Smart, J. F. (2012). Counseling individuals with physical, cognitive, and psychiatric disabilities. In C. C. Lee (Ed.), *Multicultural issues in counseling: New approaches to diversity* (pp. 151–170). Alexandria, VA: American Counseling Association.

Smith, L. (2005). Psychotherapy, classism, and the poor: Conspicuous by their absence. *American Psychologist, 60*(7), 687–696.

Super, D. E. (1955). Transition from vocational guidance to counseling psychology. *Journal of Counseling Psychology, 2*, 3–9.

Super, D. E. (1980). A life-span, life-space approach to career development. *Journal of Vocational Behavior, 13*, 282–292.

Super, D. E. (1990). A life-span, life-space approach to career development. In D. Brown & L. Brooks (Eds.), *Career choice and development: Applying contemporary theories to practice* (2nd ed., pp. 197–261). San Francisco, CA: Jossey-Bass.

Sutter, M., & Perrin, P. (2016). Discrimination, mental health, and suicidal ideation among LGBTQ people of color. *Journal of Counseling Psychology, 63*(1), 98–105. https://doi.org/10.1037/cou0000126.

United States Census Bureau. (2018). *Older Americans month: May 2017.* Retrieved from https://www.census.gov/newsroom/facts-for-features/2017/cb17-ff08.html

Ward, J. (2008). White normativity: The cultural dimensions of whiteness in a racially diverse LGBT organization. *Sociological Perspectives, 51*(3), 563–586. https://doi.org/10.1525/sop.2008.51.3.563.

Watson, M. (2013). Deconstruction, reconstruction, co-construction: Career construction theory in a developing world context. *Indian Journal of Career and Livelihood Planning, 2*, 3–14.

The Salve and the Sting of Religion/ Spirituality in Queer and Transgender BIPOC

David Ford

1 The Salve and the Sting of Religion/Spirituality in Queer and Transgender BIPOC

For some lesbian, gay, bisexual, transgender, and queer (LGBTQ+) individuals, their concept of religion/spirituality is a source of strength, refuge, peace, fellowship, and meaning. It can also be a source of marginalization, trauma, and pain. Clay Cane's 2015 documentary *Holler if You Hear Me: Black and Gay in The Church* gives accounts of several queer Black men and women who view The Black church as both their refuge and as a traumatic experience. Similarly, many Muslim LGBTQ+ individuals, coming out to family members and their religious communities can cause anxiety (Burke, 2019). Burke further states that young Muslims who are queer may receive threats from family or are afraid to reveal their affectional orientation. Religious spaces can be alienating, and some are not comfortable attending a mosque; if they do, they remain deeply closeted (Burke, 2019). For Jewish members of the LGBTQ+ community, views on same-sex relationships have shifted (My Jewish Learning, n.d.-a, n.d.-b). While Orthodox congregations may reject same-sex behavior, Conservative and Reform congregations have adopted a more liberal and inclusive stance regarding same-sex relationships. For LGBTQ+ individuals who are Buddhist, LGBTQ+ individuals experience compassion and inclusion in Buddhist communities (Cheng, 2018). This chapter discusses the role that religion/ spirituality play in the lives of LGBTQ+ individuals. The author will discuss the perspectives of LGBTQ+ Black people in The Black Church, Catholicism, in The Muslim Faith, in the Jewish Faith, and in the Buddhist Faith. The author will also discuss LGBTQ+ individuals who have Indigenous spiritualities and Pagan identities or who are atheist/agnostic (Fig. 1).

D. Ford (✉)
Department of Professional Counseling, Monmouth University, West Long Branch, NJ, USA
e-mail: dford@monmouth.edu

K. L. Nadal and M. R. Scharrón-del Río (ed.), *Queer Psychology*,
https://doi.org/10.1007/978-3-030-74146-4_15

275

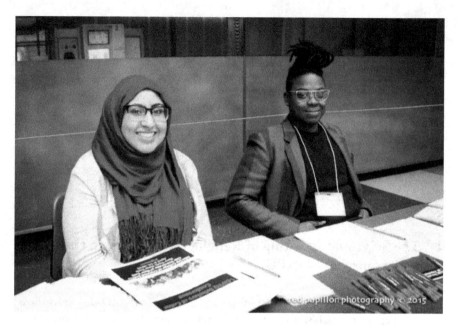

Fig. 1 Two students volunteering at the LGBTQ Scholars of Color National Conference. Photo Courtesy of Riya Ortiz/Red Papillon Photography

2 LGBTQ+ in Spiritual/Religious Traditions

2.1 The Black Church and the LGBTQ+ Community

Robertson and Avent (2016) posited that most Black people consider religion important and the culture of the Black Church influences their worldview and perspective. They further state that 59% of Black Americans are members of predominantly Black congregations. Douglas (2006) refers to the amalgamation of Black congregations as "The Black Church." According to Douglas, the Black Church is

> a multitudinous community of churches, diversified in origin, denomination, doctrine, worshiping culture, spiritual expression, class, size, and no doubt other less obvious factors. Though disparate, Black churches share a unique history, culture, and role in Black life that attest to their collective identity as the Black Church. (p. 1301).

The Black Church provides social bonding and fictive kinship (Robertson & Avent, 2016). Church members refer to each other as family and they share in each other's successes and may feel disappointment and vulnerability when a member goes against social mores (Robertson & Avant, 2016). As such, many consider The Black Church as "the cornerstone of the Black community." Robertson and Avant go on to say that Black churches have been prominent and influential in advocacy and social justice efforts in the Black community. Their legacy of fighting oppression has made The Black Church integral in The Civil Rights movement. The Black

Church has championed causes like voting rights and education inequality (Robertson & Avent, 2016).

According to Greer (2016), like gay nightclubs, Black churches give those who attend something other institutions cannot—a place where attendees can be themselves, especially when the outside world feels hostile. For LGBTQ+ members, The Black Church serves as the same refuge and place of inspiration and social gathering. Black men in the LGBTQ+ community attend church for the same reasons other Black people do (Pitt, 2010). Pitt further says Black churches fulfill social roles, are spiritual resources, and allow them to use their talents to serve the Black community (2010). The Black Church would not survive without gay people (Cane, 2015). Black men have consistently high levels of involvement in The Black Church, like that of heterosexual women (Pitt, 2010). The same can be said for other Black members of the LGBTQ+ community. Members of the LGBTQ+ community pay tithes, teach Sunday school, and head the music ministry. People will come to a church if they know that the music is good and often someone who is gay is over the music. They are playing the instruments, directing choir, and in the pulpit. Some LGBTQ+ members of The Black Church are closeted while some are out. Nonetheless, they are serving, and they are called to ministry. Members of the LGBTQ+ community have been faithfully serving, attending, and supporting The Black Church since there was a Black Church (Cane, 2015; Pitt, 2010). Black members of the LGBTQ+ community are integral to the survival and thriving of The Black Church.

The Black Church has marginalized members of the LGBTQ+ community and assails them with anti-gay rhetoric (Pitt, 2010). This marginalization can and does lead to *church hurt* or the pain inflicted by churches that distances people from their communities and from God (Zauzmer, 2017). For members of the LGBTQ+ community, church hurt results from not being received by their churches, hearing anti-LGBTQ+ messages, and not being allowed to be their full, authentic selves while worshipping and leading worship. For some Black members of the LGBTQ+ community, Black churches present one of the most oppressive environments they encounter (Pitt, 2010; Robertson & Avent, 2016).

While Black members of the LGBTQ+ community have been integral to The Black Church, they have not been afforded the privilege of being their authentic selves or have been afforded full membership (Cane, 2015). The concept of "love the sin but hate the sinner" may present some Black churches to as welcoming to LGBTQ+ members, but still posits same-sex attraction as sinful or deviant and can be cured (Quinn & Dickson-Gomez, 2014). Even though The Black Church has a history of fighting oppression and advocating for equality, many Black congregations work against antidiscrimination efforts for LGBTQ+ communities (Robertson & Avent, 2016). Some Black churches may join and/or ally with other conservative religious groups to condemn same-sex attractions, which could further alienate members of the LGBTQ+ community. Maxwell (2013) posited that because of the anti-LGBTQ+ messages in The Black Church, Black members of the LGBTQ+ community have denied their affectional orientation resulting in the Black families breaking down and the rise of HIV/AIDS in the Black community. The Black

Church could not confront AIDS in Black communities because it could not confront homosexuality and sexuality (Harris, 2009). Black men in the LGBTQ+ community who are HIV positive receive AIDS-phobic messages that increase feelings of stigma and castigation in the Black Church (Miller, 2007). As such, Black churches, although claiming to be welcoming to all and using LGBTQ+ members for their gifts and their financial contributions, continue to bring trauma and be a source of church hurt for the Black people in the LGBTQ+ community.

Despite the church hurt, many Black members of the LGBTQ+ community choose to remain in their churches. The Black Church is important and is like a pseudo-family for some Black people. Because of this importance, leaving a church abruptly because of religious homophobia is just as difficult as disconnecting from your family despite familial incidents of homophobia (V. Allen, personal communication, August 31, 2020). Staying true to their religious/spiritual beliefs can cause anxiety among members of the LGBTQ+ community. As such, they may employ one of three strategies to work through this anxiety (Pitt, 2010). They may reject their religious identity. Black members of the LGBTQ+ community are less likely to utilize this strategy because of the connection they feel from their membership in The Black Church. In fact, they will involve themselves more deeply into their church work by actively participating and attending services. Secondly, they may affiliate with gay-affirming religious institutions or those that are gay-tolerant and silent on gay issues. For many Black members of the LGBTQ+ community, these places of worship are predominately White and may not be compatible with their own cultural experiences. They prefer the homophobia of The Black Church over the racism of predominately White gay-affirming congregations (Griffin, 2006). For Black LGBTQ+ people, the third strategy, attacking the stigma, involves restructuring their beliefs about what being gay means and replacing negative religious rhetoric with neutral or positive beliefs. They focus on the illegitimacy of the messenger rather than the message. The fault lies in the speaker's interpretation of God's message, not in God or the message (Pitt, 2010). These strategies could explain why Black members of the LGBTQ+ community still attend and are active in The Black Church.

2.2   Catholicism and the LGBTQ+ Community

The Roman Catholic Church is the largest denomination in the US and has welcomed celibate members of the LGBTQ+ community but has become increasingly more intolerant of this population (Human Rights Campaign, n.d.). Many LGBTQ+ people from various ethnocultural backgrounds (i.e., Latin American countries, Philippines) have been raised in The Roman Catholic Church, whether in the U.S. or in their countries of origin, and may have attended catechism (religious instruction within the church) or Catholic schools. Many cultural festivities are tied to religious festivities, making the Catholic religion very present in people's lives.

The Roman Catholic Church views same sex acts as intrinsically immoral and contrary to natural law and calls same sex tendencies objectively disorder. Same-sex affectional orientation is not sinful (which is a break from other more fundamentalist Christian traditions), but The Roman Catholic Church views it negatively. Same sex affectional orientation is commonly seen as an intrinsic moral evil. Because The Roman Catholic Church does not view same sex affectional orientation as sinful, it has not officially approved of conversion therapy. The Roman Catholic Church states that members of the LGBTQ+ community are called to chastity and they must be accepted with respect and sensitivity. The Catholic Church has been called to avoid every sign of unjust discrimination (Human Rights Campaign, n.d.). Horowitz (2020) posited that Pope Francis, in a break from previous popes, expressed support for same-sex civil union. He views members of the LGBTQ+ community as children of God. Internal and external advocates for members of the LGBTQ+ community within the Catholic Church believe this community should be accepted—not excommunicated, shunned, or stigmatized—and have a right to form a family.

2.3   Judaism and the LGBTQ+ Community

Jewish members of the LGBTQ+ community may also find refuge and trauma in religious communities. According to Beagan and Hattie (2014), Judaism, Aboriginal traditions, Buddhism, and Hinduism tend to be the most welcoming for members of the LGBTQ+ community. Jewish views toward the LGBTQ+ community have evolved, but these views differ depending on the denomination (My Jewish Learning, n.d.-a, n.d.-b). Orthodox communities believe *The Torah's* inflexible rejection of same-sex acts. Orthodox rabbis use Levitical law as the foundation of their prohibition of same-sex acts and label them an abomination. Like Christians' view of "hate the sin, love the sinner," Orthodox Rabbis believe Levitical law does not reject LGBTQ+ individuals, but the same-sex acts. In 2010, Orthodox rabbis wrote and signed a statement fully welcoming Jews who were gay into synagogue life while reiterating traditional Orthodox opposition to same-sex acts and same-sex marriage. There are numerous grassroots for LGBTQ+ Orthodox Jews and their families (My Jewish Learning, n.d.-a, n.d.-b).

Ultra-Orthodox Jews (which include the Hasidic and Yeshivish traditions) adhere to traditional and rigid gender roles and norms where men and women study in separate schools that focus on studying *The Torah* (Nove, 2018; Shapiro Sanfran, 2013). Studying in secular institutions is discouraged. Known as *shidduchim*, marriage is often arranged through facilitated dating (Shapiro Sanfran, 2013). In the documentary *Trembling Before G-d* (DuBowski, 2001), LGBTQ+ members of the Ultra-Orthodox tradition are conflicted and must reconcile their affectional orientation with their religious beliefs. Many of the people featured in the documentary had to have their identities hidden and voices disguised for fear of the repercussions if their identities were revealed. One subject had been expelled from two Yeshivas for his affectional orientation, contracted HIV, decided to re-embrace The Orthodoxy, blamed his expulsion for contracting HIV, and wanted to relearn his Torah. A lesbian couple, who were high-school sweethearts at an Ultra-Orthodox all-girl's school, were disowned by their families. Many members of Ultra-Orthodox communities cannot live their authentic lives and resort to celibacy or living in heterosexual relationships (DuBowski, 2001).

There are resources for Orthodox Jews in the LGBTQ+ community. Eshel seeks to create a future for Orthodox LGBTQ+ individuals and their families ("Eshel Online," n.d.). Eshel supports members in this community and opens hearts, minds, and doors in Orthodox communities through its innovative and culturally sensitive programming. Eshel has twelve locations for in-person meetups in the US and two in Canada. They also have three national virtual/phone-in groups. Their website (www.eshelonline.org/resources-2/lgbtq-organizations/) provides resources for LGBTQ+ Jewish organizations in North America and in Israel ("Eshel Online," n.d.)

The Reform Movement, the first of the major denominations to have liberal views towards members of the LGBTQ+ community, began advocating for the LGBTQ+ community in 1965 and adopted the first of many resolutions support the community in 1977 (My Jewish Learning, n.d.-a, n.d.-b; ReformJudaism.org, n.d.). This denomination's rabbis endorsed same-sex marriage in 1996 and the congregations did in 1997. According to ReformJudaism.org (n.d.), Reform Jews are committed to LGBTQ+ civil rights and believe that all human beings are created in the Divine image. They believe that Levitical law prohibits promiscuous relations but does not directly address loving, monogamous same-sex couple. The Reform Jewish Movement passed resolutions calling for the inclusion of LGB individuals in the rabbinate and the cantorate and supported marriage equality. In 2015, members of the Reform Jewish Movement released a "Trans Inclusion Guide" that helped members of this denomination include transgender and gender non-conforming individuals and their family into the synagogue (ReformJudaism.org, n.d.).

In 2006, the Conservative movement adopted two contradicting opinions regarding the LGBTQ+ community: one upholds the movement's previous rejection of same-sex relationship and another upholding *The Torah's* prohibition of anal sex between men but allowing other forms of same-sex sexual intimacy (My Jewish Learning, n.d.-a, n.d.-b). Those in the latter opinion endorsed ordaining LGB members as rabbis and cantors. Both opinions are equally valid and rabbis in Conservative denominations may choose which opinion to follow (Fig. 2).

2.4 Islam and the LGBTQ+ Community

According to Beagan and Hattie (2014), Islam and Christianity were the least welcoming to LGBTQ+ individuals. While some debate exists regarding the extent to which Islam condemns same-sex acts between men, it is highly intolerant towards homosexuality culturally and legally (Beagan & Hattie, 2015). The lack of research in this area indicates that LGBTQ+ individuals who are Muslim experience tremendous identity conflict because of the religious and cultural condemnation. The group

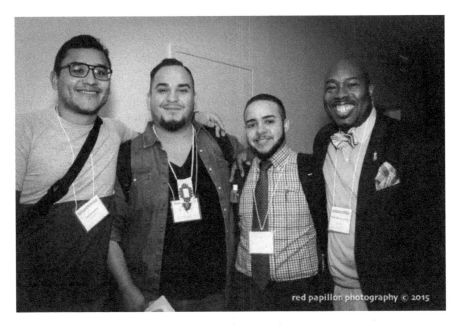

Fig. 2 Dr. David Ford (far right) with other participants at the 2015 LGBTQ Scholars of Color National Conference. Photo Courtesy of Riya Ortiz/Red Papillon Photography

Muslims for Progressive Values has created eight inclusive communities in the United States (Burke, 2019).

Muslims for Progressive Values (MPV) provides a progressive Muslim voice on contemporary issues and voices its perspectives with policy briefs and through civil discourse ("Muslims for Progressive Values," n.d.). MPV advocates for human rights, social justice, and inclusion in the US and globally. MPV is guided by ten principles rooted in Islam: collective identity, equality, separation of religious and state authorities, freedom of speech, universal human rights, gender quality, LGBTQI inclusion, critical analysis and interpretation, compassion, and diversity. Some of the main issues that MPV tackles are interfaith families, LGBTQI, race and racism, Sharia Law, Women's rights, and sexual diversity ("Muslims for Progressive Values," n.d.).

2.5   Hinduism and Buddhism and the LGBTQ+ Community

Buddhism and Hinduism are seemingly more welcoming to members of the LGBTQ+ community than some other religious/spiritual traditions (Beagan & Hattie, 2014). Cheng (2018) posited that Buddhist culture cultivates compassion towards the LGBTQ+ community. Buddhists that are LGBTQ+ can cultivate self-acceptance through Buddhist teachings like clarification of nature and manifestation, Buddhist equality, and proper interpretation of Buddhist precepts. Buddhist teachings also encourage inclusiveness. Hinduism does not explicitly forbid same-sex activity, but cultural norms could mean the Hindus who are LGBTQ+ fear the loss of family and community (Cheng, 2018).

Hijra are transgender people in the Hindu tradition that are neither male nor female and experience social exclusion (Khan et al, 2009). In Bangladesh, *hijra* are extremely excluded with no sociopolitical space where they can lead a life with dignity. Their exclusion is based in not being recognized as a separate gender beyond the male-female dichotomy. Because they live on the extreme margin of exclusion, they cannot hold space in the greater society with human potential and security. They experience physical, verbal, and sexual abuse and because of their social exclusion, they experience diminished self-esteem and sense of social responsibility. Khan et al. (2009) suggest that *hijra* should be recognized within the gender continuum and are a part of Bangladesh's diversity and have gender, sexual, and citizenship rights that should be protected.

2.6 Paganism and Atheism/Agnosticism and the LGBTQ+ Community

Pagan spiritual traditions are typically accepting of gender and sexual diversity and some LGBTQ+ youth have left nonaccepting religious traditions to become Pagan (Higa et al, 2014). Like Pagan traditions, those who are nonreligious (Atheist/ Agnostic) are typically accepting of members of the LGBTQ+ community. According to the Pew Research Center (2020a), 2020b), 94% of Atheists and Agnostics believe same-sex acts should be accepted. For LGBTQ+ BIPOC, while leaving their non-accepting religious/spiritual traditions is an option, many choose to remain in their respective traditions because the benefits outweigh the anxiety caused by anti-LGBTQ+ messages (Pitt, 2010; Robertson & Avent, 2016).

2.7 Indigenous Traditions and the LGBTQ+ Community

According to Picq and Tikuna (2019), sexual diversity has been the norm among indigenous communities and native terminologies referring to same-sex acts and non-binary and gender fluid identities existed long before LGBTQ+ frameworks. In the Juchitán District of Mexico, the Zapotec society recognizes *muxes*, people who are biologically male but embody a third gender that is neither male nor female, as a blessing from the gods. The *muxes* are biologically male and who refuse to be translated as transvestite. Alternative genders exist in several indigenous cultures and are viewed as sacred or have spiritual powers (Picq & Tikuna, 2019).

Two-Spirit refers to non-binary definitions of gender and affectional orientation in Native American traditions (Davis-Young, 2019). Terminology in the Obijwe language used for men who don women's roles in society and women who don men's roles in society inspires the Two-Spirit identity. Many of North American indigenous traditions include a non-binary/fluid idea of gender but hundreds of years of forced assimilation have erased many of their traditions and customs. Two-Spirit powwows are a way to challenge rigid notions of gender and sexuality, which are the unfortunate remnants of colonization. Navajo traditions have at least four genders. The powwows are a way to learn about and celebrate these traditions and not be bound by rigid gender roles (Davis-Young, 2019).

3   Mental Health Applications

The Multicultural and Social Justice Counseling Competencies (MSJCC) (Ratts et al, 2016), provide a framework that mental health professionals can use to guide their work with LGBTQ+ individuals experiencing church hurt from their respective faith-based institutions. The first step is becoming aware of your own biases, prejudices, and assumptions. When working with LGBTQ+ BIPOC with strong religious/spiritual views, mental health professionals should become aware of their biases regarding race/ethnicity, regarding LGBTQ+ individuals, and regarding religion/spirituality. Doing so would assist the professional with building a strong relationship with the client and not letting those biases impede that relationship. Next, the mental health professional understands the client's worldview. Worldview includes how the client views the world and how the client believes the world views them. When working with this population, the mental health professional must understand the worldview regarding the client's desire to retain their religious/spiritual views, what those views mean to them, and the desire to remain in their respective places of worship. The professional must also understand how the client believes their religious/spiritual community views them, especially if the client is receiving anti-LGBTQ messages from their spiritual leader and/or cannot be their full authentic selves (Ratts et al, 2016).

The next domain in the MSJCC is the counseling relationship (Ratts et al, 2016). The mental health professional, in collaboration with the client, must determine what culturally responsive interventions and strategies need to be implemented. One such strategy is cultural broaching. Day-Vines et al. (2007) describes cultural broaching as the counselor's ability to consider how race and other sociopolitical factors influence the client's counseling concerns. Broaching culture facilitates client's empowerment, strengthens the counseling relationship, and enhances counseling outcomes. Broaching begins at the onset of the therapeutic relationship and is a consistent, ongoing process (Day-Vines et al.). Mental health professionals counseling this population must broach at the onset of the relationship so that the clients will feel comfortable presenting their authentic selves. When broaching, the professional should pay special attention to concepts of race/ethnicity, affectional orientation and gender identity/expression, and religion/spirituality in the client. Professionals must also work through any discomfort they may have with discussing these concepts.

The final domain is counseling and advocacy interventions. Once the client and professional collaboratively develop culturally responsive interventions, these interventions can be implemented. These interventions include learning about the client's religion and religious/spiritual rituals, learning about the client's place of worship, finding information about open and affirming congregations in the client's tradition, or in other traditions. As the professional, you should not suggest the client leave their faith-based community, but if the client asks for those resources, the professional will already have them. Another intervention is assisting clients in attacking the stigma (Griffin, 2006) by empowering the client and helping them to reframe their relationship with their higher power. Doing so will help them place more emphasis on the message they receive from their higher power and less emphasis on the message interpreted through the lens of their spiritual leader (Griffin, 2006).

4   Conversion "Therapy"

The premise of conversion "therapy" is that LGBT affectional orientation is a mental illness and is an unhealthy deviation from accepted social norms (McGeorge et al, 2015), and thus, needs to be changed. Conversion "therapy" is erroneously supported by the notion that LGBT affectional orientation is immoral based on the religious belief that heterosexual affectional orientation is the only acceptable orientation and any deviation from this norm is sin. This intervention approach strives to eliminate unwanted same-sex attraction by allegedly helping individuals develop their heterosexual potential. Central to conversion "therapy" is the premise that LGBT affectional orientation is not a true orientation but is a lifestyle choice or set of sexual attractions able to be changed or controlled using behavioral therapy (McGeorge et al, 2015). Individuals may seek conversion "therapy" because of their religious orientation and internalized homophobia (Tozer & Hayes, 2004). Oftentimes, it is family members and/or church communities who push LGBTQ+ people (including minors) to attend practitioners who peddle this practice.

Conversion "therapy" is harmful, unethical, and lacks empirical evidence regarding its efficacy (McGeorge et al, 2015; Tozer & Hayes, 2004); therefore, the description of this approach as "therapy" is inaccurate and misleading. According to the American Medical Association (AMA, 2019), 18 states and the District of Columbia have banned conversion "therapy" and all mental health professional organizations have issued statements opposing this intervention approach. Conversion "therapy" is in direct violation of the ethical imperative of all mental health professions called "nonmaleficence" or "do no harm" (McGeorge et al, 2015). In 2018, The American Psychiatric Association (APA) reaffirmed its recommendation that attempts to change an individual's affectional orientation are unethical, and encouraged legislation that would prohibit conversion "therapy" (APA, 2018a). The APA further states that affectional orientation is something that should not and need not be changed, and efforts to do so are significantly harmful.

Subjecting LGBTQ+ individuals to forms of treatment that are not scientifically supported and that have been documented to cause harm, severely impacts the physical, mental, emotional, and spiritual well-being of whoever is subjected to this practice. There is no credible evidence that any mental health intervention can reliably and safely change affectional orientation; nor, from a mental health perspective does affectional orientation need to be changed (APA, 2018b). The American Psychological Association (APA) concluded that there is insufficient evidence supporting conversion "therapy" and mental health professionals should avoid misrepresenting the efficacy of this intervention approach (Anton, 2010). The American Counseling Association (ACA) opposes promoting conversion "therapy" as a cure for LGBTQ+ individuals, and further stated that conversion therapy is ineffectual, causes harm, violates fraud-protection law, and is a significant and serious violation of its ethical code (ACA, 2017). The National Association of Social Workers (NASW) states that conversion "therapy" harms an individual's mental health and cannot/will not change affectional orientation or gender identity (NASW, 2015). NASW (2015) further states that conversion "therapy" violates their code of ethics. The AMA (2019) stated that conversion "therapy" lacks evidence supporting its efficacy and may cause significant psychological distress.

Conversion therapy may also increase suicidal behaviors in this population, where suicide is already disproportionally prevalent. Conversion "therapy" is in violation of ethical codes (AMA, 2019). The American Association of Marriage and Family Therapists (AAMFT) posited that same-sex attraction is not a disorder that requires treatment and thus sees no need for any intervention that attempts to do so (McGeorge et al, 2015). Like other medical and mental health organizations, the American Mental Health Counselors Association (AMHCA, 2014) purported that conversion "therapy" has no scientific evidence supporting its use. AMHCA further stated that conversion "therapy" poses critical health risks like depression, shame, lower self-esteem, social withdrawal, substance abuse, risky behavior, and suicidal ideation. Conversion "therapy" reinforces homonegativity and increases stress by reaffirming stigma (AMHCA, 2014). The Substance Abuse and Mental Health Services Administration (SAMHSA, 2015) issued a statement about ending conversion "therapy" in LGBTQ youth and posited that conversion therapy is not evidenced-based, has no scientific support, and perpetuates antiquated views of gender and homonegativity. In sum, all major health and mental health professional organizations agree that (1) there is no scientific evidence that conversion approaches can change affective orientation; (2) there is no need to change affective/sexual orientation or gender identity; (3) that this practice is harmful to physical, emotional, and mental health of those who are subjected to it; (4) that this practice is in violation of their code ethics; and (5) support a ban on this harmful practice (Fig. 3).

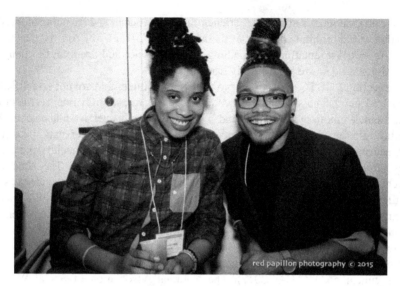

Fig. 3 Two community members at an LGBTQ community event. Photo Courtesy of Riya Ortiz/ Red Papillon Photography

5   Case Study

Diontré is a multiethnic, 25-year-old, same-gender-loving (SGL) cisgender man. His mother is White, and his father is Black. Phenotypically, he is Black and self-identifies as Black. He has developed a strong Black identity and is a member of a historically Black Greek-letter Organization. He attended a prestigious Southeastern Predominantly White Institution (PWI) for his undergraduate and graduate degrees. All throughout his life, he has felt isolated. Other Black people have questioned his Blackness, especially with him being SGL and out. He has been the subject of bigotry from White people. He has experienced homophobia from all ethnic groups. He has experienced this ostracism and bigotry in college and in the workplace. Diontré is very active in his church. He attends a strict Pentecostal church with very traditional views, especially regarding same-sex feelings, acts, and relationships. He has always been active in his church, especially with the music ministry. He sings in the choir and has been told he has the voice of an angel. He is also the choir director. Even though his pastor constantly preaches against homosexuality, he still attends his church, loves his church, and loves his music ministry. Lately, he has experienced depression because of these experiences and has started using crystal meth to fit in with a community and to address his feelings of isolation. One evening after partying and using, he was sexually assaulted by someone at the party who is also a fellow church member. A few weeks later, he developed flu-like symptoms and noticed his lymph nodes were swollen. He went to the clinic and found out he was HIV positive.

In working with Diontré, a mental health professional may consider using the Multicultural and Social Justice Counseling Competencies (MSJCC) (Ratts et al, 2016). First, they must identify how their biases, prejudices, or assumptions would affect their work with him. How have their past experiences influenced their experiences with Black same-gender-loving men, as well as people living with HIV/AIDS? Next, the practitioner would need to understand the client's worldview. They would need to explore with him how his Pentacostal religion, his Blackness, his sexuality, and all of his experiences affect the ways that he sees and interprets the world. In doing so, the practitioner may need to assist Diontré in unpacking any of the negative messages he has learned about all of his identities, especially his historically marginalized identities (i.e., his Black and SGL identities). Specific to religion, the practitioner may assist Diontré in examining any anti-LGBTQ messages that have been learned by preachers or other religious leaders, and how that may have affected his perceptions of his own sexuality and his own relationships. Further, in developing counseling and advocacy interventions, the practitioner may be mindful of a number of factors—including Diontré's love for his church, as well as the conflict that this commitment may cause. Finally, the practitioner must keep all of these cultural and social justice factors in mind, while also monitoring Diontré's, depressive symptoms and his ability to function, particularly as he comes to terms with his HIV diagnosis. Perhaps it would be helpful to refer him to support groups or organizations of other queer Black men (or men of color) living with HIV, or to brainstorm people and spaces who csn be helpful in serving as social support as he adjusts to his new serostatus and the experiences that come with it.

6 Conclusion

Religion and spirituality continue to be important to LGBTQ BIPOC and mental health professionals must be culturally sensitive to the needs of this community, especially when they have experienced trauma and marginalization in their faith communities. Mental health professionals must educate themselves about the history and rituals of various religious/spiritual traditions, educate themselves about the stigma, trauma, and marginalization that LGBTQ BIPOC experience in their faith communities, and be able to provide resources for members of this community. They must also advocate for affirmative counseling interventions and join/initiate efforts to ban conversion therapy. The Multicultural and Social Justice Counseling Competencies (MSJCC) (Ratts et al, 2016), cultural broaching (Day-Vines et al, 2007), and attacking the stigma (Griffin, 2006) provide mental health professionals with the tools to intervene while honoring the client's autonomy. The preceding case study will allow you to implement these interventions.

References

American Counseling Association. (2017). *Resolution on reparative therapy/conversion therapy/sexual orientation Change Efforts (SOCE) as a significant and serious violation of the ACA code of ethics.* Retrieved from https://www.counseling.org/docs/default-source/default-document-library/reparative-therapy-resoltution-letter-head_edited.pdf?sfvrsn=8ed562c_4

American Medical Association. (2019). *LGBTQ change efforts (So-called "conversion therapy").* Retrieved from https://www.ama-assn.org/system/files/2019-12/conversion-therapy-issue-brief.pdf

American Mental Health Counseling Association. (2014). *AMHCA statement on reparative or conversion therapy.* Retrieved from https://www.amhca.org/HigherLogic/System/DownloadDocumentFile.ashx?DocumentFileKey=eae41719-9650-cec8-c247-655d9ef45c37&forceDialog=0

American Psychiatric Association. (2018a). *Position statement on conversion therapy and LGBTQ patients.*

American Psychiatric Association. (2018b). *APA reiterates strong opposition to conversion therapy.* Retrieved from https://www.psychiatry.org/newsroom/news-releases/apa-reiterates-strong-opposition-to-conversion-therapy

Anton, B. S. (2010). Proceedings of the American Psychological Association for the legislative year 2009: Minutes of the annual meeting of the Council of Representatives and minutes of the meetings of the Board of Directors. *American Psychologist, 65*(5), 385–475. https://doi.org/10.1037/a0019553.

Beagan, B., & Hattie, B. (2014). LGBTQ experiences with religion and spirituality: Occupational transition and adaptation. *Journal of Occupational Science, 9*(2), 92–117. https://doi.org/10.1080/14427591.2014.953670.

Beagan, B., & Hattie, B. (2015). Religion, spirituality, and LGBTQ identity integration. *Journal of LGBT Issues in Counseling, 9*(2), 92–117. https://doi.org/10.1080/15538605.2015.1029204.

Burke, D. (2019). *In a survey of American Muslims, 0% identified as lesbian or gay. Here's the story behind that statistic.* CNN. Retrieved from https://www.cnn.com/2019/05/28/us/lgbt-muslims-pride-progress/index.html

Cane, C. (Director) (2015). *Holler if you hear me: Black and gay in the church* [Film]. BET.

Cheng, F. K. (2018). Being different with dignity: Buddhist inclusiveness of homosexuality. *Social Sciences, 7*(4), 51. https://doi.org/10.3390/socsci7040051.

Davis-Young, K. (2019, March 29). *For many native Americans, embracing LGBT members is a return to the past.* Washington Post. Retrieved from https://www.washingtonpost.com/national/for-many-native-americans-embracing-lgbt-members-is-a-return-to-the-past/2019/03/29/24d1e6c6-4f2c-11e9-88a1-ed346f0ec94f_story.html

Day-Vines, N. L., Wood, S. M., Grothaus, T., Craigen, L., Holman, A., Dotson-Blake, K., & Douglass, M. J. (2007). Broaching the subjects of race, ethnicity, and culture during the counseling process. *Journal of Counseling and Development, 85*(4), 401–409. https://doi.org/10.1002/jcad.12069.

Douglas, K. B. (2006). Sexuality and the Black church. In R. S. Keller & R. R. Ruether (Eds.), *Encyclopedia of women and religion in North America* (pp. 1300–1304). Bloomington: Indiana University Press.

DuBowski, S. S. (Director) (2001). *Trembling before g-d* [Film]. Cinephil.

Eshel Online. (n.d.). *Eshel online.* Retrieved from https://www.eshelonline.org/

Greer, B. (2016). *Gay nightclubs and Black churches are sanctuaries. Here's how to make them safer.* The Washington Post. Retrieved from https://www.washingtonpost.com/news/soloish/wp/2016/06/13/gay-nightclubs-and-black-churches-are-sanctuaries-heres-how-to-make-them-safer/

Griffin, H. L. (2006). *Their own receive them not: African American lesbians and gays in Black churches.* Cleveland, OH: Pilgrim Press.

Harris, A. C. (2009). Sex, stigma, and the holy ghost: The black church and the construction of AIDS in new York City. *Journal of African American Studies, 14*(1), 21–43. https://doi.org/10.1007/s12111-009-9105-6.

Higa, D., Hoppe, M. J., Lindhorst, T., Mincer, S., Beadnell, B., Morrison, D. M., Wells, E. A., Todd, A., & Mountz, S. (2014). Negative and positive factors associated with the well-being of lesbian, gay, bisexual, transgender, queer, and questioning (LGBTQ) youth. *Youth & Society, 46*(5), 663–687. https://doi.org/10.1177/0044118X12449630.

Horowitz, J. (2020). *In shift for church, Pope Francis voices support for same-sex civil unions*. The New York Times. Retrieved from https://www.nytimes.com/2020/10/21/world/europe/pope-francis-same-sex-civil-unions.html

Human Rights Campaign. (n.d.). *Stances of faiths on LGBTQ issues: Roman Catholic church*. Retrieved from https://www.hrc.org/resources/stances-of-faiths-on-lgbt-issues-roman-catholic-church

Khan, S. I., Hussain, M. I., Parveen, S., Bhuiyan, M. I., Gourab, G., Sarker, G. F., Arafat, S. M., & Sikder, J. (2009). Living on the extreme margin: Social exclusion of the transgender population (*Hijra*) in Bangladesh. *Journal of Health, Population, and Nutrition, 27*(4), 441–451. https://doi.org/10.3329/jhpn.v27i4.3388.

Maxwell, C. (2013). *Writer discusses the Black church and anti-gay sentiment*. Windy City Times. Retrieved from https://search-proquest-com.ezproxy.monmouth.edu/docview/1412851352?OpenUrlRefId=info:xri/sid:summon&accountid=12532

McGeorge, C. R., Carlson, T. S., & Toomey, R. B. (2015). An exploration of family therapist' beliefs about the ethics of conversion therapy: The influence of native beliefs and clinical competence with lesbian, gay, and bisexual clients. *Journal of Marital and Family Therapy, 41*(1), 42–56. https://doi.org/10.1111/jmft.12040.

Miller, R. L. (2007). Legacy denied: African American gay men, AIDS, and the Black church. *Social Work, 52*(1), 51–61. https://doi.org/10.1093/sw/52.1.51.

Muslims for Progressive Values. (n.d.). *Muslims for progressive values*. Retrieved from https://www.mpvusa.org/

My Jewish Learning. (n.d.-a). *Judaism and LGBTQ issues: An overview*. Retrieved September 5, 2020, from https://www.myjewishlearning.com/article/judaism-and-the-lgbtq-community-an-overview/

My Jewish Learning. (n.d.-b). *Orthodox Judaism and LGBTQ issues*. Retrieved September 5, 2020, from https://www.myjewishlearning.com/article/orthodox-judaism-and-lgbtq-issues/

National Association for Social Workers. (2015). *Sexual orientation change efforts (SOCE) and conversion therapy with lesbians, gay men, bisexuals, and transgender persons*. Retrieved from https://www.socialworkers.org/LinkClick.aspx?fileticket=IQYALknHU6s%3D&portalid=0

Nove, C. R. (2018). Becoming un-orthodox: Stories of ex-Hasidim. By Lynn Davidman. *Jewish History, 31*(3–4), 395–398. https://doi.org/10.1007/s10835-018-9300-x.

Pew Research Center. (2020a). *Views about homosexuality among agnostics*. Retrieved September 3, 2020, from https://www.pewforum.org/religious-landscape-study/religious-family/agnostic/views-about-homosexuality/

Pew Research Center. (2020b). *Views about homosexuality among atheists*. Retrieved September 3, 2020, from https://www.pewforum.org/religious-landscape-study/religious-family/atheist/views-about-homosexuality/

Picq, M. L. & Tikuna, J. (2019). *Indigenous sexualities: Resisting conquest and translation*. Retrieved from https://www.e-ir.info/2019/08/20/indigenous-sexualities-resisting-conquest-and-translation/

Pitt, R. N. (2010). "Killing the messenger": Religious Black gay men's neutralization of anti-gay religious messages. *Journal for the Scientific Study of Religion, 49*(1), 56–72. https://doi.org/10.1111/j.1468-5906.2009.01492.x.

Quinn, K., & Dickson-Gomez, J., (2014) *"Love the sinner, hate the sin": Examining Black faith leaders' perception of homosexuality and HIV* [Paper presentation]. American Public Health Association 142nd Annual Meeting & Expo, New Orleans, LA, United States.

Ratts, M. J., Singh, A. A., Nassar-McMillan, S., Butler, S. K., & McCullough, J. R. (2016). Multicultural and social justice counseling competencies: Guidelines for the counseling profession. *Journal of Multicultural Counseling and Development, 44*(1), 28–48. https://doi.org/10.1002/jmcd.12035.

ReformJudaism.org. (n.d.) *Reform Jewish views on LGBTQ equality.* Retrieved September 5, 2020, from https://reformjudaism.org/reform-jewish-views-lgbtq-equality

Robertson, D. L., & Avent, J. R. (2016). African American counselors-in-training, the Black church, and lesbian-, gay-, and bisexual-affirmative counseling: Considerations for counselor education programs. *Counseling and Values, 61*(2), 223–238. https://doi.org/10.1002/cvj.12039.

Shapiro Sanfran, R. (2013). *A multidimensional assessment of Orthodox Jewish attitudes toward homosexuality* (3520925) [Doctoral dissertation, Seton Hall University]. ProQuest Dissertation Publishing.

Substance Abuse and Mental Health Services Administration. (2015). *Ending conversion therapy: Supporting and affirming LGBTQ youth.* Retrieved from https://store.samhsa.gov/product/Ending-Conversion-Therapy-Supporting-and-Affirming-LGBTQ-Youth/SMA15-4928?print=true

Tozer, E. E., & Hayes, J. A. (2004). Why do individuals seek conversion therapy? The role of religiosity, internalized homonegative, and identity development. *The Counseling Psychologist, 32*(5), 716–740.

Zauzmer, J. (2017). *Damaged by the church? This pastor has a congregation full of 'recovering Christians.'* The Washington Post. Retrieved from https://www.washingtonpost.com/news/acts-of-faith/wp/2017/03/08/amid-a-wave-of-church-hurt-one-boston-pastor-tries-to-repair-christians-relationship-with-god/

Queering Forensic Psychology: What Intimate Partner Violence and Sex Trafficking Can Tell Us About Inclusivity

Kendra Doychak and Chitra Raghavan

1 Queering Forensic Psychology: What Intimate Partner Violence and Sex Trafficking Can Tell Us About Inclusivity

Forensic psychology—although present in the early development of psychology as a science—expanded rapidly in the eighties with increased offerings in higher education, formal guidelines, and forensic publication outlets (American Psychological Association, n.d.; Brigham, 1999; Heilbrun & Brooks, 2010; Loh, 1981) and has continued through the new millennium (Bull, 2011). Most psychologists agree that forensic psychology is broadly defined as an application of psychology to legal areas and that psychologists from a wide variety of disciplines can engage in forensic applications (e.g., Brigham, 1999; Blackburn, 1996; Heilbrun & Brooks, 2010; Nadal, 2020; Otto & Heilbrun, 2002). Blackburn, (1996) cautions that this field should not be confused as a separate branch of psychology, such as developmental or neuropsychology. Rather, it is the application of psychological principles to issues that arise in law (Fig. 1).

Some of the earliest forays of medical personnel and psychologists into legal arenas involved providing protection for the mentally ill and arguing against discriminatory state practices (Brigham, 1999; Regina v. M'Naghten, 1843). Specifically, psychologists and other mental health professionals used social science knowledge to provide information on legal issues—which corresponds closely to contemporary calls for social justice. Impressively, in its earliest manifestations, forensic psychology addressed class and gender (Muller v. Oregon, 1908) and race discrimination (Brown v. Board of Education, 1954).

Despite forensic psychology's early progressive beginnings, contemporary focus in forensic psychology has not grappled with racial and gender discrimination—nor

K. Doychak (✉) · C. Raghavan
John Jay College of Criminal Justice—CUNY Graduate Center, New York, NY, USA
e-mail: kdoychak@jjay.cuny.edu; craghavan@jjay.cuny.edu

K. L. Nadal and M. R. Scharrón-del Río (ed.), *Queer Psychology*,
https://doi.org/10.1007/978-3-030-74146-4_16

Fig. 1 A young queer
Black man raises his fist
for racial justice. Photo
Courtesy of Nicholas
Swatz

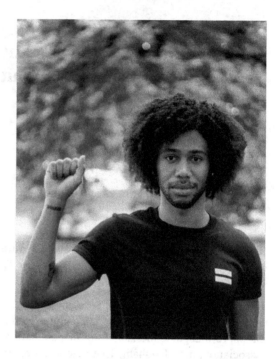

homophobia and transphobia—in American society. Instead, within clinical practice, this field has continued to emphasize criminalizing and pathologizing offenders with clinical psychologists battling out issues of competency, dangerousness,
and the credibility of defendants. Indeed, numerous psychologists have devoted
their lives to trying to catch "dangerous liars" with little critical insight into how
power, politics, and culture have shaped who decides what is a truth and what is a
lie. This dangerous lack of insight has very real implications. It has resulted in, for
example, repeated assaults on women's credibility when describing sexual assaults
or intimate partner violence (IPV), while men's denials are viewed as honorable
(Hempel, 2004).

This lack of critical awareness has also blinded forensic psychology to queer
issues—almost nothing is known of how queer populations experience and negotiate interpersonal forensic settings, nor what their most pressing needs are. This lack
of critical awareness also undergirds research; forensic psychology research has
remained limited with a focus on eyewitness issues, violence recidivism, malingering, psychopathy, and jury selection. Few forensic psychologists study race-related
trauma, microaggressions that queer populations endure daily, hate crimes, rehabilitation of queer offenders, spiritual healing for queer offenders and victims, and IPV
and sex trafficking in the queer community—all areas of inquiry with deep and
meaningful intersections in the fields of psychology and law. As American society
becomes more multicultural and accepting of multiple sexualities and genders, so
has the backlash against sexual minorities increased (e.g., see FBI crime statistics,
which likely underestimate rates and yet, still report a steady increase in hate crimes
against LGBTQ individuals since 2014).

The field of forensic psychology is not immune from perpetuating this same discrimination. Non-majority sexual and gender identities previously overtly criminalized (e.g., sexual psychopath and sodomy laws; Sutherland, 1949), continue to face harmful and false assumptions about their propensity for crime rooted in homo- and trans-phobias. For example, despite evidence that perpetrators of child sexual assault are largely male with female victims (Puzzanchera et al., 2018), stereotypes about gay and lesbian sexual "predators" still exist. These harmful assumptions are influenced by theories and data with little to no LGBTQ representation. For example, typologies regarding serial/spree killers often include the notion of the "homosexual serial killer" despite the fact that a small minority of these murders involve male perpetrators and exclusively male victims (e.g., 7 out of 92 offenders; Morton et al., 2015). Forensic psychology has perpetuated the notion of the "homosexual crime," rather than challenging it through new research or the consideration of existing—albeit limited—data, the role of toxic masculinity, gender role socialization, internalized oppression, and histories of trauma and systemic oppression (Nadal, 2020).

Forensic psychology has remained colorblind and genderblind, critically aware of deep-seated racial, gender, and sexual prejudice within psychology and yet reacting turgidly to how such prejudices bleed into forensic applications. As such, forensic psychology is marginally involved in social justice issues through individual actors, rather than as a field. In contrast, other branches of psychology are breaking boundaries and redefining existing Western-centric, masculine, and industrialized world assumptions, often in radical ways, drawing from non-Western cultures. For example, the study of dreams—once viewed as unscientific—has received renewed interest in neuroscience (Blechner, 2018), and dream work from Tibetan traditions is being explored for its utility in personal growth (Ricard & Singer, 2017). The use of psychotropic drugs and their history in traditional shamanic medicine is being acknowledged in the treatment of addictions and trauma (Holland, 2020). Forensic psychology remains shackled to narrow Western traditions with its punitive and authoritarian outlook.

This chapter is a call for mental health practitioners and scholars—for those who are contemplating a forensic career and even, for those who do not regard themselves as forensic—to begin engaging more critically with issues that affect queer individuals with intersectional identities who are caught up in the criminal justice system. We begin the process of queering forensic psychology via the lens of intimate partner violence (IPV) and sex trafficking, two issues that affect queer Americans in profound and debilitating ways. To illuminate, queer couples experience IPV at equal or even higher rates than heterosexual or gender binary individuals and face unique elements of such abuse (e.g., threats of "outing"), as well as additional stigmatization in seeking help. One study found that transgender individuals comprised a disproportionate rate of sex trafficking victims, accounting for 3% of the total sample (Nichols et al., 2019); yet, a mere 0.39% of respondents identified as transgender in a large-scale general population survey (Meerwijk & Sevelius, 2017). We hope this chapter serves as encouragement to pursue research and practice that has previously been neglected in forensic arenas, drawing from multiple branches of psychology—and not just Western branches.

1.1 Sexist and Heterosexist Biases in IPV and Sex Trafficking

To begin, we utilize IPV and sex trafficking research and practice—issues that deeply affect everyday life of queer folk. IPV, sex trafficking, and traumas that arise from these abuses are not subject areas that are routinely taught in forensic classes; yet, a disproportionate number of individuals entangled in the legal system report IPV and trauma. The lack of information and criminalization of heterosexual IPV survivors contributes to the continuing ignorance and revictimization of queer survivors.

A sexist framework is, in part, a way of ordering the world though binary categories of masculine and feminine, and attributing stereotypic gender roles and sexual activities to each sex. Heterosexual women survivors are often seen as vengeful liars, exaggerating or dramatizing the violence (Bryant & Spencer, 2003; Fischel-Wolovick, 2018). Even if there is clear evidence of IPV, women are blamed for not leaving earlier; and when they do leave, they are charged with neglect for exposing their children to violence (e.g., see Nicholson v. Scoppetta, 2004). In 2020, women who kill their abusers in self-defense are being sentenced to decades in prison.

For the queer population, sexism is compounded by heterosexism (i.e., the belief that heterosexuality is "superior" or the social and cultural "norm") and further, homophobia (e.g., fear, disgust, or prejudice toward non-heterosexual individuals). These culturally prescribed and hurtful ideals are perpetrated through the media, sex role socialization, and traditional religious values (Sherkat, 2002), leading to the stigmatization and discrimination of non-heterosexual behavior and identities (Herek, 1990). Related to IPV, heterosexist biases also influence how IPV situations are interpreted. For example, abuse dynamics against male partners may be trivialized as unimportant or disregarded as a "tiff" (Brown, 2008; p. 459).

Furthermore, because many constructs (and subsequent measures in forensic psychology) are not normed on LGBTQ populations, many traditional forensic psychologists might wonder if more forensic psychology research should be expanded to include gay men (or LGBTQ people in general). As an example, there is a lack of research on LGBTQ people and malingering, which is defined as the ability to exaggerate or feign illness (Rogers, 2008); it is a tactic that is often used to assess people who are deemed as psychopaths who may malinger as a way of achieving more favorable legal outcomes. While forensic psychology researchers may be interested in exploring how psychopathy might manifest among LGBTQ "liars," it is also critical to deconstruct why we need to use malingering as a legal defense at all. Further, we must question why and how many queer populations are stigmatized and disbelieved, and how this harms them. Thus, instead of moving automatically and robotically to create more norms in the name of cultural competency, we must deconstruct the overuse of malingering—among other norms—as a standard forensic practice and identify when and how queer and vulnerable populations involved in IPV are being targeted (Fig. 2).

Fig. 2 A young woman at a #BlackLivesMatter rally in Hawai'i. Photo Courtesy of Daniel Torobekov

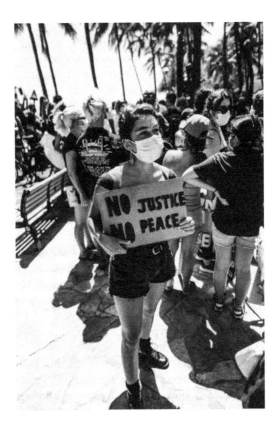

2 A Case of IPV and Sex Trafficking

In this case study, we will illustrate how lack of forensic representation, homophobia/heterosexism, and reliance on traditional forensic ideas of malingering and psychopathy were used to evaluate a survivor of IPV and trafficking. While the case study involves a gay cisgender man, many of the depressing and harassing encounters he experienced are likely to apply to other queer and trans individuals involved in the legal system.

2.1 Presenting Information

Armand[1] was in his late thirties when he initially met the second author (who was his evaluating psychologist). He was light skinned, strikingly beautiful, tall, and well-mannered—attributes that would initially prejudice his case. He was also

---

[1] Names, places, and identifying information altered to protect confidentiality.

numb and depressed. He moved slowly and struggled to speak but was determined
to tell his story, no matter how painful. Armand was gay and was raised in a wealthy
rural farming family in South America that was conservative, homophobic, and very
Catholic. Growing up, he had been physically abused by his father who found him
"effeminate" and therefore, offensive. He witnessed his father also severely abuse
his mother and older brother—which as a young child scared him so much that he
began to dissociate early in life to cope with these incidents.

When Armand was 14, his father ordered him to sleep with a prostitute—a
woman who was about 10 years older. He dared not refuse and managed to achieve
coitus, creating confusion and self-hatred for many years. His father would regularly encourage him to purchase sex; on his second or third visit with each, the
women would tell Armand that he was probably gay, but that she and her friends
would lie to his father to protect him. As his first open confrontations with his sexuality, Armand was scared, yet relieved; the women kept their word, and he would
visit with them (to merely smoke or hang out) for several years until he left for college. By his mid-twenties, Armand began identifying as gay in private circles. He
noted that if his father had known, he had no doubt that he would have ordered his
son killed, maimed, or punished in some very violent way.

When Armand was in his late twenties, he moved to the United States, and he
quickly became involved in a romantic relationship with another Latinx man.
Deprived of being able to openly express his sexuality throughout his life, Armand
was thrilled and fully engaged with his boyfriend. Although highly educated,
Armand could not use his degree in the U.S. and worked in small menial jobs. When
his boyfriend suggested that he engage in sex work, Armand was horrified and
refused. But eventually, terrified of losing him and eager to prove that he was a
capable caretaker, he agreed. He worked as a high-end escort for several years.

Initially, Armand was flattered because he was in high demand but soon began
despising escorting. He tried to express it but could not. Armand noted that he was
integrated into a gay community openly for the first time in his life and this community was sacred to him. His gay world—many of them escorts—normalized and
glamorized his lifestyle; and he did not want to alienate them. Later, he would
encounter other gay communities who were supportive of his choices, understood
his entrapment, and would help him navigate the lines between celebrating sexuality and objectifying it. However, as a new immigrant who was building his gay
identity and trying to survive, he did not think he had other choices.

Armand also struggled with understanding what healthy norms were; he did not
know if he was indeed repressed or sexually conservative because of his father's
abuse and his homophobic family, or if escorting was genuinely harming him.
Rapidly, he began using dissociation techniques that he had employed as an abused
child. And when dissociation alone could not emotionally protect him, Armand
began ingesting molly, cocaine, and ecstasy. Drugs were also part of the requirement during his escorting work, and Armand noted that he played the role of the
"happy hooker" so well that demand for his services increased.

In his late twenties, Armand met his future husband, Leo, during a paid sex party.
Leo was a millionaire working in big city finance; he was highly educated, Asian,

smaller in stature (particularly in comparison to Armand), and generally soft spoken. Leo began courting him, and he eventually suggested that Armand quit sex work and move in with him. He also promised to further his education and help him get into an Ivy League school to complete his advanced degree. Armand (who was single at this point) was thrilled by this turn of events; because he was so desperate to leave escorting, he agreed after a short courting period.

Initially, Leo was controlling, and very jealous, but not violent. Armand attributed this behavior to Leo's low self-esteem and difficultly with his own gay identity. Indeed, Armand was empathetic and compassionate—applying his own difficult childhood and his continual need to be closeted from his family as explanations for Leo's progressively erratic and violent behavior. Over time, Leo became severely physically abusive. Armand was physically beaten and choked; he was ridiculed, demeaned, called names daily, and sexually exploited. He was required to perform sexual acts daily; if he did not abide, his husband would withhold finances. He was prevented from continuing his education, and instead was forced into cooking and cleaning.

Armand's freedom was curtailed. He had no friends and little freedom in movement. Leo had cameras installed in the apartment, and whenever Armand left or returned, his visits would have to be explained. At the behest of Leo, Armand participated in group sex and initially enjoyed it; however, he later grew tired of this and refused. When he did, Leo would fly into rages—physically hitting him or withdrawing affection and sometimes finances. Eventually, Armand unwillingly surrendered. He was frequently directed by his husband during these orgies and forced to sleep with important business associates and closeted political allies in the U.S. and internationally. During these humiliating sexual encounters, Leo would degrade Armand and refer to him as "a prostitute whom he married." After almost a decade of physical and sexual exploitation, Armand fled from his husband and sought legal protection.

2.2   Initiating the Legal Process

When filing the divorce papers, Armand discovered that Leo had never filed his permanent residency papers. If they were to divorce, Armand would be deported. Leo, furious at Armand's departure, accused him of lying about the abuse and emphasized that Armand was nothing more than a high-end escort. Government lawyers appeared to agree; they demanded evidence that Armand was not lying about the IPV or sexual exploitation. In communicating with Armand's legal team, they noted that government lawyers had difficulty believing that a 6-foot tall man with an advanced degree could not defend himself against his much smaller husband. They posed as evidence that if there had been abuse, why would Armand have remained for such a long time. They also expressed nervousness around the allegations of forced sexual behavior—largely because Armand had not brought it up in great detail at their initial meetings. Why was he alluding to sexual abuse now when the stakes were higher? And, if Armand had willingly participated in group sex multiple times and worked as an escort in the past, why was he calling it rape later in the marriage?

As Armand's evaluating psychologist, the second author was not surprised by the legal team's prejudice, but was flummoxed by the depth of it. Prejudice abounds in heterosexual IPV cases, and sexism pervades research and practice regarding partner violence. In Armand's situation, these biases impacted the way the government viewed him and judged his behavior. From their point of view, Armand was a disgruntled gay party boy, too lazy to work, enjoying a glamorous life of sex and drugs. Now, discarded, he was seeking revenge. Further, there was serious doubt whether the violence had even occurred—could someone like this be a victim or was he malingering? And worse, the kiss of death legally—given his partying, drugs, sex, and now possible lying about violence—did he have Anti-Social Personality Disorder? Was he just an "exotic" malingering psychopath, good looking and charming to boot?

2.3   The Question of Malingering

Armand spoke English well, but it was not his first language. As a result, standardized tools to assess malingering—different assessments that help psychologists decide the extent to which someone is being truthful—were not an option. While non-verbal assessments exist, their utility is questionable. Eventually, the second author decided against such an assessment. She noted that she would have probably conducted the assessment only because it is the "party line" and it could have easily satisfied the technical demands of the government. But because the entire discriminatory process of disbelieving Armand and asking for a malingering evaluation was a harmful one, the psychologist did not conduct one. By labeling Armand as a potential malingerer, the discussion took a troubling path, and reinforced heterosexist beliefs as a legitimate starting point for a forensic investigation. One simple solution to this is mainstreaming research on partner violence and how it intersects with gender and sexuality, supported by easily accessible data.

In constructing a response to the possibility that he was faking IPV, the second author began considering how oppressive this accusation was and how forensic psychology was playing into it. Both authors have frequently encountered cases in which women, of all races and backgrounds, are viewed as lying about IPV—especially when they are not "perfect" victims (i.e., they have other circumstances or factors that are used to discredit their claims). Similar types of prejudice were used towards Armand; so although he had privileged identities as a middle class, Hispanic-white, and educated man, he was also queer, an immigrant, a former escort, used heavy drugs, and engaged in "kinky" or "deviant" sex. The prejudice that runs deep in our society around IPV intersected with homophobia led to a traditional forensic solution—questioning Armand's truthfulness and attributing his "lifestyle" to a gay version of psychopathy.

Similarly, there are multiple relevant explanations as to why Armand disclosed his sexual abuse later, why he didn't define it as abuse initially, and his personal pathways into and out of drugs. But, none of these questions were posed—instead, questions about his credibility arose. And indeed, little research exists in forensic psychology that examines disclosure—although, researchers in counseling psychology have examined how traumatized respondents conceal disclosure for various reasons (Ahrens et al., 2010; Larson et al., 2015; Sorsoli, 2010). The government had only one explanation for his behavior—that he must be lying. When other reasons—including data supporting why survivors don't disclose sexual abuse, Armand's beliefs that he was to blame, his deep shame, his sexual abuse history, and initial lack of recognition that he was abused—were offered, suspicions around his truthfulness dissipated.

Again, diversifying forensic psychology research to explore creatively why narratives are delayed, take different forms, and are fragmented, and how these are further shaped by intersectional marginalization would offer multiple models for legal actors to select and test. Imagine if the government had said, "Oh, of course, sexual abuse is rarely self-disclosed. I've read about it, and Armand's behavior is consistent with the data. Could you help figure out if it's related to lack of identification, shame, fear, or trauma-related memory?" Instead, they asked if Armand could be lying–demonstrating the White heterosexual cisgender male lens that is used in approaches to violence and abuse.

2.4   Queering Conceptualizations of Violence

Another issue that arose was even if there was violence towards Armand, was it all that bad? Isn't it true that men can rough each other up and neither get really hurt? And, if it was all that bad, why did Armand stay for almost 10 years? Further, there was the question of Armand's husband—an erudite, soft spoken, highly educated, and wealthy East Asian man. Could someone this refined really be this crude? Heterosexism and homophobia playing out through sex, gender, race, and class all became central to obscuring Armand's true suffering.

In Armand's case, one key to understanding his abuse was coercive control—an abuse dynamic intended to rob the victim of power and autonomy. Critical elements of these controlling behaviors include an ongoing strategy of intimidation, isolation, and control of access to financial resources, employment, and education (Stark, 2006). Perpetrators also obtain compliance through monitoring the victim's activities and through the use of (or threats of) physical and sexual violence (Dutton & Goodman, 2005; Stark, 2007); but, these more overt tactics are not always present or even necessary, especially in chronic violence. The studies examining coercive control are generally limited in how they define and organize these issues with close to no attention to sexuality, physicality, and its role or its lack of a role. One study of male same-sex relationships found that 6 of the 69 participant relationships exhibited control and dominance exclusively of one partner over another partner

(Stanley et al., 2006), and concluded that coercive control was unimportant in this population. Frankland & Brown (2014) found that about a quarter of their combined male and female same-sex sample used coercive controlling behaviors and the particular combinations of control and violence differed from those identified by Johnson (2008)—this was at least a good start.

But, the second author had to go further than simply demonstrating that violence had occurred. She had to demonstrate the ways in which this violence was profoundly damaging, had created fear in Armand, and led to debilitating posttraumatic stress disorder. This violence was not just because "boys were being boys." Similar to heterosexual cases, we explained that once fear is induced, physical violence is not necessary (Raghavan et al., 2019). The relative invisibility of microregulation (i.e., relentless control of small mundane daily activity and tasks) from outside the relationship, coupled with its critical role in achieving control over Armand, underscored how undetectable, yet powerful, these behaviors were. Throughout the report, absurdly basic arguments needed to be made, including that being queer doesn't protect you from violence; gender does not equate sex; and while men are more likely to be abusive than are women in heterosexual relationships, this latter statistic has no meaningful bearing on queer couples. These simple equations, drawn from existing heterosexist beliefs, almost derailed Armand's quest for justice.

Another problem arose when trying to work out confused links between gender, sex, race, and class. IPV in LGBTQ populations remains understudied and there is little by way of forensic work. Thus, there were very few sources to cite, potentially discrediting the report as flimsy and biased. Yet, the lack of forensic scholarship on queer and trans people is a forensic reality. Government lawyers were probably not familiar with same-sex IPV because gay men rarely report their victimization to the police (Finneran & Stephenson, 2013; Langenderfer-Magruder et al., 2016), thereby limiting arrest and conviction (or perpetrator) data. Further, even if seriously injured and hospitalized, male victims may not identify the injury as IPV-related (Kuehnle & Sullivan, 2003; Letellier, 1994; Loveland & Raghavan, 2014) even though prevalence data indicate that partner violence is more prevalent among gay, lesbian, and bisexual partners, compared to heterosexual couples (Messinger, 2011). This dearth of knowledge was clearly noted as a meta-fact. That is, if one doesn't think Armand was abused, it is just as much about one's lack of experience with LGBTQ communities, as it is about the field of forensic psychology.

2.5   Forensic Pathology

There are many different stories that Armand could tell—of his resilience, courage in seeking legal redress, moving from a luxury apartment to a homeless shelter, his continued love for his mother who could not protect him, understanding why his first entry into gay America was the way it had been. But none of these tales would help him legally.

Legal requirements aside, there is no pathway in forensic psychology that charts growth, resilience, and compassion mingled with pain as evidence of abuse or ill-treatment. Indeed, the only acceptable outcome is bleak pathology. This either-or requirement not only pathologizes survivors, it forces them to lie or delete moments of strength and growth from their narratives—lest authorities think they have not suffered enough. Yet, psychologically, years of research tells us that deep suffering leads to different levels of growth, which exist alongside scars. We told a simpler story to the government.

Years of abuse had left Armand with severe untreated Posttraumatic Stress Disorder and depression. Pathologizing Armand with labels of PTSD and depression were in his favor—they gave his story credence and a stamp of realism. Of course, female survivors are also asked to provide evidence of harm as a result of trafficking. But in Armand's case, it seemed to tip the scale from viewing him as a pathological liar to a "true" victim. If several mental health professionals diagnosed him with trauma, then the sexual abuse must have been really bad, Indeed, for a grown *masculine* man to be diagnosed with PTSD, must mean serious business.

Forensic psychologists shape what knowledge is important in legal arenas. If we take a stand, identify how suffering is complex and multi-faceted and includes trauma and growth, and shape its importance in documenting abuse, we can tell the full story. When considering shame, trauma, and victimization, those subjected to these hardships already face so many difficult—at times, unanswerable—questions. What took you so long to come forward? Why does your story not add up? How do you explain that missing detail? Why did you stay? All of these questions are produced from a simplistic and limited understanding of trauma and victimization, predefined by what the field has deemed interesting or important and are deeply impacted by racism, sexism, homophobia, and xenophobia. They force cookie-cutter applications of psycho-legal inquiry and explanation. By expanding the framework, allowing nuance, and even seeming contradiction, we can tell valid stories of victimization and of healing. And, we can begin to challenge the notion that one must be suffering and broken to be worthy of legal salvation or protection. In doing this, we too challenge sexist and homophobic notions of victimhood (Fig. 3).

2.6   Sex Work Versus Sex Trafficking

Armand described the sexual torture he had endured, often weeping quietly. He was filled with self-loathing and didn't blame the government for not believing his stories because he himself could not believe that he had endured such abuse, let alone married the abuser. Intelligent and thoughtful, he wondered why he had escorted

Fig. 3 Protestors holding
up signs at a protest in
Brooklyn, New York.
Photo Courtesy of
Kelly Lacy

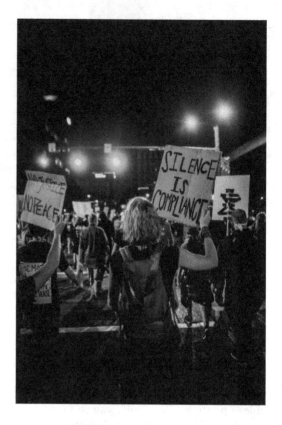

even when he hated it. He believed that his early escorting had led to exploitation and that in some way, he deserved such abuse.

The earliest research on men engaged in prostitution emerged in the late 1940s, framing this activity as psychopathological (Browne & Minichiello, 1996; Butts, 1947; Freyhan, 1947; Minichiello et al., 2013), unnatural, and socially problematic (Scott, 2003).[2] Commercial sex is currently understood as a profession that is rationally chosen by an individual for financial gain (Bimbi, 2007; Scott et al., 2005). Those who endorse this view, otherwise known as the empowerment paradigm (Weitzer, 2010), argue that violence, coercion, and other harms are not intrinsically linked to commercial sex (Comte, 2014; Scott et al., 2005), thereby assuming a reduced risk of violence during commercial sex. The desire to frame commercial sex as empowering is completely understandable, given the history of blame, stigmatization, prejudice, and debasement experienced by individuals involved in the industry. This desire is even further understood for the queer population, which has historically faced harsher abuses in childhood, increased rates of homelessness, and

---

[2] For a full review of history of male commercial sex, see: Minichiello, V., Scott, J., & Callander, D. (2013). New pleasures and old dangers: reinventing male sex work. *Journal of Sex Research*, *50*(3–4), 263–275.

sometimes additional barriers to employment or access to healthcare—all contributing to a potential increased need to engage in commercial sex as a means of survival. However, in Armand's particular case, peer pressure presented him with a false dichotomy—criticize commercial sex and lose his friends or maintain his newfound social support and conflate the necessity to enter commercial sex with an absence of emotional harm.

The government seemed to have little interest in (or perhaps knowledge of) this history, which easily explained Armand's initial cultural encounters with one of many slices of gay community. Neither were they particularly interested in the idea that Armand might have engaged in escorting because his community—accessed for the first time in his life—meant a great deal to him at a time when he was isolated. This is, perhaps, because so little of forensic psychology even broaches the questions of sexual identity and commercial sex. Whereas the identity of heterosexual alliances is rarely subject to definition, men and women in same-sex relationships are defined in part by a shared sexual minority identity (Mohr & Kendra, 2011; Warner & Shields, 2013) and must make conscious decisions about whether to conceal or reveal their sexual preferences (Chrobot-Mason et al., 2001). Groups become crucial in helping navigate identity, especially for someone with Armand's history of oppression. This kind of information—crucial to Armand's decisions— was not available in much of forensic writing, although it is available in other branches of queer studies and psychology.

If the government didn't understand his trafficking pattern, it was simply because they had very little access to these data. They wanted more information on what made legal sense to them—were his activities with Leo consensual or coerced? As it was, on this matter, the government was puzzled; Why would Armand regularly engage in paid and then later, unpaid group sex—then change his mind? And if he continued to ingest party drugs before the event and admitted to enjoying some of the events, surely this indicated consent? To be fair, consent is another underdeveloped issue in forensic psychology—one that raises its murky head whenever sexual assault or sexual coercion with female survivors emerge. Misunderstanding Armand was both a failure to understand the role of homophobia, coming out later in life, and queer sexuality and also a general failure of understanding sexual consent.

Armand entered a relationship with hope but was eventually sexually trafficked—that is, coerced into sleeping with wealthy and powerful men, rewarded when he did, and punished when he did not. Failing to recognize the broad scope of experiences within forced sexual exploitation leads to a dichotomization of victims' experiences (Doychak & Raghavan, 2018). Trafficked survivors are viewed as either consenting and "fallen" or physically abused and "innocent." In addition, government initially viewed with incredulity that someone who admitted to enjoying group sex could then change his mind. Dangerous and harmful stereotypes of queer men as party "animals" with enviable and voracious sexual appetites—and therefore, invulnerable to harm—raised their multiple heads. Interestingly, these are some of the same sexual stereotypes many of us have encountered when working with young black trafficked girls.

Again, forensic psychology can take a stand and start redefining how crucial matters of consent and coercion should be understood—by context steeped in sound understanding of intersectionalities of sexuality, race, gender, class, and immigration status.

2.7 Strategic Opportunities to Navigate Oppressive Systems

Despite the suspicion that the IPV could not have really been all that bad and some reluctance to accept the sexual abuse and exploitation, a strange opportunity presented itself. The case was "legally messy" but there was much interest in prosecuting sex trafficking in the U.S. Armand's team, a brilliant duo of lawyers (some of whom were gay), saw a potential exit for Armand. They reframed the legal argument from an IPV case, to a sex trafficking encounter, positioning Leo as a pimp. Psychologically, it made little sense to Armand. He viewed himself as a survivor of IPV who had been sexually exploited—the entirety of his terrible ordeal contributed to his current suffering. He wanted us to know that he had loved Leo and that Leo had tried to love him but could not. He wanted us to know that he had stayed with Leo because of strength, not weakness. He did not see Leo as a pimp but rather, a sexually damaged man who could only be intimate if he demeaned Armand.

But legally, many of Leo's actions met the Federal Government definition of sex trafficking.[3] While the government hemmed and hawed over whether Armand had been in a truly violent relationship, they eventually found it much easier to swallow that Armand had been sexually exploited and harmed by this exploitation. Armand's intense fears of being killed in his hometown did not resonate intuitively at all for the same patriarchal and heterosexist reasons that the IPV narrative did not—but they did fit a convenient legal requirement. Further, his immigration status was familiar to them; many women are exploited because they do not have permanent residency status in both sex trafficking and IPV cases. And of course, once divorced, Armand was willing to testify in open court against his rich and powerful husband—something that very few survivors dared to do. Armand's social class and education continued to baffle them, but they seemed to not dwell upon it.

In part, this case was a political opportunity. In part, the government's ultimate approach seemed to come from a genuine place—they saw Armand as a victim but could not understand quite how. This confusion highlights shortcomings of our current forensic frameworks and of not understanding sub-cultural norms—the kinds of incidents that Armand described fit better into narratives of gay life than they did

---

[3] The comprehensive federal statute aimed at combatting human trafficking through protection, prosecution, and prevention efforts— The Victims of Trafficking and Violence Protection Act (TVPA; 2000, 2003, 2005, 2008, 2013)—defines sex trafficking as "the recruitment, harboring, transportation, provision, or obtaining of a person for labor or services, through the use of force, fraud, or coercion for the purpose of subjection to involuntary servitude, peonage, debt bondage, or slavery."

in dominant heterosexual ones. Ironically, the government perhaps saw an opportunity to demonstrate how deleterious the effects of sex trafficking are, which they struggled to do without good data. And, since opportunities to litigate sex trafficking are fewer than IPV, they took it.

Ultimately, Armand applied for legal rights to remain in this country based on sex trafficking and the harms that ensued from it and was granted permanent residency and the opportunity to start his life over. I have heard from his lawyers that he is doing well, in recovery, and living a quiet life in the country. While he courageously pressed charges against his abuser, at the time of this case, Leo was not investigated.

3 Implications for Psychology

This chapter is a call to action regarding the many fundamental issues in forensic psychology—which have never been critically examined or deconstructed—and how they arise in harmful and sometimes absurd ways when working with queer populations. Forensic psychologists have a grave responsibility, as they bridge psychology and law. When legal actors try to understand a psychological context, they reach out for what is most central and easily available in forensic psychology print. The government had at its disposal volumes of forensic information on psychopathy and malingering, but nothing on queer sexuality, queer identity, trauma, and same-sex IPV or commercial sexual exploitation. When no easier explanation presented itself, they leaned on what was available.

Fortunately, the question as to whether Armand might have an Anti-Social Personality Disorder—the go-to diagnosis in forensic psychology—disappeared. Perhaps Armand's legal team imagined this fear, or perhaps the government recognized how absurd it was when they had spent hours questioning him. But, the fact that the question was even raised is a problematic reality of what many people in the criminal justice system are presumed to be. We shudder to think of the injustice Armand might have severely suffered had he been labelled as a malingering psychopathic drug-addicted gay escort.

Though currently limited in its pathways for resolve, forensic psychology can improve the way cases like Armand's are approached, understood, and litigated. Forensic psychology is broadly defined and thus, requires no additional definition to meet these goals. However, we must reevaluate what is important within forensic psychology and how to move toward more inclusive training and application. Though psychology rests upon personality development and identity formation, forensic psychology does little to consider identity of any kind. Intersectional queer identity is particularly important; marginalized groups must forge their own histories and these histories shape who we are. The histories of queer identity, how queer identities develop (which would have furthered Armand's case quickly), and how these could intersect with forensic issues should be part of a standard forensic curriculum. Gender and sexuality in cultural contexts—altogether ignored in forensic psychology—should be frontally confronted. The intersectionalities of gender, ethnicity, immigration status, social class, language, and sexuality should begin the introduction to forensic psychology class, not be added as a footnote.

Further, in addition to improving *how* we educate and practice, *who* is overseeing the training of forensic psychology matters for the way in which it is conceptualized. Representation in the classroom—as well as lab rooms and court rooms—matters in a field grappling with a white, dominant framework for understanding intersections of psychology and law. Herein lies a self-fulfilling prophecy. We must consider the accessibility and attractiveness of forensic psychology to POC/LGBTQ psychologists. After all, why would budding POC/LGBTQ students—who themselves or whose communities have been seen as unreliable, incompetent, potentially dangerous, and subject to sexist and heterosexist microaggressions daily—line up to engage in perpetuating more of the same in the name of science?

Without a strong understanding of gender, sex, and culture, the deep heterosexist prejudices that Armand encountered in the legal system, will continue. And, Armand was luckier than many—while his case dragged for years, his team was experienced, committed, and queer. Forensically-relevant data on LGBTQ communities should be collected or, if it exists, disaggregated and made easily available. How many queer folks are incarcerated and why? Do they encounter homophobia and microaggressions in correctional settings? Was the trial process free of prejudice? Was their arrest even justified or an example of profiling?[4] How does their trauma history—if it exists, and it so often does—interact with their current presentation, or their history of offending? This utter lack of inclusion harms forensic psychologists' ability to do their work—as we found when trying to cite Armand's report. Lack of data is yet another self-fulfilling prophecy, as it discourages queer research. But if there is to be new research, it should be thoughtful. Merely replicating and expanding existing forensic research, adding queerness as a solo variable, will only reinforce heterosexism and white hegemonic empiricism. We need to deconstruct forensic psychology's reliance on old concepts of malingering, dangerousness, and the overuse of psychopathy as the only explanatory variable.

Overall, the government wanted to be helpful but they too were dealing with standard adversarial forensic tools. Deconstruction of these tools, which are used to harm those of marginalized sexual and gender identities, should become an important topic of discussion. Why do we study malingering and not truthfulness? How do heterosexist, homophobic, or transphobic ideals impact the way we arrive at answers? Why do we not explore other reasons that queer men like Armand may have concealed aspects of his private life, other than lying? Understanding the misuse of standard forensic tools while being critically aware of queer history and identity will advance and queer forensic psychology.

---

[4] For example, advocates argue that New York's Loitering for the Purpose of Prostitution Law (colloquially referred to as the Walking While Trans Ban) effectively allows police to make arrests based on the visual suspicion of engagement in commercial sex and disproportionately impacts transgender women of color (LGBTQ Rights Committee et al., 2020).

Trauma—and its presentation in the courts—must also be reconsidered, as an overwhelming number of those involved in the legal system bear trauma histories. The trauma literature speaks much of pain and growth, and exhorts psychologists to not minimize one for the other but to understand the interconnectedness. For many abused individuals, surviving the experience leads them to strength. But in forensic contexts, this would be technical suicide. For good results—whether civil or criminal—only the terrible, bad, and very bad should be presented. But this is not reality; it is simplistic, non-psychological thinking. We don't propose that forensic psychologists stop evaluating negative outcomes of victimization; but rather, that we find ways to explain to our clients or lawyers why we use certain terms and language, while seeking ways to decolonize the pathological labels that are applied so freely.

The scope and application of forensic psychology has been focused around three large issues, which play out in the court system. The first roughly corresponds to establishing the mental status of a defendant at the time a crime was committed and how to manage this through the legal process. The second focuses on psychological information to protect children in the case of IPV and/or divorce. A third largely non-clinical strand includes research (and court testimony) on how legal actors such as police, judges, and eyewitnesses interact in court. Much more queer and intersectional research needs to enter the field, which is relevant to sexual and ethnic non-majority populations. Applying microaggression, race-related trauma, and gender discrimination to not only legal processes, but as predictors of violence and violence resistance would increase the relevance of this field.

While we have only spoken of an immigrant queer cisgender man, trafficking of trans and queer women is a serious issue and is little researched or considered. In making these larger changes toward queering forensic psychology, IPV and sex trafficking researchers and practitioners offer us a model on how to begin challenging dominant value systems and harmful frameworks for understanding human behavior. We must systematically strive for inclusivity while confronting oppressive systems; we must do this not by developing forensic research or teaching forensic curricula that attempts to fit queer narratives into current forensic models—which pathologize, ignore, or marginalize the experience of certain groups and not others—but by dismantling these frameworks and reconstructing new ones.

References

Ahrens, C. E., Rios-Mandel, L. C., Isas, L., & del Carmen Lopez, M. (2010). Talking about interpersonal violence: Cultural influences on Latinas' identification and disclosure of sexual assault and intimate partner violence. *Psychological Trauma: Theory, Research, Practice, and Policy, 2*(4), 284–295. https://doi-org.ez.lib.jjay.cuny.edu/10.1037/a0018605.

American Psychological Association. (n.d.). *Division 41: American Psychology-Law Society.* Retrieved from http://www.apa.org/about/division/

Bimbi, D. (2007). Male prostitution: Pathology, paradigms, and progress in research. *Journal of Homosexuality, 53*(1/2), 7–35.

Blackburn, R. (1996). What is forensic psychology? *Legal and Criminological Psychology*, *1*, 3–15.

Blechner, M. J. (2018). *The mindbrain and dreams: An exploration of dreaming, thinking, and artistic creation*. New York, NY: Routledge.

Brigham, J. (1999). What is forensic psychology, anyway? *Law and Human Behavior, 23*(3), 273–298. Retrieved July 20, 2020, from www.jstor.org/stable/1394354.

Brown, C. (2008). Gender-role implications on same-sex intimate partner abuse. *Journal of Family Violence, 23*(6), 457–462.

Brown v. Board of Education. (1954). 347 US 483.

Browne, J., & Minichiello, V. (1996). Research directions in male sex work. *Journal of Homosexuality, 31*(4), 29–56.

Bryant, S. A., & Spencer, G. A. (2003). University students' attitudes about attributing blame in domestic violence. *Journal of Family Violence, 18*, 369–376. https://doi.org/10.102 3/A:1026205817132.

Bull, R. (2011). *Forensic psychology*. Thousand Oaks, CA: Sage Publications.

Butts, W. H. (1947). Boy prostitutes of the metropolis. *Journal of Clinical Psychopathology, 8*, 673–681.

Chrobot-Mason, D., Button, S. B., & DiClementi, J. D. (2001). Sexual identity management strategies: An exploration of antecedents and consequences. *Sex Roles, 45*(5–6), 321–336.

Comte, J. (2014). Decriminalization of sex work: Feminist discourses in light of research. *Sexuality & Culture, 18*(1), 196–217.

Doychak, K., & Raghavan, C. (2018). "No voice or vote:" Trauma-coerced attachment in victims of sex trafficking. *Journal of Human Trafficking*. https://doi.org/10.1080/23322705.201 8.1518625.

Dutton, M. A., & Goodman, L. A. (2005). Coercion in intimate partner violence: Toward a new conceptualization. *Sex Roles, 52*(11–12), 743–756.

Finneran, C., & Stephenson, R. (2013). Intimate partner violence among men who have sex with men: A systematic review. *Trauma Violence Abuse, 14*(2), 168–185.

Fischel-Wolovick, L. (2018). *Traumatic divorce and separation: The impact of domestic violence and substance abuse in custody and divorce*. Oxford University Press.

Frankland, A., & Brown, J. (2014). Coercive control in same-sex intimate partner violence. *Journal of Family Violence, 29*(1), 15–22.

Freyhan, F. A. (1947). Homosexual prostitution: A case report. *Delaware State Medical Journal, 19*, 92–94.

Heilbrun, K., & Brooks, S. (2010). Forensic psychology and forensic science: A proposed agenda for the next decade. *Psychology, Public Policy, and Law, 16*(3), 219–253. https://doi.org/10.1037/a0019138.

Hempel, C. L. (2004). Battered women who strike back: Using expert testimony on battering and its effects in homicide trials. In B. J. Cling (Ed.), *Sexualized violence against women and children: A psychology and law perspective* (pp. 71–97). New York: The Guildford Press.

Herek, G. M. (1990). The context of anti-gay violence: Notes on cultural and psychological heterosexism. *Journal of Interpersonal Violence, 5*(3), 316–333. https://doi.org/10.1177/088626090005003006.

Holland, J. (2020). *Good chemistry: The science of connection, from soul to psychedelics*. New York: HarperCollins Publishers.

Johnson, M. P. (2008). *A typology of domestic violence: Intimate terrorism, violent resistance, and situational couple violence*. Boston: Northeastern University Press.

Kuehnle, K., & Sullivan, A. (2003). Gay and lesbian victimization: Reporting factors in domestic violence bias incidents. *Criminal Justice and Behavior, 30*, 85–96. https://doi.org/10.1177/0093854802239164.

Langenderfer-Magruder, L., Whitfield, D. L., Eugene Walls, N., Kattari, S. K., & Ramos, D. (2016). Experiences of intimate partner violence and subsequent police reporting among lesbian, gay, bisexual, transgender, and queer adults in Colorado: Comparing rates of cisgender and transgender victimization. *Journal of Interpersonal Violence, 31*(5), 855–871. https://doi.org/10.1177/0886260514556767.

Larson, D. G., Chastain, R. L., Hoyt, W. T., & Ayzenberg, R. (2015). Self-concealment: Integrative review and working model. *Journal of Social and Clinical Psychology, 34*(8), 705–e774. https://doi.org/10.1521/jscp.2015.34.8.705.

Letellier, P. (1994). Gay and bisexual male domestic violence victimization: Challenges to feminist theory and response to violence. *Violence and Victims, 2*, 96–106.

LGBTQ Rights Committee, Civil Rights Committee, Criminal Justice Operations Committee, Immigration & Nationality Law Committee, and Sex & Law Committee. (2020). Repeal the "Walking While Trans" Ban Committee Report (Report No. A.654 M. of A. Paulin, S.2253 Sen. Hoylman). New York City Bar. Retrieved from https://www.nycbar.org/member-and-career-services/committees/reports-listing/reports/detail/repeal-the-walking-while-trans-ban

Loh, W. D. (1981). Perspectives on psychology and law. *Journal of Applied Social Psychology, 11*, 314–355.

Loveland, J. E., & Raghavan, C. (2014). Near-lethal violence in a high-risk sample of men in same-sex relationships. *Psychology of Sexual Orientation and Gender Diversity, 1*(1), 51–62.

Meerwijk, E. L., & Sevelius, J. M. (2017). Transgender population size in the United States: A meta-regression of population-based probability samples. *American Journal of Public Health, 107*(2), e1–e8. https://doi.org/10.2105/AJPH.2016.303578.

Messinger, A. (2011). Invisible victims: Same-sex IPV in the National Violence against Women Survey. *Journal of Interpersonal Violence, 26*(11), 2228–2243. https://doi.org/10.1177/0886260510383023.

Minichiello, V., Scott, J., & Callander, D. (2013). New pleasures and old dangers: Reinventing male sex work. *Journal of Sex Research, 50*(3–4), 263–275.

Mohr, J. J., & Kendra, M. S. (2011). Revision and extension of a multidimensional measure of sexual minority identity: The lesbian, gay, and bisexual identity scale. *Journal of Counseling Psychology, 58*(2), 234.

Morton, R. J., Tillman, J. M., & Gaines, S. J. (2015). *Serial murder: Pathways for investigations. National center for the analysis of violent crime*. Washington, DC: Federal Bureau of Investigation. Retrieved from http://www.fbi.gov/news/stories/2014/october/serial-killers-part-8-new-research-aims-to-help-investigators-solve-cases/serial-murder-pathways-forinvestigations.

Muller v. Oregon. (1908). 208 US 412.

Nadal, K. L. Y. (2020). *Queering law and order: LGBTQ communities and the criminal justice system*. New York: Lexington Books.

Nichols, A. J., Preble, K. M., & Cox, A. (2019). *Human trafficking in Missouri and Metro East St. Louis: Provider based needs assessment and demographic snapshot*. Retrieved from https://marillacmissionfund.org/application/files/2915/7678/4013/Needs_Assessment_Report11.15.19FINAL.pdf

Nicholson v. Scoppetta (2004). 820 NE 2d 840.

Otto, R. K., & Heilbrun, K. (2002). The practice of forensic psychology: A look toward the future in light of the past. *American Psychologist, 57*, 5–19.

Puzzanchera, C., Smith, J., Kang, W. (2018). *Easy access to NIBRS victims, 2016: Victims of domestic violence*. Retrieved from https://www.ojjdp.gov/ojstatbb/ezanibrsdv/.

Raghavan, C., Beck, C. J. A., Menke, J. M., & Loveland, J. E. (2019). Coercive controlling behaviors in intimate partner violence in male same-sex relationships: A mixed-methods study. *Journal of Gay and Lesbian Social Services, 31*(3), 370–395. https://doi.org/10.1080/10538720.2019.1616643.

Regina v. M'Naghten. (1843). 10 Cl. & Fin. At 203, 8 Eng. Rep. at 720.

Ricard, M., & Singer, W. (2017). *Beyond the self: Conversations between Buddhism and neuroscience*. Cambridge, MA: The MIT Press.

Rogers, R. E. (2008). *Clinical assessment of malingering and deception*. New York: Guilford Press.

Scott, J. (2003). A prostitute's progress: Male prostitution in scientific discourse. *Social Semiotics, 13*(2), 179–199.

Scott, J., Minichiello, V., Marino, R., Harvey, G. P., Jamieson, M., & Browne, J. (2005). Understanding the new context of the male sex work industry. *Journal of Interpersonal Violence, 20*(3), 320–342.

Sherkat, D. E. (2002). Sexuality and religious commitment in the United States: An empirical examination. *Journal for the Scientific Study of Religion, 41*(2), 313–323. https://doi.org/10.1111/1468-5906.00119.

Sorsoli, L. (2010). 'I remember', 'I thought', "I know I didn't say": Silence and memory in trauma narratives. *Memory, 18*(2), 129–141. https://doi-org.ez.lib.jjay.cuny.edu/10.1080/09658210903168046.

Stanley, J., Bartholomew, K., Taylor, T., Oram, D., & Landolt, M. (2006). Intimate violence in male same-sex relationships. *Journal of Family Violence, 21*, 31–41. https://doi.org/10.1007/210896-005-9008-9.

Stark, E. (2006). Commentary on Johnson's "conflict and control: Gender symmetry and asymmetry in domestic violence". *Violence Against Women, 12*(11), 1019–1025.

Stark, E. (2007). *Coercive control: How men entrap women in personal life.* New York, NY: Oxford University Press.

Sutherland, E. H. (1949). The sexual psychopath laws. *Journal of Criminal Law & Criminology, 40*, 543–554.

Warner, L. R., & Shields, S. A. (2013). The intersections of sexuality, gender, and race: Identity research at the crossroads. *Sex Roles, 68*(11–12), 803–810.

Weitzer, R. (2010). Sex work: Paradigms and policies. In R. W. (Ed.), *Sex for sale: Prostitution, pornography, and the sex industry* (pp. 1–43). New York: Routledge.

Future Directions and Queer Activism

María R. Scharrón-del Río and Kevin L. Nadal

1 Conclusion: Future Directions and Queer Activism

Within academic writing, locating oneself and writing about our own realities have often been frowned upon. In the name of scientific "objectivity", the self has needed to remain hidden, promoting the illusion of impartiality and neutrality. This Cartesian dichotomy between the self and the object of study, is part of what Martín-Baró (1998) called the *parcialization* of human experience in positivist science. Reducing the study of an object to its parts erases the interactions between them and the object's context, as well as the relationship between the scholar and what their focus of study (Scharrón-Del Río, 2010). Queer, Feminist, and Critical Race theory eschew the illusion that our production of knowledge can come from a neutral/objective stance: as stated eloquently in one of our chapters, we are always in relation to whom and what we study (Cerezo & Renteria, 2022) (Fig. 1).

This book, *Queer Psychology*, was conceptualized and written because of our relationship to the field. The editors and most of the authors identify as queer or trans, and a large majority of the authors also identify as Black, Indigenous, and other People of Color (BIPOC). As graduate students, clinicians, practitioners, advocates, emergent and established scholars in our respective fields, many of us knew firsthand about the erasure, gaps in research, limited and/or ill-fitting theory, educational/health/mental health disparities, and lack of training of traditional psychology—especially as it relates to queer and multiple-marginalized communities.

M. R. Scharrón-del Río (✉)
Brooklyn College—City University of New York, School of Education, Brooklyn, NY, USA
e-mail: MariaRS@brooklyn.cuny.edu

K. L. Nadal
Department of Psychology, John Jay College of Criminal Justice—City University of New York, New York, NY, USA
e-mail: knadal@jjay.cuny.edu

Fig. 1 A young queer
person wrapped in a
rainbow flag at a Pride
Parade. Photo Courtesy of
Ronê Ferreria

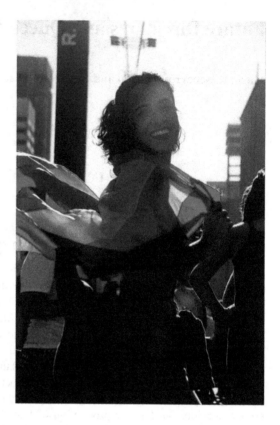

Many of our contributors are "queering psychology" on an everyday basis, sometimes just by showing up and claiming space, in systems and institutions that were
not built for us.

In the introduction of this book (Nadal & Scharrón-del Río, 2022), we state that
"queering" means to challenge the status quo. Queering is an intentional reflection
about what we know—or what we think we know—in order to choose expansion
instead of constriction and limitation (Scharrón-Del Río, 2020a; b). Queering challenges the oppressive structures and categories that are imposed on our communities. The process also acknowledges our interconnectedness with each other, while
celebrating and affirming our differences. Queering, in its true sense, involves an
epistemic stance that leads towards action (Hunt & Holmes, 2015).

The authors in this book present many avenues for queering and challenging
traditional psychology, in areas such as research, training, clinical work, policy, and
epistemics/theory. They also provide direction for queer activism to engage in liberating praxis. While the authors' contributions are many, we wish to summarize a
few before offering brief concluding remarks.

1.1 Research

> *To the extent that a specific theory of psychotherapy is developed, constructed, and tested in a particular cultural group, packaged as empirically sound, and imposed on another, there may be a new form of cultural imperialism.* (Bernal & Scharrón-del Río, 2001, p. 333).

In their chapter on queering research methods, Cerezo and Renteria (2022) remind us that research and psychometric instruments in psychology have primarily focused on people who are Western, Educated, and from Industrialized, Rich and Democratic (WEIRD) countries (Henrich et al., 2010). Psychological research devoid of the examination of its context and source can easily be used as yet another form of cultural imperialism (Bernal & Scharrón-del Río, 2001). Decolonizing and queering research involves understanding the limitations of its applicability, as well as its history of misuse as an instrument of European imperialism, colonialism, oppression and subjugation (Smith, 1999; Trimble et al., 2014). Thus, it is imperative to queer psychology, so that it expands the populations where psychological research, interventions, and instruments are developed and validated (Cerezo & Renteria, 2022). Queering psychology also requires us to be knowledgeable about the history of research-induced trauma in marginalized communities, while challenging concepts and approaches that have contributed to the pathologization, stigmatization, and systemic oppression of queer and BIPOC communities (Trimble et al., 2014).

Research needs to also include "non-Eurocentric and indigenous perspectives", as Puzio and Forbes (2022) describe eloquently in Chap. 3. Queering psychology means to acknowledge the work of queer scholars of color who have taken the lead on examining the experiences of multiply marginalized communities—often using a plurality of methods, from autoethnographic to empirical approaches (Cerezo & Renteria, 2022; Puzio & Forbes, 2022). Queering psychology means to celebrate and value the works of other disciplines, such as Ethnic Studies, Queer Studies, and Gender Studies, as such fields have been at the forefront of social justice movements for much longer than the field of psychology. Further, while traditional interventions (developed with mostly White samples and in WEIRD countries) are often used on queer and BIPOC communities, more research is needed on how and when to adapt interventions for queer and BIPOC communities and especially queer BIPOC communities (Freeman-Coppadge & Farhadi Langroudi, 2022; Trimble et al., 2010).

Traditional psychology often continues to rely on dichotomous/binary models regarding identity, pathologizing difference, and divergence from what is considered "normal". It is crucial to first question who gets to control what is considered normalized and standard, and who then is deemed abnormal or inferior. In perpetrating WEIRD standards, psychology is perpetuating colonial standards which we all are socialized to follow or adhere too. In this way, when psychologists who come from historically marginalized groups are taught the Western psychology is superior and that other practices and approaches are inferior, they may internalize such messages that they may then pass onto their students, mentees, trainees, and so forth.

Further, it is very important to advance research that includes expansive models of gender, particularly in how we look at the experiences of people who identify outside binary and traditionally normative categories, and how we can develop more holistic assessments (Puzio & Forbes, 2022). In addition, it is paramount to increase attention to the strengths, coping strategies, and resilience of queer and BIPOC community (Singh et al., 2022), expanding and challenging what are often deficit and pathologizing models—a common trend particularly when we describe LGBTQ and BIPOC health and mental health (Mereish & Taylor, 2022; Velez et al., 2022). Research must also incorporate intersectionality, particularly in how we address the negative impacts of multiple marginalization on LGBTQ communities of color (Estrellado et al., 2022; Freeman-Coppadge & Farhadi Langroudi, 2022). Further, as stated in our introduction, we must also expand intersectional research to include LGBTQ people with disabilities—as such experiences have been minimal and/or erased in the field of psychology. We recognize a need for psychologists to become more aware of, and actively supportive of, the Queer Crip movements, especially in the ways that we learn about social justice and the ways that we can advocate for the holistic needs of historically marginalized people.

Some of our chapters addressed particular subfields of study, and our authors made specific recommendations regarding the dearth/gaps of research in their areas. In their chapter, Estrellado et al. (2022) make a case about the importance to include other family structures other than the heteronormative couple in research around parenting and families. According to these authors, research on queer families must include single-parent families, other-than couple parenting arrangements, families with bisexual parents (who constitute the largest percentage of queer parents), and queer BIPOC families (especially since there are higher percentages of BIPOC couples are parenting than there are White couples who are parenting). Meanwhile, in their chapter on queer youth, Torre and Avory (2022) exhort psychologists to center research about queer youth (and BIPOC queer youth in particular) on their perspectives, needs, and challenges. Their chapter—along with the chapter on gender identity and sexual orientation identity—remind us that more research is needed on queer childhood development. In its current state, what we know about queer identity is from retrospective narratives, as opposed to research conducted with LGBTQ children themselves.

Finally, Doychak and Raghavan (2022) state that research on issues involving queer people in Forensic Psychology needs to increase and that there is a need for more data collection (or access to disaggregated data) on forensic statistics regarding queer and trans people. These authors challenge forensic psychology to queer its methodology—letting go of its "reliance on old concepts of malingering, dangerousness, and the overuse of psychopathy as the only explanatory variable" (Doychak & Raghavan, 2022).

1.2 Training

To eliminate health and mental health disparities, part of what is needed is to improve the training of our health and mental health providers. Training programs must improve training around queer communities and issues in order to improve intervention outcomes and quality of treatment, while reducing bias, stigma, and barriers to services (Chan & Silverio, 2022; Mereish & Taylor, 2022; Velez et al., 2022). Training should also include knowledge on the history of systems of oppression and an understanding of intersectionality (Ford, 2022; Singh et al., 2022; Freeman-Coppadge & Farhadi Langroudi, 2022). Syndemics theory and its implications on health and mental health should also be included in the training of health and mental health professionals (Chan & Silverio, 2022; Velez et al., 2022).

Training programs for health and mental health professionals must challenge the emphasis on pathologization of queer and BIPOC communities by engaging in education to reduce bias (i.e., anti-racist education) and replace deficit models with an emphasis on strengths, resiliency factors, and affirming identity development (Velez et al., 2022; Freeman-Coppadge & Farhadi Langroudi, 2022). Curriculum needs to be improved to counter "queer erasure" and invisibility: readings and experiences need to be incorporated to learn about our queer communities' affective, romantic, sexual, and familiar relationships (Doychak & Raghavan, 2022; Estrellado et al., 2022; Freeman-Coppadge & Farhadi Langroudi, 2022; Rider et al., 2022). Finally, providers must receive training in LGBTQ-affirmative therapies/interventions, adapted to consider additional marginalized identities (Baquet et al., 2022); Freeman-Coppadge & Farhadi Langroudi, 2022) (Fig. 2).

1.3 Clinical Work

What is most needed at this time are evidence-based practices that utilize intersectional and social justice lenses to apply to sexual and gender minorities (SGMs) with multiple marginalized identities at individual, interpersonal, and institutional levels. (Freeman-Coppadge & Farhadi Langroudi, 2022)

Many of the recommendations proposed by our chapter authors around clinical work complement the above recommendations towards improving training. Our queer and BIPOC communities need practitioners committed to liberation and that can engage in radical models of healing (Comas-Díaz et al., 2019; Doychak & Raghavan, 2022; Martín-Baró, 1998). Health and mental health professionals might need to make up for the invisibility of queer issues ("queer erasure") and intersectionality in their training (Chan & Silverio, 2022; Estrellado et al., 2022; Freeman-Coppadge & Farhadi Langroudi, 2022; Rider et al., 2022). Clinicians need to be able to discuss racism (as well as other systems of oppression) and how it impacts queer BIPOC (Freeman-Coppadge & Farhadi Langroudi, 2022). Health and mental health providers must be able to understand how cultural differences (i.e., being part

Fig. 2 A "Love is love" mural painted on the side of a building. Photo Courtesy of Annette Dawn

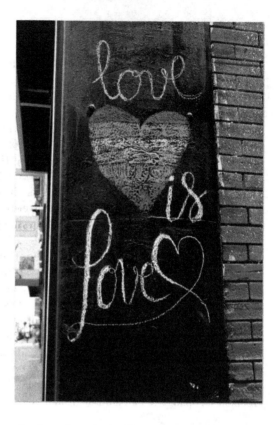

of a collectivistic culture, acculturation/enculturation) affect queer individuals differently according to the intersection of their identities (Chan & Silverio, 2022; Freeman-Coppadge & Farhadi Langroudi, 2022). Moreover, practitioners need to be knowledgeable about the impact of historical and transgenerational trauma in queer BIPOC (Freeman-Coppadge & Farhadi Langroudi, 2022).

While many health and mental health practitioners have received training around multicultural competence, this might not have included an understanding of intersectionality. Clinicians must understand how multiple-marginalized identities affect their clients, starting with acknowledging that LGBTQ clinical competence is not synonymous with intersectional LGBTQ clinical competence. Intersectional affirming care is sorely needed in our communities (Freeman-Coppadge & Farhadi Langroudi, 2022). Mental health interventions need to recognize and address the impact of systemic oppression in queer communities, particularly in people who have multiple marginalized identities. As an example, Velez, Zelaya, and Scheer mention an intervention (Effective Skills to Empower Effective Men, ESTEEM), that actively addresses the stress that oppression has on gay and bisexual men's syndemic conditions. Chan and Silverio also emphasize how health and mental health providers have a duty to assess and address "the accumulating effects sustained by health inequities and overlapping forms of oppression" in queer communities (p. # **). Practitioners also need to be knowledgeable about community resources for queer people, particularly for those that belong to multiple marginalized communities.

Various chapters stress the need for clinicians to include in their evaluations thorough assessments of strengths, resiliencies, and coping strategies of queer communities (Singh et al., 2022), as well as of the impact of the intersection of their identities (Freeman-Coppadge & Farhadi Langroudi, 2022). It follows then that interventions need to include self-advocacy as part of the skills to strengthen/develop. Singh, Estevez, and Truszczynski suggest incorporating role-play opportunities as part of clinical work with queer communities, as a way of ensuring that LGBTQ+ people and BIPOC know their rights. Aligned with the emphasis on self-determination advocated by indigenous communities (Smith, 1999), such practices are vital to community members' empowerment and healing processes (Trimble et al., 2014).

Intersectional approaches not only consider racial, ethnic, gender, class, and sexual identity. Often overlooked, age, spirituality, and (dis)ability are important dimensions for queer people. While some needs and challenges of queer youth and young queers are shared by older queer people, the cumulative effect of historical events in our older generation—in addition to changes regarding (dis)abilities and earning potential—need to be considered when assessing queer older adults (Chan & Silverio, 2022).

Clinicians must be also able to assess and include in their interventions discussions about religion/spirituality, particularly for queer BIPOC (Ford, 2022; Freeman-Coppadge & Farhadi Langroudi, 2022). Mental health practitioners need to understand that belonging to a religious/spiritual community means something different for queer people according to their racial/ethnic identity (Ford, 2022). Religion/spirituality can be simultaneously a source of resiliency and trauma for queer people. Mental health professionals need to be knowledgeable about the history and rituals of various religious/spiritual traditions, educate themselves about the stigma, trauma, and marginalization that LGBTQ BIPOC experience in their faith communities, and be able to provide appropriate resources (Ford, 2022).

1.4 Policy Work

There are numerous policy implications in the knowledge contained in this book. Queering psychology means that we must use research to develop and support policies that address the structural and institutional barriers that impact queer people's lives and well-being (Mereish & Taylor, 2022). Since all oppressions are interconnected, queer advocacy should pursue policies that will impact our society as a whole, such as access to universal health care, increasing available resources and countering racist, sexist, heterosexist, anti-immigrant, and anti-disability policies/laws (Singh et al., 2022). Universal healthcare is necessary to bridge health and mental health disparities in our queer communities, and such care must include and facilitate access to mental health treatments, gender-affirming interventions, and assisted reproductive technology, among many other services (Estrellado et al., 2022).

Queer advocacy must also seek to impact training guidelines and accreditation standards. Curricula for health and mental health practitioners must include instruction in systemic oppression, intersectionality, and how oppression of people with multiple-marginalized identities affect communities, including our queer community. In addition, it should also include training in intersectional and LGBTQ-affirming interventions.

Some chapters include policy recommendations specific to subgroups within queer communities. Estrellado, Felipe, Nakamura, and Breen address issues related to queer parenting and families. These authors urge us to support policies that recognize and protect the rights of queer parents in all aspects of society, from de-facto inclusion in official records such as birth certificates, to protecting their rights to adopt and foster children. Baquet et al. (2022) remind us that policy changes are still needed to fully protect the rights of queer people in the workplace, ensuring that both gender identity and sexual orientation are protected classes in current and future laws. Ford reminds us that we must continue our efforts to ban conversion "therapies". Finally, Doychak and Raghavan challenge traditional forensic psychology to advocate for deconstructing and challenging standard adversarial forensic tools, which adversely impact queer and multiple marginalized identity people.

Queer advocacy needs to be intersectional. We need to be advocating for BLM, immigration reform, (dis)ability rights, children/youth/elder welfare, universal healthcare, food security, housing justice/rights, sex workers' rights, elderly rights, workplace protections, prison reform, stopping to school-to-prison pipeline, and the dismantling of all systemic/institutional oppression (Baquet et al., 2022; Chan & Silverio, 2022; Freeman-Coppadge & Farhadi Langroudi, 2022; Mereish & Taylor, 2022; Rider et al. 2022; Singh et al., 2022). Queering psychology means centering the margins, writing and supporting policies that challenge systemic oppression and the inequities it perpetuates.

1.5   Epistemic

Our contributors queer psychology by challenging many of its hegemonic assumptions, definitions, and stances. As mentioned earlier, they challenge the assumption of generalizability of theories and instruments developed for and with people from WEIRD countries (Cerezo & Renteria, 2022). Ferguson challenges the prevailing epistemological approach to identity models and research ("single-axis" analysis), which has historically focused on one-dimensional considerations of identity. Intersectionality upends this approach, centering analysis in the interaction between social identities in relation to their positionality within systems of privilege/oppression. Queering psychology challenges us to examine our reality taking into consideration our multiple positions within these systems, all of which are interrelated in complex ways that create different lived experiences within single-axis identity communities. Thus, our LGBTQ community is not a monolithic group, but a collection of communities.

Psychological theory and research need to reflect this plurality and complexity in order to better capture and address our realities. This epistemic shift involves a decentering of the historical hegemonic discourse, as well as centering what has traditionally been considered marginalized. It also urges our field to look outside of the US/Eurocentric reality and acknowledge the contributions to queer psychology from other regions and countries (Freeman-Coppadge & Farhadi Langroudi, 2022; Scharrón-Del Río, 2020b). Queering psychology also means to welcome interdisciplinary scholarship, such as the work of social scientists and indigenous scholars outside of psychology (Puzio & Forbes, 2022).

Many chapters challenge dichotomous categories and perspectives, including gender identity (Doychak & Raghavan, 2022; Puzio & Forbes, 2022) and sexual orientation (Adames & Chavez-Dueñas, 2022). At the same time, they challenge the pathologizing discourses and approaches that stem from traditional hegemonic discourses (e.g., Eurocentric, heteronormative), including the identification of gender identities outside of the binary as part of what is to be expected within normative gender identity development (Puzio & Forbes, 2022). Eurocentric cis-het hegemonic discourses erase queerness, and along it, our queer communities affective, romantic, sexual, and familiar relationships (Doychak & Raghavan, 2022; Estrellado et al., 2022; Rider et al., 2022).

Queering psychology also involves challenging the focus on the decontextualized individual person as it relates to identity development and their well-being. In their chapter regarding gender, Puzio and Forbes enumerate various contemporary theories on gender identity that include the impact of immediate social and cultural factors (i.e., typicality, felt pressure, available gender categories) and their dynamic between the person as part of the process of gender identity development. Adames and Chavez-Dueñas incorporate in their Racial Queer Identity (RQI) Framework the impact that affirming and non-affirming messages regarding our identities affect their development. Challenging the idea that the different aspects of our identity develop separately from the others, the RQI Framework transcends single-axis identity theories in order to showcase how "racism, heterosexism, and cissexism overlap" (p. **) and their impact in identity formation among Queer People of Color (QPOC).

Acknowledging that our well-being entails more than our individual present experiences, Freeman-Coppadge and Farhadi Langroudi highlight the importance of recognizing historical/transgenerational trauma, as well as how psychology must incorporate indigenous healing practices and approaches. Similarly, by incorporating syndemics theory, some of our authors also challenge individualistic and traditional views regarding well-being: queer and multiply marginalized people may at times engage in health-risk behaviors as a way of coping with the effect of minority stress in their lives (Mereish & Taylor, 2022; Velez et al., 2022).

2   Queering Psychology Is Liberatory Praxis

In order to truly queer psychology, to genuinely challenge the institutional barriers and systems of oppression that keep our psychological theories, research, and interventions representative of mainly WEIRD (Western, Educated, and from Industrialized, Rich and Democratic) countries–therefore excluding and marginalizing our queer and BIPOC communities—we must engage in intersectional liberatory praxis. We must capture the voices of the marginalized (Torre & Avory, 2022) using multiple methods (Cerezo & Renteria, 2022). We must recognize indigenous knowledge and the contribution of queer BIPOC. We must train health and mental health providers how to provide intersectional affirming care. Our policies and advocacy need to procure liberation from all members of our queer communities, particularly at the intersection of additional oppressions. We must continue to challenge dichotomous/binary, decontextualized, and pathologizing theories and approaches, and engage in decolonization of our field and in liberation praxis. There is much to be done.

To queer psychology we need a greater amount of queer BIPOC psychologists, counselors, health and mental health professionals, and researchers. To achieve this, we must address educational disparities that keep BIPOC youth out of undergraduate and graduate education. These disparities are a consequence of the racism, ethnocentrism, classism, and the pervasive underfunding of public P-12 and higher education, among other factors. We need to challenge the intersection of systems of oppression that stacks layers of barriers against the success of queer BIPOC and non-traditional students (Brim, 2020).

Queer BIPOC students often do not see themselves in the research (Scharrón-Del Río, 2020a; b), an academic invisibility that compounds queer erasure. We need to challenge academia to recognize poor queer studies (Brim, 2020): to look at the production of queer scholarship and research that is produced by scholars, advocates, and communities outside of elite institutions. Within these poor queer studies, we often find the intersectional scholarship that the field sorely needs, often produced by multiply marginalized students, advocates, and scholars.

In addition to a greater amount of queer BIPOC psychologists, we also need more psychologists of all sexual orientations, gender identities, racial and ethnic groups, and others to be more willing to stand up and advocate for justice. People with more historically privileged identities (e.g., White people, cisgender people, men, educated people, academics with tenure) need to be more willing and vocal in advocating for equity. People with less privileged identities must strategize to create opportunities to advocate for justice too—whether they get involved in community organizing, collective actions, or even subtler ways of infusing justice into their practice. Either way, it will take people across all walks of life to work collectively together in order for us to decolonize and queer psychology in the way that it needs to be.

Some of the common threads in the epistemic shifts contained in the chapters of this book include topics that are also part of decolonization and liberation efforts within psychology. As Hunt and Holmes (2015) state:

> Decolonization involves actively challenging or disrupting systems of knowledge that do not fully account for the lives of Indigenous people, queer and trans people, and many others whose lives are erased through epistemic and material violence. (p. 159).

Recognizing and resisting hegemonic Euro-centric discourses (Adames & Chavez-Dueñas, 2022; Freeman-Coppadge and Farhadi Langroudi, 2022), including indigenous knowledge and practices (Adames & Chavez-Dueñas, 2022; Puzio & Forbes, 2022; Ford, 2022), embracing intersectionality (Adames & Chavez-Dueñas, 2022; Baquet et al., 2022; Cerezo & Renteria, 2022; Chan & Silverio, 2022; Doychak & Raghavan, 2022; Estrellado et al., 2022; Ferguson, 2022; Ford, 2022; Freeman-Coppadge & Farhadi Langroudi, 2022; Mereish & Taylor, 2022; Rider et al., 2022; Singh et al., 2022; Torre & Avory, 2022; Velez et al., 2022), reclaiming our space and history—despite invisibilization and erasure—(Adames & Chavez-Dueñas, 2022; Baquet et al., 2022; Cerezo & Renteria, 2022; Estrellado et al., 2022), and supporting self-determination (Puzio & Forbes, 2022; Singh et al., 2022; Torre & Avory, 2022) are part of the process of decolonizing psychology.

Moreover, queering psychology requires us to embrace solidarity, embracing interconnection across multiple dimensions of oppression (Scharrón-del Río & Aja, 2020). This dynamic of solidarity is a revolutionary resistance to the process of "othering" that propelled colonialism and that is the basis of all systems of oppression. Thus, solidarity across "interconnected identities and positionalities" is key to decolonizing and liberatory praxis (Hunt & Holmes, 2015; Martín-Baró, 1998).

Queering psychology involves a commitment to a psychology of liberation (Martín-Baró, 1998; Singh, 2016). Thus, we must center our scholarship around conscientization and liberation: acknowledging and challenging oppressive approaches, systems, and institutions, and engaging communities in processes and interventions that will assist in their liberation. As we move towards a queer and liberatory psychology, Martín-Baró (1998) offers our field some direction: "to examine not only *what we are* but *what we could have been*, and most importantly, *what we could be* regarding the needs of our peoples" (p. 167). The editors and contributing authors in this book have undertaken this call, providing the field with a review of its contributions and limitations, to finally propose concepts, models, theories, methods, interventions, and approaches that intend to better represent and serve our queer and BIPOC communities. It is our hope that readers and future psychologists, practitioners, and scholars will also do the same.

3   A Final Note to LGBTQ Readers

To end this text, we offer a final note to our LGBTQ readers—particularly our queer and trans youth who may have happened upon this text. We hope that you continue to not just queer psychology, but to queer society however, whenever, and wherever you can. We hope you have grown up in a world that has been a little bit easier because of the people who sacrificed their lives for you to have the things they never

Fig. 3 A same-sex couple enjoying a moment of queer love and joy. Photo Courtesy of Ketut Subiyanto

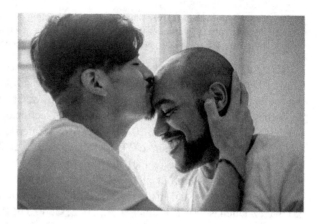

did. Please remember that loving yourself is a revolutionary act. Loving each other is revolutionary act. Having the audacity to live in your truest and most authentic ways is a revolutionary act.

We also hope that you use all of the opportunities that you have to always fight for justice. Please always remember that even if you have it easier than others— whether it be privileges that you were born into or love and support that you were lucky or fortunate enough to have or come across—we hope that you will always pay it forward to others. Be kind to each other. Be as supportive as you can be. Do not ever inflict the pain onto others that has been inflicted onto our communities. Always strive to be your best self, and please encourage others to be too. And if we all can commit to this, we do not only make the world a queerer place for everyone to live, but we can also make the world a kinder and safer place for all of us too (Fig. 3).

References

Adames, H., & Chavez-Dueñas, N. Y. (2022). Reclaiming all of me: The racial queer identity framework. In K. L. Nadal, & M. Scharron-del Río (Eds.) *Queer psychology: Intersectional perspectives* (pp. 59–80). Springer.

Baquet, S., Marasco, V., & Hill, J. (2022). Queer vocational and workplace considerations. In K. L. Nadal, & M. Scharron-del Río (Eds.) *Queer psychology: Intersectional perspectives* (pp. 257–274). Springer.

Bernal, G., & Scharrón-del Río, M. R. (2001). Are empirically supported treatments (EST) valid for ethnic minorities? *Cultural Diversity and Ethnic Minority Psychology, 7*, 328–342.

Brim, M. (2020). Poor queer studies: Class, race, and the field. *Journal of Homosexuality, 67*(3), 398–416. https://doi.org/10.1080/00918369.2018.1534410.

Cerezo, A., & Renteria, R. (2022). Queering psychology research methods. In K. L. Nadal, & M. Scharron-del Río (Eds.) *Queer psychology: Intersectional perspectives* (pp. 138–158). Springer.

Chan, C., & Silverio, N. (2022). Issues for LGBTQ elderly. In K. L. Nadal, & M. Scharron-del Río (Eds.) *Queer psychology: Intersectional perspectives* (pp. 237–256). Springer.

Comas-Díaz, L., Hall, G. N., & Neville, H. A. (2019). Racial trauma: Theory, research, and healing: Introduction to the special issue. *American Psychologist, 74*(1), 1–5. https://doi.org/10.1037/amp0000442.

Doychak, K. & Raghavan, C. (2022). Queering forensic psychology: What intimate partner violence and sex trafficking can tell us about inclusivity. In K. L. Nadal, & M. Scharron-del Río (Eds.) *Queer psychology: Intersectional perspectives* (pp. 291–310). Springer.

Estrellado, J., Felipe, L., Nakamura, N., & Breen, A. (2022). LGBTQ parenting: Building families on the margins. In K. L. Nadal, & M. Scharron-del Río (Eds.) *Queer psychology: Intersectional perspectives* (pp. 119–216). Springer.

Ferguson, A. (2022). Intersectional approaches. In K. L. Nadal, & M. Scharron-del Río (Eds.) *Queer psychology: Intersectional perspectives* (pp. 15–32). Springer.

Ford, D. (2022). The salve and the sting of religion/spirituality in queer and transgender BIPOC. In K. L. Nadal, & M. Scharron-del Río (Eds.) *Queer psychology: Intersectional perspectives* (pp. 275–290). Springer.

Freeman-Coppadge, D., & Farhadi Langroudi, K. (2022). Beyond LGBTQ-affirmative therapy: Fostering growth and healing through intersectionality. In K. L. Nadal, & M. Scharron-del Río (Eds.) *Queer psychology: Intersectional perspectives* (pp. 159–180). Springer.

Henrich, J., Heine, S. J., & Norenzayan, A. (2010). The weirdest people in the world? *Behavioral & Brain Sciences, 33*(2/3), 61–135.

Hunt, S., & Holmes, C. (2015). Everyday decolonization: Living a decolonizing queer politics. *Journal of Lesbian Studies, 19*(2), 154–172. https://doi.org/10.1080/10894160.2015.970975.

Martín-Baró, I. (1998). In A. Blanco Abarca (Ed.), *Psicología de la liberación*. Madrid, Spain: Editorial Trotta.

Mereish, E., & Taylor, M.S. (2022). Sexual and gender minority people's physical health and health risk behaviors. In K. L. Nadal, & M. Scharron-del Río (Eds.) *Queer psychology: Intersectional perspectives* (pp. 81–102). Springer.

Nadal, K. & Scharrón-del Río, M.R. (2022). Introduction to queer psychology. In K. L. Nadal, & M. Scharron-del Río (Eds.) *Queer psychology: Intersectional perspectives* (pp. 1–14). Springer.

Puzio, A. & Forbes, A. (2022). Gender identity as a social developmental process. In K. L. Nadal, & M. Scharron-del Río (Eds.) *Queer psychology: Intersectional perspectives* (pp. 33–58). Springer.

Rider, N., Cai, J., & Candelario-Pérez, L. (2022). Queering sex and romance: Considerations of gender diversity, sex, and relationships. In K. L. Nadal, & M. Scharron-del Río (Eds.) *Queer psychology: Intersectional perspectives* (pp. 181–198). Springer.

Scharrón-Del Río, M. R. (2010). Supuestos, explicaciones y sistemas de creencias: Ciencia, religión y psicología. *Revista Puertorriqueña de Psicología, 20*, 85–112.

Scharrón-Del Río, M. R. (2020a). Intersectionality is not a choice: Reflections of a queer scholar of color on teaching, writing, and belonging in LGBTQ studies and academia. *Journal of Homosexuality, 67*(3), 294–304.

Scharrón-Del Río, M. R. (2020b). Burning out at the intersections: Reflections on teaching multicultural competencies as a queer and genderqueer Puerto Rican educator. In K. LaFollette & N. Santavicca (Eds.), *Queer approaches: Emotion, expression and communication in the classroom* (pp. 7–39). Charlotte, NC: Information Age Publishing.

Scharrón-del Río, M. R., & Aja, A. (2020). Latinxs: Inclusive language as liberation praxis. *Journal of Latinx Psychology, 8*(1), 7–20.

Singh, A. A. (2016). Moving from affirmation to liberation in psychological practice with transgender and gender nonconforming clients. *American Psychologist, 71*(8), 755–762. https://doi-org.brooklyn.ezproxy.cuny.edu/10.1037/amp0000106.

Singh, A., Estevez, R., & Truszczynski, N. (2022). LGBTQ+ people and discrimination: What we have and continue to face in the fight for our lives. In K. L. Nadal, & M. Scharron-del Río (Eds.) Queer psychology: Intersectional perspectives (pp. 119–138). Springer.

Smith, L. T. (1999). *Decolonizing methodologies: Research and indigenous peoples*. Zed Books.

Torre, M. & Avory, S. (2022). "My wings may be broken, but I'm still flying": Queer youth negotiating expansive identities, structural dispossession, and acts of resistance. In K. L. Nadal, & M. Scharron-del Río (Eds.) *Queer Psychology:Intersectional Perspectives* (pp. 217–236). Springer.

Trimble, J., Scharrón-del Río, M. R., & Bernal, G. (2010). The itinerant researcher: Ethical and methodological issues in conducting cross-cultural mental health research. In D. C. Jack & A. Ali (Eds.), *Silencing the self across cultures: Depression and gender in the social world* (pp. 73–98). New York, NY: Oxford University Press.

Trimble, J. E., Scharrón-del Río, M. R., & Casillas, D. M. (2014). Ethical matters and contentions in the principled conduct of research with ethnocultural communities. In F. L. Leong, L. Comas-Díaz, G. C. Nagayama Hall, V. C. McLoyd, & J. E. Trimble (Eds.), *APA handbook of multicultural psychology, Vol. 1: Theory and research* (pp. 59–82). Washington, DC: American Psychological Association. https://doi.org/10.1037/14189-004.

Velez, B., Zelaya, D., & Scheer, J. (2022). LGBTQ mental health. In K. L. Nadal & M. Scharron-del Río (Eds.) *Queer psychology: Intersectional perspectives* (pp. 103–118). Springer.

Correction to: Queer Psychology

Kevin L. Nadal and María R. Scharrón-del Río

Correction to:
K. L. Nadal and M. R. Scharrón-del Río (ed.),
Queer Psychology, https://doi.org/10.1007/978-3-030-74146-4

This book was inadvertently published with few typos in "Abstracts" in chapter 3, without the separation of 1st and 2nd authors in chapter 10 and without updating the figure captions in chapter 10.

This has now been amended throughout the book to the correct format as should be "has been described by the social sciences." and "a case study will be used." The chapter authors name has to be separated with comma G. Nic Rider, Jieyi Cai in chapter 10 and the figure captions has to be corrected as shown below:

P. 21 - "From Stonewall Riots" to "Stonewall Uprisings".

P. 182 – Fig1: From "A moment of queer love and friendship at a trans couple's wedding" to "A moment of queer love and friendship between a couple and their officiant at their wedding."

P. 246 – Fig 2: From "Dr. Debra Joy Perez at the LGBTQ Scholars of Color National Conference with a participant" to "Dr. Debra Joy Perez and Billy Fields share a moment at the 2015 LGBTQ Scholars of Color National Conference in New York City".

The updated version of the chapters can be found at
https://doi.org/10.1007/978-3-030-74146-4
https://doi.org/10.1007/978-3-030-74146-4_2
https://doi.org/10.1007/978-3-030-74146-4_3
https://doi.org/10.1007/978-3-030-74146-4_10
https://doi.org/10.1007/978-3-030-74146-4_13

Index

E

Early sexual orientation models, 17
e-cigarettes, 86
Ecological momentary assessment
(EMA), 154
Effective Skills to Empower Effective Men
(ESTEEM), 110
Elite white males, 15, 18, 19, 22, 23
Emergency medical technicians (EMTs), 93
Empathy, 231, 232
Empirical research, 139–141
Empowering Queer Identities in
Psychotherapy (EQuIP), 110
Equal Employment Opportunity
Commission, 259
Ethical commitments, 220
Ethics in psychology research, 142–144
*Ethnic and cultural diversity among lesbians
and gay men*, 6
Ethnicity, 224, 225

F

Family formation, LGBTQ parenting
assisted reproductive technology, 205–207
children from previous relationships,
207, 208
family structure, 203–205
foster parenting and adoption, 205
Family of choice, 204
Family structure, 203, 204
Fatphobia, 128, 130, 131
Feminine Ideology Scale (FIS), 48
Financial issues, 243
Foster parenting, 205

G

Gay identity theory, 17
Gay in the Church, 275
Gay Liberation Movement, 65, 66
Gender, 223, 224
binary, definition, 35
intersectionality and, 23, 24
and sexuality, 305
Gender bundle
birth-assigned gender category, 44
current gender identity, 44
gender evaluations, 44
gender roles and expectations, 44
gender social presentation, 44
Gendered sexual socialization, 70, 71
Gender expression, 61

Gender identity, 61, 201, 202
definition, 35
Gender identity development
"adaptive/natural" process of human
development, 36, 37
compatibility, 42
core gender identity, 37
current perspectives on gender identity, 38
early adulthood, 53, 54
early childhood, 51
favoritism, 42
five-dimension model, 40
gender bundle, 42
birth-assigned gender category, 44
current gender identity, 44
gender evaluations, 44
gender roles and expectations, 44
gender social presentation, 44
gender norm adherence, 39
gender schema theory, 38
gender typicality and felt pressure, 41
historical timeline of transgender
identity, 50
indigenous, historical, and cross-cultural
perspectives, 45
burrnesha, 45
hijra, 45
Muxes of Juchitán, 45
late adolescence, 52, 53
measurement of gender identity
AFIS, 48
AMRIS, 47
BSRI, 46
CFNI, 48
changes, 48
CPAQ, 47
CSRI, 47
FIS, 48
MRAS, 47
MRNS, 47
PAQ, 47
Medicaid and Medicare, 50
membership knowledge, 41
middle childhood, 52
non-pathological model, 49
self-identification and labels, 35, 36
social-learning theory, 39
TGNC community, 50
white cisgender children, 34
Gender identity disorder in childhood
(GIDC), 49
Genderism, 261–262
Gender minority stress, 125

CPSIA information can be obtained
at www.ICGtesting.com
Printed in the USA
LVHW080052260822
726871LV00003B/92

9 783030 741457